Avicenna in Renaissance Italy

AVICENNA
in Renaissance Italy

The *Canon* and Medical Teaching
in Italian Universities
after 1500

Nancy G. Siraisi

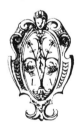

PRINCETON UNIVERSITY PRESS

PRINCETON, NEW JERSEY

Copyright © 1987 by Princeton University Press

Published by Princeton University Press, 41 William Street, Princeton, New Jersey 08540
In the United Kingdom: Princeton University Press, Guildford, Surrey

Library of Congress Cataloging in Publication Data will be found on the last printed page of this book

ISBN 0-691-05137-2

Publication of this book has been aided by a grant from the Publications Program of the National Endowment for the Humanities, an independent Federal agency

This book has been composed in Linotron Bembo

Clothbound editions of Princeton University Press books are printed on acid-free paper, and binding materials are chosen for strength and durability. Paperbacks, although satisfactory for personal collections, are not usually suitable for library rebinding

Printed in the United States of America by Princeton University Press, Princeton, New Jersey

IN MEMORY OF
Charles B. Schmitt

Contents

Illustrations follow page 116.

vii

Acknowledgments

It is a pleasure to be able to record my gratitude for all the help of various kinds that I have received while working on this book. My greatest debt is to the late Charles B. Schmitt, whose encouragement to pursue this topic, generosity in sharing his learning, and kindness in reading much of the manuscript before publication helped me at every stage. My ideas on the Renaissance fortuna of the *Canon* of Avicenna took shape in the light thrown on sixteenth-century academic culture by his work on Aristotelianism. Anthony Grafton and Vivian Nutton read the manuscript for Princeton University Press, providing invaluable comments and saving me from many errors. Although I was not able to follow every one of Vivian Nutton's suggestions, I have nonetheless benefited greatly from his advice. Special thanks are also owed to Richard Palmer for drawing my attention to the collection of documents in the Archivio di Stato of Venice discussed in Chapter 4.

Others who have given me the benefit of their criticism, advice, or other assistance on particular topics or sections of the book include Constance Barrett, Jerome J. Bylebyl, Adriano Carugo, Bruce Chandler, F. Edward Cranz, Luke Demaitre, John Elliott, John B. Friedman, Bernard R. Goldstein, Tamara Green, Danielle Jacquart, Robert Jones, David C. Lindberg, Herbert Matsen, Per-Gunnar Ottosson, Noel Swerdlow, Katherine Tachau, and Linda Voigts. I am, as always, grateful to Paul Oskar Kristeller for his encouragement and to the women scholars of a previous generation who taught me: Beryl Smalley and Pearl Kibre. Over the last four years, I have presented early drafts of some chapters as papers at seminars at the History of Science Department, Harvard University; the Program in the History of Science, Princeton University; the Johns Hopkins Institute of the History of Medicine; the Warburg Institute; and the Conference on Sixteenth-Century Medicine held at Corpus Christi College, Cambridge. The discussion on these occasions was useful to me, and I wish to express my gratitude to the organizers and to all those who took part. Naturally, none of those mentioned is responsible for any of my mistakes or misapprehensions.

Part of Appendices 1 and 2 appeared in my article "Renaissance Commentaries on Avicenna's *Canon*, Book 1, Part 1, and the Teaching of Medical *Theoria* in the Italian Universities," *History of Universities* 4

(1984), 47–97; and part of Chapter 5 appeared as a chapter in *The Medical Renaissance of the Sixteenth Century*, ed. A. Wear, R. K. French, and I. M. Lonie (Cambridge, 1985), pp. 16–41, 279–96. Thanks are due to *History of Universities* and to Cambridge University Press for permission to reprint this material.

Research for this book has taken me to numerous libraries in this country and abroad (most of them are indicated by the manuscript locations specified in Appendix 2 and the bibliography). I retain pleasant memories of these travels, and am grateful to the staffs of the various libraries and archives that I visited in Italy and elsewhere. Especially extensive help was given me by librarians at the Wellcome Historical Medical Library, the Warburg Institute, the History of Medicine Division of the National Library of Medicine, the Rare Book Room of the New York Academy of Medicine, and by the archivists of the Archivio Antico dell'Università, Padua. I am also grateful to Special Collections, Columbia University, the Wellcome Library, and the New York Academy of Medicine for providing reproductions of illustrations from early printed books in their collections.

My research was supported at various stages by the John Simon Guggenheim Memorial Foundation, the National Endowment for the Humanities, and the Research Foundation of the City University of New York. Most recently, a year at the Institute for Advanced Study, Princeton (in conjunction with a fellowship leave from Hunter College), provided ideal conditions in which to finish the work. I am grateful to those members of the Institute's secretarial staff who helped in manuscript preparation, especially Sandra Lafferty and Margaret Van Sant.

I should also like to express my thanks to Naomi C. Miller, chairperson of the Department of History, Hunter College, who has over many years consistently encouraged my research.

What I owe to my husband and sons extends far beyond the making of this book.

May 1986

Abbreviations

Throughout the text and footnotes that follow, early editions of the *Canon*, and manuscripts and printed editions of commentaries thereon, are cited under abbreviated titles. The reader will find full descriptions of these items in Appendices 1 and 2. Other abbreviations used throughout this book are as follows.

AAUP	Archivio Antico dell'Università, Padua
ASB	Archivio di Stato, Bologna
ASF	Archivio di Stato, Florence
ASP	Archivio di Stato, Pisa
ASV	Archivio di Stato, Venice
Biogr. Lex.	*Biographisches Lexikon der hervorragenden Aerzte aller Zeiten und Völker*, ed. A. Wernich and August Hirsch, 6 vols. (Vienna and Leipzig, 1884–88)
BL	British Library, London
BNC	Biblioteca Nazionale Centrale, Florence
comm.	commentary
CTC	*Catalogus translationum et commentariorum: Medieval and Renaissance Latin Translations and commentaries*, ed. Paul Oskar Kristeller and F. Edward Cranz, 1– (Washington, D.C., 1960–)
DBI	*Dizionario biografico degli Italiani* (Rome, 1960–)
DSB	*Dictionary of Scientific Biography*, ed. Charles C. Gillispie, 16 vols. (New York, 1970–80)
IA	*Index aureliensis; catalogus librorum sedecimo saeculo impressorum*, 1– (Orleans, 1965–)
Klebs	Arnold C. Klebs, *Incunabula scientifica et medica* (Bruges, 1938; reprint ed., Hildesheim, 1963)
Kühn	*Claudii Galeni Opera omnia*, ed. C. G. Kühn, 20 vols. (Leipzig, 1821–33)
NLM	National Library of Medicine, Bethesda, Maryland, History of Medicine Division
NYAM	New York Academy of Medicine, Rare Book Room
TK	Lynn Thorndike and Pearl Kibre, *A Catalogue of Incipits of Mediaeval Scientific Writings in Latin*, 2nd ed. (Cambridge, Mass., 1963)
WL	Wellcome Historical Medical Library, London

In citations of and quotations from Latin works printed before 1700, abbreviations have been expanded and some capitalization, punctuation, and uses of *i, j, u,* and *v* have been silently modernized. I have followed the nineteenth-century biographer of G. B. Da Monte in using the form Giambatista for his first name.

Following current English usage, I have employed the term "university" to translate the Latin *studium* and the Italian *studio* and to signify an entire academic community of teachers, students, and administrators. However, from time to time "university" is also used to translate *universitas* in the earlier sense of a corporation forming a legal entity within a larger academic community (e.g., "the university of arts and medicine at Padua" was the corporation to which students of those subjects belonged).

PART I

The *Canon* as a Latin Medical Book

I

Text, Commentary, and Pedagogy in Renaissance Medicine

The fortunes of the *Canon* of Avicenna in Renaissance and early modern medical schools provide a case study of university science and medical teaching, an enterprise that has often been contrasted unfavorably either with contemporary innovations within academia (for example, the revival of anatomy) or with burgeoning scientific activities and interests outside the academic milieu. To the extent that continued use of this medieval Islamic medical encyclopedia, in Latin translation, as a textbook or reference work in western European universities after the end of the Middle Ages has been the object of attention, such use has usually been treated as a negative symbol of extreme conservatism, traditionalism, or medieval scholasticism in medical teaching.[1] The evidence for Renaissance interest in Avicenna's medical writings—between 1500 and 1674 at least sixty editions of the complete or partial text of the *Canon* in Latin were printed and a substantial body of new commentary was composed[2]—seems, however, to call for a new evaluation of the subject. The more closely one looks at the written output of Renaissance medicine, the more difficult the delineation of "conservative" and "progressive" areas becomes. Rather than attempt any such delineation, it may be preferable to inquire what this material has to tell us about the intellectual formation provided in university faculties of medicine, institutions that in the period under consideration helped to shape the minds of a large proportion of those who interested themselves in the life sciences. Such an inquiry is the purpose of the present work.

I have set out, first, simply to map the extent of Renaissance interest in the *Canon*: to determine as completely as possible (though doubtless still incompletely) the number and provenance of editions of, commentaries on, and treatises about the work, and to relate them to specific academic, professional, or commercial milieus. Most of these

[1] See, for example, George Sarton, "Query No. 134—Was any attempt made by the editors of the late Latin editions of Avicenna's *Canon* to modernize it?" *Isis* 43 (1952), 54.
[2] These editions and commentaries are listed in Appendices 1 and 2.

3

books were the product of, and found their audience in, university circles. But Renaissance medical practitioners also drew on Avicenna, or on works based on his teaching; and the production and dissemination of editions of the *Canon* and the literature it engendered are part of the history of Renaissance printing and publishing.

Second, I have tried to trace aspects of the intellectual history contained in these works and to accompany editors and authors as they strove to set down and set in order their attitudes to the various currents that shaped their ideas or demanded their attention: Avicenna and Arabo-Latin medicine; medieval Latin scholastic medicine; contemporary Galenism and medical humanism; controversies between Aristotelians and Galenists; contemporary philosophical eclecticism; the idiosyncrasies of Renaissance encyclopedic naturalism and occultism; and the accumulation of new theories and new data in medicine, anatomy, and botany. *Canon* editions and commentaries yield much information about general trends in Renaissance medicine and the response to innovation among the academic medical community. Tracing the impact and interaction of these developments by way of successive publications of a single text and works related to it offers one path through a complex and often confusing area of intellectual history and history of science. The *Canon* is indeed only one of a number of texts that might profitably be followed in this way. Recent studies of Renaissance commentaries on philosophical texts have begun to reveal both the full extent of this literature, and also its richness, diversity, and significance for the history of philosophy and of philosophy and science education.[3] Similarly, aspects of the history of medieval and Renaissance cosmology and physical theory have been traced through the literature of commentary.[4] Medical commentaries, which have so far been less explored, are equally informative about the intellectual environment in which they were produced.[5]

---

[3] See Charles H. Lohr, "Renaissance Latin Aristotle Commentaries: Authors A-B," *Studies in the Renaissance* 21 (1974), 228–89, and subsequent parts in *Renaissance Quarterly* 28 (1975), 689–741; 29 (1976), 714–45; 30 (1977), 681–741; 31 (1978), 532–603; 32 (1979), 529–80; 33 (1980), 623–734; 35 (1982), 164–256; and Charles B. Schmitt, *Aristotle and the Renaissance* (Cambridge, Mass., and London, 1983), pp. 34–63, 121–33.

[4] Recent examples are Edward Grant, *Much Ado about Nothing: Theories of Space and Vacuum from the Middle Ages to the Scientific Revolution* (Cambridge, 1981), pp. 1–181; and idem, *In Defense of the Earth's Centrality and Immobility: Scholastic Reaction to Copernicanism in the Seventeenth Century*, Transactions of the American Philosophical Society, 74, pt. 4 (Philadelphia, 1984).

[5] Among the few recent studies, mention may be made of Danielle Jacquart, "Le regard d'un médecin sur son temps: Jacques Despars (1380?–1458)," *Bibliothèque de l'Ecole des Chartes* 138 (1980), 35–86; and Gundolf Keil "Roger-Urtext und Roger-Glosse vom

Third, I have been interested in the way in which the *Canon* was used as a teaching text and, in particular, in the question of how the teaching of a scientific subject by means of commentary on a medieval text synthesizing ancient sources was actually accomplished in the Renaissance classroom. Here commentaries must be approached with caution, since they do not necessarily reflect classroom practice directly.[6] Although almost all Latin medical commentaries of the fourteenth to the seventeenth centuries probably originated in university lectures, the surviving body of material has not only undergone undetermined amounts of subsequent editing, but also represents only a fraction of all the lectures delivered over the centuries. That fraction is likely to be the work of the more ambitious and energetic (and hence uncharacteristic) professors. (The latter supposition explains why the publication of commentaries on parts of the *Canon* by living or recently deceased authors tapered off long before the texts themselves disappeared from statutory university curricula or lectures on them ceased to be given; new commentaries stopped appearing in print at the point publication of expositions of traditional texts became unlikely to enhance scholarly or scientific reputations.)

Nonetheless, the surviving commentaries offer a good deal of information about the goals, methods, and assumptions of university medical teaching. They cast light on the balance between exposition of the author and exposition of the subject, on the extent to which the content of teaching was determined by the medieval tradition of commentary on the same text, and on the degree to which lectures on the *Canon* varied according to the interests of individual teachers. As for the permeation of lectures on the *Canon* by current intellectual and scientific concerns, the question is not whether this occurred, since the flexibility of commentary as a form had always made such permeation inevitable, but how, and to what extent. Mordechai Feingold has recently shown with regard to Oxford in the later sixteenth and first half of the seventeenth century that the reputed conservatism of university teaching needs to be carefully delimited, in that teachers whose announced conclusions remained conservative might nonetheless choose to inform

---

12. bis ins 16. Jahrhundert," and Peter Dilg, "Die botanische Kommentarliteratur in Italien um 1500 und ihr Einfluss auf Deutschland," both in *Der Kommentar in der Renaissance*, ed. August Buck and Otto Herding (Boppard, 1975), pp. 209–24, 225–52.

[6] Commentaries are unlikely to have the immediacy, for example, of the students' annotations of classical texts from the University of Paris in the second half of the sixteenth century, discussed in Anthony Grafton, "Teacher, Text, and Pupil in the Renaissance Class-Room: A Case Study from a Parisian College," *History of Universities* 1 (1981), 37–70.

their students of the existence and implications of alternative views. In the second decade of the eighteenth century, according to another recent study, lectures on Aristotle's *Meteorology* delivered at Padua included accounts of seventeenth-century discoveries in pneumatics and of Cartesian physics.[7] The reduction of commentary to a mere shell for teaching of another kind—exemplified in medicine by Morgagni's ingenious use of his prescribed lectures on *Canon* 1.1, at Padua in 1713, to teach seventeenth-century physiology (see Chapter 6)—had not yet occurred a century earlier; instead, the sixteenth- and early seventeenth-century commentaries that form a large part of the subject of this book maintain an uneasy balance between scholastic tradition, the Renaissance enthusiasm for all things Greek in medicine, philosophical eclecticism, and (often unaccepting) presentation of new scientific data and theories. Although in lectures on the *Canon* the bent toward scholastic tradition is naturally considerable, teaching based on the *Canon* evidently had much in common with some of the other approaches to medical and natural philosophical subject matter in the same epoch. These commentaries cannot be written off as the product of a scholastic backwater unrepresentative of the culture of the age.

The period between about 1500 and about 1625, which is the principal focus of this book, constitutes only one phase of long history of the use of Avicenna's eleventh-century medical encyclopedia in western Europe. I have chosen to concentrate on this time span because, despite Avicenna's justified reputation as a medieval school author, the later period is arguably that in which the most thorough study of the *Canon* was undertaken by scholars in the Latin West. It is also that in which the work aroused most controversy, and in which the process resulting in the obsolesence of Avicenna's place in Western medicine began. For about the first two hundred years after its introduction into university curricula in the thirteenth century, the *Canon*, although subjected to occasional criticism, was generally and on the whole rightly esteemed as a sophisticated systematization and summary of almost all available medical learning. By about the mid-seventeenth century, despite the *Canon*'s great historical importance, its irrelevance to current developments in European physiology was clearly apparent; its long survival thereafter in various university curricula (at Bologna part of the work retained a nominal position until 1800) must be attributed

---

[7] Mordechai Feingold, *The Mathematicians' Apprenticeship: Science, Universities and Society in England, 1560–1640* (Cambridge, 1984), esp. pp. 20, 102–3, 215; Brendan Dooley, "Science Teaching as a Career at Padua in the Early Eighteenth Century: The Case of Giovanni Poleni," *History of Universities* 4 (1984), 115–51.

chiefly to academic inertia, as eighteenth-century educational reformers were not slow to point out.

But in the sixteenth and early seventeenth centuries, notwithstanding the emergence of powerful and indeed ultimately revolutionary forces of change in science and philosophy, the *Canon*, like other textbooks used in medieval universities, could reasonably be regarded as having a valid place in science education. The Galenic medicine and Aristotelian natural philosophy on which Avicenna's synthesis was based retained their hold over the minds of most educated men; in and outside the schools the approach to nature was still in large measure book-oriented, classicizing, and scholastic; and teaching scientific disciplines by means of commentary on ancient texts remained common practice. Hence, rather than constituting a reactionary rear guard, those university teachers who continued to show an active interest in the *Canon* by publishing commentaries upon it and by collaborating in the preparation of editions of the work fell within the mainstream of contemporary intellectual life. Their commentaries and editions reveal the history of successive attempts to modernize the presentation of Avicenna's text and the teaching of his ideas, attempts that served to shore up the position of the work in some university curricula in the short run and also contributed to its subsequent obsolescence.

The inspiration for these attempts was derived from the importation of some of the ideals of Renaissance humanism into medicine beginning in about the last quarter of the fifteenth century. The humanist insistence upon attention to original texts in the original languages stimulated a closer attention to Avicenna's relation to his Greek (especially his Galenic) sources than had hitherto been undertaken; and despite the limitations of Arabic studies in sixteenth-century Europe, some efforts were made to approach the Arabic text directly. The humanist desire for more accurate, or at any rate more elegant and readily understandable, translations lay behind various revisions of the Latin text and partial translations into Latin from a Hebrew version. And the vigorous humanist polemic against the medieval translators of Greek and Arabic works, and against Arabic medicine in general and Avicenna in particular, both penetrated some commentaries on the *Canon* itself and engendered reactive efforts to defend Avicenna's work. Perhaps somewhat paradoxically, therefore, the long life of the *Canon* in the schools of the West seems at least in part due to the efforts of sixteenth-century scholarly editors and commentators who, far from being oblivious to such phenomena as Renaissance Galenism and the humanist attack on Arab medicine and Latin medical scholastics, attempted to approach the *Canon* itself in the spirit of medical humanism. Thus, although

7

Renaissance interest in Avicenna's medical writings is a phenomenon much smaller in scale than Renaissance Aristotelianism or Renaissance Galenism, it has much in common with these larger intellectual movements.[8] In all three cases, there is obvious and important continuity with an antecedent scholastic tradition; but at the same time the reality and significance of change are also undeniable. Indeed, the interest in Avicenna was intimately associated with contemporary Galenism, since Avicenna tended to be judged, by friend and foe alike, on the basis of his adequacy as a summarizer and interpreter of Galen's thought.

The survival of the *Canon* in sixteenth-century and later academic medical curricula was not confined to any one region of Europe. But regional intellectual traditions ensured that active interest in providing and publishing improved versions of the Latin text accompanied by a modern body of commentary was predominantly an Italian and (though to a somewhat lesser extent) Iberian undertaking. For the most part, this book deals with the *Canon* in the Italian universities. This emphasis was partly dictated by the numerical predominance of commentaries and editions of Italian provenance—professors from Padua and Bologna predominated in the writing of commentaries, and Venetian presses in the publication of both commentaries and editions—and partly by my own earlier studies of Italian scholastic medicine, which made me want to trace later stages of the regional academic medical tradition of which Taddeo Alderotti was a leading early representative.[9] Medieval and Renaissance Italian universities have for the most part been studied on an individual rather than a comparative basis; this book essays a comparative approach to one restricted area of medical teaching in these institutions. Yet among the Italian universities Padua was in the sixteenth and early seventeenth century an international center famous among contemporaries as among modern historians of medicine for innovative work in anatomy and physiology and for the teaching of practical medicine. It was also, as is equally well known,

---

[8] For the scope of Renaissance interest in Galen, see Richard J. Durling, "A Chronological Census of Renaissance Editions and Translations of Galen," *Journal of the Warburg and Courtauld Institutes* 24 (1961), 230–305; no complete bibliography of Renaissance commentaries on Galen so far exists. A picture of the extent of Renaissance Aristotelianism is provided by F. Edward Cranz, *A Bibliography of Aristotle Editions, 1501–1600*, 2nd ed. with addenda and revisions by Charles B. Schmitt, Bibliotheca Bibliographica Aureliana 38★ (Baden-Baden, 1984); and Lohr's catalogue of commentaries (n. 3, above). The count of editions of the *Canon* is easily, and substantially, exceeded by the count of editions of some individual works of Aristotle; see, e.g., the editions of the *Physica* listed in Cranz and Schmitt, pp. 212–13.

[9] Nancy G. Siraisi, *Taddeo Alderotti and His Pupils: Two Generations of Italian Medical Learning* (Princeton, N.J., 1981).

still a notable center of Aristotelian natural philosophy. Although Padua's preeminence seems more due to general liveliness and productivity and to sociopolitial factors than to any peculiarly Paduan ideas or attitudes (which, if they existed, have proved singularly hard to track down), the investigation of the position of the *Canon* in such a milieu seemed a task of particular interest.

At Padua and Bologna, universities that had been centers of medical instruction since the thirteenth century, a standard and highly traditional curriculum of lectures on set books was in the course of the sixteenth century supplemented and consequently reduced in importance by the expansion and development of private medical teaching and of public anatomical and botanical instruction.[10] And anatomy at Padua in particular early produced very striking and widely celebrated scientific results in the shape of the achievement of Vesalius. Although the lectures on set books were in important respects slow to change, they were in fact affected in a variety of ways by the local and immediate scientific, professional, and institutional context. Thus, at Padua neglect of statutory lectures on the *Canon* and demands for curricular reform of a kind that would remove Avicenna from the schools were counterbalanced by other reform proposals that proposed sections of the *Canon* as the appropriate text for a unified overview of medicine (see Chapter 4). In this way, the history of the *Canon* becomes intertwined with that of university reform and with that of the antecedents of medical textbooks of the variety known as the "institutes of medicine." Furthermore, those who accepted the statutory obligation to lecture on portions of the *Canon* at Padua included at least two men who themselves made significant contributions to the development of medical education and the introduction of new standards of demonstration, evidence, and proof into medicine and physiology, namely Giambatista Da Monte (d. 1551), well known for his emphasis upon clinical instruction in a hospital setting and his role in the founding of the Paduan botanic garden, and Santorio Santorio (d. 1636), who is remembered for his part in developing physiological measurement, instrumentation, and quantification. The commentaries on the *Canon* of these men, and also those of their less distinguished colleagues, reflect the authors' encounters with the ideas, activities, and controversies of the Paduan medical milieu.

Analysis of all the content of all the Renaissance commentaries on the

---

[10] Summary and interpretation of these developments is provided by Jerome J. Bylebyl, "The School of Padua: Humanistic Medicine in the Sixteenth Century," in *Health, Medicine and Mortality in the Sixteenth Century*, ed. Charles Webster (Cambridge, 1979), pp. 335–370.

Canon would be a task as daunting as it is pointless. I have instead elected to concentrate on the role of the first part of the first book as a textbook of medical philosophy and physiology, and to confine the analysis of specific medical, scientific, and philosophical content to six commentaries on this portion of the work. The brief text of *Canon* 1.1 occupies a position of considerable significance in the history of ways of thinking about the philosophy of medicine and of physiology. For several hundred years, this section of the work provided medical students and others with a coherent and well-crafted survey of the fundamentals of a largely Galenic physiology set in the context of Aristotelian natural philosophy, and with a concise expression of some of the key concepts of scholastic medical thought. In university medical curricula, the first book of the *Canon*, and especially the first section of that book, was early adopted as a textbook of *theoria*, the branch of medicine that acquainted the neophyte with the nature of medical science, the position of medicine in the hierarchy of arts and sciences, and the proper relationship of medicine and philosophy, as well as with the basic principles of physiology, pathology, and regimen. So long as the Aristotelian world view survived, so long as physiology was generally Galenic, and so long as the exposition of texts remained an accepted mode of scientific investigation and discourse, *Canon* 1.1 was deservedly esteemed by physicians. On particular points Avicenna's opinion might be disputed, but *Canon* 1.1 as a whole constituted one of the clearest available short statements of the principles underlying the entire system of medical learning taught in the universities of medieval and Renaissance Europe.

Insofar as an overview of physiology was presented to medical students in public lectures at Renaissance Padua or Bologna, this was accomplished in the course on *theoria* for which *Canon* 1.1 provided the text. (Other courses in *theoria* were based on the Hippocratic *Aphorisms* and the Galenic *Ars*, or *Microtechne*, neither of which provided the comprehensive and systematic overview of physiology found in *Canon* 1.1). Sixteenth-century critics and their modern successors have rightly perceived the division into *theoria* and *practica* as one of the main weaknesses of the Renaissance university medical curriculum. Nevertheless, the topics discussed in courses on *theoria* were by no means isolated from current debate and contemporary scientific interests. For instance, physiological and anatomical debates overlapped in many areas, so that discussions of the implications of sixteenth-century anatomical findings could without incongruity or inappropriateness find their way into commentaries on *Canon* 1.1. Similarly, a whole range of topics of debate, usually having to do with differences between Aristotelian and Galenic physiology, which had been standard since the thirteenth century in expositions of *Canon* 1.1 and other scholastic medical works, continued to arouse lively interest among working anatomists in the sixteenth and early seventeenth centuries, who, however, began to opt for experimental rather than dialectical solutions. Among these topics it is sufficient to name the controversy over Aristotelian and Galenic views of the function of the heart. Moreover, dialectical controversy among physicians had by no means vanished in the sixteenth century, and the commentaries on *Canon* 1.1 provide some excellent insights into the course and assumptions of such disputes. Furthermore, it was in the courses on *theoria* that the relationship claimed between medicine and philosophy was real, so commentaries on *Canon* 1.1 can add to our knowledge of the way in which general philosophical and scientific information was presented to and disseminated among medical students and of the reactions to scientific change within the medical community; the discussions of Copernican theory found in some of the commentaries are a striking case in point.

The account in this book of the medical, philosophical, and scientific content of commentary on *Canon* 1.1 is of necessity selective, since these works are diffuse by nature and often heterogeneous in content. I have tried to focus on themes of some general significance for the history of scientific thought during the transition from the medieval to the early modern world, but the arguments I have chosen to follow in detail are by no means necessarily the only ones worth examining.

Teaching based on *Canon* 1.1 was, I think, a major aspect of the meaning of Avicenna's work for Renaissance medical culture, but such teaching far from encompasses the whole story of Avicenna in Renaissance medicine. Other sections of the *Canon* were used to teach medical *practica* and by actual practitioners. Thus, it has recently been demonstrated that Avicenna's summary of Galen's teaching on fevers was considered as useful for teaching pathology in university courses designated *practica* as was *Canon* 1.1 for physiology in courses on *theoria*.[11] (The terms "physiology" and "pathology" are not, strictly speaking, anachronistic, since cognate Latin words came into use among physicians during the sixteenth century; obviously, however, they do not connote the conceptions and methodology of the modern sciences.) And the attentive reader of this book will come across numerous contemporary expressions of the idea that the *Canon* constituted a valuable

---

[11] Iain M. Lonie, "Fever Pathology in the Sixteenth Century: Tradition and Innovation," in *Theories of Fever from Antiquity to the Enlightenment*, ed. W. F. Bynum and V. Nutton, *Medical History*, Supplement no. 1 (London, 1981), pp. 19–44.

resource for practitioners, especially as regards *materia medica*. Although I have brought together evidence for the practical uses of the *Canon*, I have not undertaken any detailed analysis of the content of lectures on sections other than *Canon* 1.1. Further study of the university teaching of medical *practica* in the sixteenth century is unquestionably called for, although here far more than in the case of *theoria* a whole range of formal and informal instruction, not just statutory lectures on one textbook, needs to be taken into account. Moreover, a challenge for future studies of Renaissance medicine remains to trace the full history of efforts to come to grips with, to interpret, and finally in large part to discard technical vocabulary of Arabic origin (although often unrecognizably distorted) in pharmacological botany and anatomy, a struggle partially reflected in some editions and critiques of the *Canon*. But the formidable task of disentangling that history is beyond the scope of the present book.

More generally, it may be questioned whether concentration upon the theoretical writings of academic physicians does not focus attention on the least significant aspects of Renaissance medicine. Academic Galenists—a designation that more or less encompasses almost all the medical writers discussed in this book—were notoriously suspicious of philosophical or practical innovation, and hostile to empiricism, Paracelsianism, certain aspects of Renaissance occultism, and the activities of non-university-trained medical practitioners. It could be argued that these professors found all the most interesting and genuinely progressive aspects of Renaissance medicine worthy only of disdain. Quite apart from the fact that some of the individual commentators discussed below were significant medical innovators in their own right, such an argument seems to me generally misconceived. Galenism was as wide, as flexible, and as variable a category in the Renaissance as Charles Schmitt has recently shown Aristotelianism to be.[12] If one ignores the broad stream of traditional natural and medical philosophies and concentrates only on ideas that are or appear to be innovative, or if one deals solely with the scientific ideas of outstanding individuals, one omits a great deal of the intellectual and scientific culture of the period.

Moreover, medical *theoria* and those who expounded it were both part of and affected by contemporary intellectual currents. Hence, the formulations of teachers of medical *theoria* are revealing of the assumptions governing a good deal of Renaissance thought on the life sciences, as well as of ways in which specific technical or practical innovations might be absorbed and interpreted within a still largely traditional

---

[12] Schmitt, *Aristotle and the Renaissance*, passim.

framework. Certainly, the views of the segment of the academic medical community engaged in teaching the most conservative part of the medical curriculum were those of a narrow elite who had a great deal invested in the perpetuation of existing systems of medical education and professional organization. Similar elites have scarcely been an insignificant feature of the social history of European and other universities. Recent sociocultural historians have created a valuable new historiography of the study of the culture of more or less powerless groups often previously excluded from historical consideration. There remains something to be said for the study of the culture of the establishment, if only as a way of understanding the difficulty and complexity of the process of replacing one system of thought by another, difficulty and complexity that is social and institutional as well as intellectual. Some of us who teach in universities today may recognize ourselves in the delays, the self-seeking, the divisional rivalries, and the proliferation of professorial opinion that accompanied the efforts to reform the medical curriculum at Padua at the end of the sixteenth century and resulted in the addition of yet another chair for the exposition of the *Canon* of Avicenna in the year 1601 (see Chapter 4).

Avicenna's *Canon* played yet another role in the Renaissance, namely as the object of attention from scholars involved in the earliest phase of the development of Arabic or Oriental studies in the West. Although in Chapter 5 a number of sixteenth- and very early seventeenth-century examples of work on the text inspired by interest of this type are noted, no attempt has been made to provide a complete picture of the place of the *Canon* in the interests of learned Arabists of the later seventeenth or eighteenth centuries. Other scholars are better equipped than I am to deal with that subject. Moreover, from the standpoint of the present work, the endeavors of the noteworthy handful of men who from the fifteenth to the seventeenth century made efforts to secure a closer acquaintance with the Arabic text of the *Canon* appear to have had very limited impact on the way the work was studied in medical schools. The *Canon* continued to be taught and studied in Latin by medical men, although with some attention to revised or partially retranslated versions of the Latin text. Thus, a somewhat revised version of the twelfth-century Latin translation of the *Canon*, produced in the light of a knowledge of Arabic by the Paduan-trained doctor Andrea Alpago (d. 1522), was widely disseminated and indeed at Padua officially adopted by the College of Philosophers and Physicians; but as the reader will see, it is doubtful whether several of the Italian scholarly physicians who subsequently involved themselves in the preparation of elaborately annotated editions of Alpago's text knew any Arabic at all.

Certainly, the Italian medical commentators showed no signs in their expositions of the *Canon* of either knowing Arabic themselves or expecting their students or readers to know it. And the impact on medical teaching of the most celebrated instance of the application of Arabist learning to the *Canon* in this period, namely the printing of the complete work in Arabic by G. B. Raimondi for the Medici press (Rome, 1593), appears to have been negligible.

My use of Avicenna's name in its Latin form throughout this book may serve as a reminder that this is an examination of a phase of Latin scientific culture.[13] To the general history of the *Canon*, an enduring monument of medieval Islamic medical science, my study is no more than a footnote. I make no claim to have contributed to such large and still largely uncharted subjects as the full analysis of the medical, philosophical, and scientific content of Avicenna's own work; its relation to its Greek or other sources; and its influence through several cultures and many centuries up to and including the present one.[14] Instead, my goal has simply been to present to the reader an exploration of aspects of the intellectual milieu of the Italian university faculties of medicine in a period in which a notable regional tradition of medical learning was undergoing partial, sometimes painful, and ultimately productive transformation.

An underlying assumption is that Latin academic medicine in Italy between about 1300 and about 1600 constitutes a relatively unified field of inquiry. I do not, of course, mean to imply either that Latin medical learning sprang into being around 1300 or that it thereafter remained unchanged for three centuries. On the contrary, the medicine taught in the schools of western Europe in the late Middle Ages derived much of its content from Greek authorities and owed much to the Latin medical teaching and learning of the earlier Middle Ages, as well as to the con-

---

[13] Some Renaissance editors of Latin versions of Avicenna's work occasionally tried to introduce closer renderings of his name (see the edition of Venice, 1523, in Appendix 1, below, for example), but by and large the usage "Avicenna" prevailed in Western medical circles.

[14] A useful overview and bibliography of the historiographical development of attitudes toward Avicenna's contribution to medicine among historians of medicine is provided by Ursula Weisser, "Ibn Sīnā und die Medizin des arabisch-islamischen Mittelalters—Alte und neue Urteile und Vorurteile," *Medizinhistorisches Journal* 18 (1983), 283–305. Weisser traces the process whereby the disdain for the medieval Islamic contribution to medicine expressed by early modern European historians of the subject gave way to a more sympathetic evaluation of Avicenna's role as a synthesizer of ancient medical science, and most recently, to efforts to demonstrate that he made valid original contributions to various specialized areas of medicine. In her view, not all the claims that have been made for Avicenna in the last category can be justified.

tribution of the Arabs. During the thirteenth century, however, traditional forms of medical learning were refined, developed, and institutionalized under the impact of Aristotelian natural philosophy, the rise of universities, and the emergence of a secular and organized medical profession. In this century, too, Latin scholars identified the great theme of scholastic medicine: the exploration and, where possible, reconciliation of the differences between the physiological teachings of Aristotle and Galen.

The importance of the north Italian schools as European centers of medical education also dates from the late thirteenth century. On the whole, despite some periods of difficulty, Bologna, and later Padua, were, from the time of Taddeo Alderotti's (d. 1295) professorship at Bologna until William Harvey's student days at Padua, rivaled in fame for medical learning only by Montpellier. Moreover, the multiplication in northern Italy of other *studia* (some of them short-lived) offering medical teaching meant that professors of medicine and medical authors, although never more than a fraction of those who engaged in healing, early came to constitute in Italy a relatively numerous group. One result was the production of a prolific medical literature, which stimulated and perpetuated pride in local achievements. From the early fourteenth century, the works of Italian professors of medicine abound in citations of local and relatively unknown predecessors. The historic predominance of the late medieval north Italian faculties of medicine was therefore derived less from any peculiarly Italian features of the medical or natural philosophical curriculum of books to be studied (since by and large the Italian schools participated in a common European cultural tradition), than from the numerous faculty members and students, large output of written works, and strong local traditions of practical and surgical training.

In the fourteenth and fifteenth centuries pride in the regional medical tradition was loudly expressed. Thus, even the humanist chancellor of Florence, Coluccio Salutati—a hostile witness, since his words occur in a work dedicated to proving the superiority of law over medicine—wrote, in 1398, of the "glory of the discoveries of medicine." Among them he listed various Arab authors and Maimonides and then passed straight to "the Italians who have treated this logical medicine with marvellous subtlety," naming various university professors of medicine famed for their scholastic learning, among them Taddeo Alderotti and Pietro d'Abano (d. ca. 1316). Salutati apparently felt no compunction in omitting any mention of either Montpellier or the once important southern Italian medical school of Salerno. One must admit that his remarks are entirely consistent with the normal pattern of citation in the writings of late medieval and early Renaissance north Italian medical authors. Other authors, medical and nonmedical, proudly stressed the philosophical attainments of leading Italian medical writers; for example, Benedetto Accolti, in a work on the outstanding men of modern times dedicated to Cosimo de' Medici, listed a group of north Italian medical authors under the general heading of philosophy alongside Averroes and Thomas Aquinas.[15] If the main achievements of north Italian medicine between 1300 and 1500 appear now to have been the pioneering of autopsy and anatomy in early fourteenth-century Bologna and the flowering of instruction in practical medicine in fifteenth-century Padua, these were not necessarily the aspects that contemporaries found most worthy of celebration.

After 1500, changes in the academic tradition thus formed were rapid and, ultimately, destructive of traditional medical learning. A major goal of this book is indeed to use the *Canon* of Avicenna as a case study of the extent to which scholastic medical learning in the sixteenth century was capable of assimilating or initiating change. Nonetheless, curricula, textbooks, pedagogical methods, and, often, subjects of debate provided a framework of substantial continuity in the teaching of medicine in the Italian, as in other, universities throughout a period extending from the thirteenth to the seventeenth century. And in Italy, the early phase of university medical education before 1500 had been, in its own terms, one of outstanding success.

The periodization of the history of medicine within this general time frame, ca. 1300 to ca. 1600, deserves closer scrutiny than it usually gets; arbitrary and stereotypical concepts of the Middle Ages and the Renaissance, seldom now found in serious works of intellectual or cultural history, have not yet wholly vanished from the history of medicine. Thus, on the one hand, scholastic medical authors who flourished in the Italian cities of the Tre- and Quattrocento tend to be classified, without qualification, as medieval; on the other, the expressions of the idea of the renewal or rebirth of medicine by writers who lived between 1300 and 1600 have seldom been subjected to the kind of critical

---

[15] Coluccio Salutati, *De nobilitate legum et medicinae. De verecundia*, ed. Eugenio Garin (Florence, 1947), pp. 70–72 (for the date, see Garin's introduction, p. xxxii); *Benedicti Accolti . . . Dialogus de praestantia virorum sui aevi*, ed. Benedetto Bacchini (Parma, 1689), in Filippo Villani, *Liber de civitatis Florentiae famosis civibus ex codice mediceo Laurentiano nunc primum editus et de Florentinorum litteratura principes fere synchroni scriptores*, ed. C. G. Galletti (Florence, 1847), pp. 122–23. On these and other contemporary evaluations of fourteenth- and fifteenth-century Italian medicine, see Nancy G. Siraisi, "The Physician's Task: Medical Reputations in Humanist Collective Biographies," in *The Rational Arts of Living*, ed. A. C. Crombie, Smith College Studies in History (forthcoming).

analysis accorded to parallel claims for arts and letters. For example, the Florentine historian Filippo Villani, in a work probably first written in the early 1380s and revised in the mid-1390s, referred to Taddeo Alderotti as "among the first of the moderns."[16] Taddeo's modernity, in Villani's view, lay in his ability to open up the profoundest secrets of medicine, which had been hidden under the words of medical authorities—in other words, to write scholastic commentaries. Writing in 1580 or shortly before, Andrea Graziolo, a Paduan-trained physician, dated the crucial transformation some time after the mid-fifteenth century. In his view, a revival of letters that followed the arrival of Greek refugees from the Ottoman conquests and the invention of printing had led to medicine being "recalled to its sources," "purified," and "restored to light." For Graziolo, the renewal of medicine apparently meant primarily fuller acquaintance with Greek sources; but his remark occurs in the preface to his scholiated edition of a revised version of the Latin text of Book 1 of the *Canon*.

We may grant the opinions of both Villani and Graziolo a measure of truth, and yet recognize that Taddeo Alderotti's commentaries on a few scattered chapters of the *Canon* (among the earliest Latin expositions of the work) and Graziolo's humanistic scholia, which parade their author's familiarity with recently edited and newly translated Greek works, belong in important ways to a common tradition. Moreover, despite the striking innovations in medicine and allied sciences in the sixteenth-century Italian university milieu, and despite floods of rhetoric attacking the "barbarism" of medieval translators and commentators, there is plenty of evidence to suggest that the medical professoriate at Padua, Bologna, and elsewhere in Italy remained to a significant extent the conscious heirs of the regional academic medical tradition. The reader of the present work will find abundant awareness of the work of such luminaries as Pietro d'Abano, Torrigiano de' Torrigiani (d. ca. 1319?), Giacomo da Forlì (d. 1414), and Ugo Benzi (d. 1439) on the part of their sixteenth- and early seventeenth-century successors. Rather than being killed once and for all by late fifteenth- or early sixteenth-century humanistic vituperation, the Italian scholastic medical tradition had as long a life as the active phase of engagement with the *Canon* itself. Elsewhere in Europe, too, medieval texts remained embedded in university curricula in medicine well into the early modern period. And Galenism, using the term as shorthand for

---

[16] Villani, *Liber de . . . famosis civibus*, pp. 26–27. On the dating of this work, see Talbot R. Selby, "Filippo Villani and His 'Vita' of Guido Bonatti," *Renaissance News* 11 (1958), 243–48.

an entire system of medical and physiological explanation, broke down only in the second half of the seventeenth century.[17] But only the Italian universities were blessed or encumbered with a local tradition of exceptionally well-known and in its day distinguished scholastic medical exposition. One wonders, for example, how broadly the rather numerous editions of the *Conciliator* of Pietro d'Abano, issued by Venetian presses throughout the sixteenth century, were disseminated in northern Europe; it seems likely that the distribution of these publications was mostly regional in character.[18] In early modern Europe in general, the long process of detachment from the old in medicine and physiology has a history as complex (and in some ways as important) as that of the introduction of the new; begun by medical humanists around 1500, the process was not completed in intellectual terms until the general acceptance of seventeenth-century innovations in physiology, and not in institutional terms until the educational reforms of the eighteenth century. Meanwhile, international predominance in medical education passed from Bologna and Padua to other, northern institutions. The history of the *Canon* recounted in this volume is therefore to be seen in the context of a regional medical culture, which for all its marked innovation and creativity in the sixteenth and early seventeenth centuries was also linked in a special way to the medieval and early Renaissance, as well as to the ancient, past.

[17] See Owsei Temkin, *Galenism: Rise and Decline of a Medical Philosophy* (Ithaca, N.Y., 1973), pp. 153–83; and Lester S. King, *The Road to Medical Enlightenment, 1650–1695* (London and New York, 1970). Temkin, p. 165, points out that Galenic therapy and dietetics survived even longer than Galenic physiology and pathology.

[18] Fourteen sixteenth-century editions of the complete work, the last published in 1595, are noted in Sante Ferrari, *Per la biografia e per gli scritti di Pietro d'Abano* (Rome, 1916), pp. 136–38. Of these, twelve were issued at Venice, one at Pavia, and one at Basel.

2

The *Canon* of Avicenna

The encyclopedic medical work written by Avicenna (d. 1037) is far too lengthy and, as the massiveness of the Latin commentaries on short sections of it testifies, far too complex to be adequately characterized in brief. The following comments are intended only to draw the reader's attention to certain features of the organization and content of the *Canon* that seem particularly relevant to its reception in the schools of the West and the emergence of a tradition of Latin commentary and, especially, to the adoption of *Canon* 1.1 as a textbook for the teaching of medical theory. Beginning with a brief overview of the *Canon* as a whole, I shall then pass to a somewhat more detailed, but still highly compressed, account of the physiological treatise in Book 1, Part 1. In the absence of full studies of Avicenna's relationship to his sources and of the relationship of the Latin to the Arabic text of the *Canon*, a summary of *Canon* 1.1 can only be, at best, sketchy and impressionistic. The immediate goal is, however, merely to indicate some of the main features of that treatise as its appears in its Latin form. A few comparisons with other ancient and medieval treatments of somewhat similar material illustrate the distinguishing characteristics of *Canon* 1.1.

The following description refers to the Latin translation of the *Canon* attributed by his pupils to Gerard of Cremona (d. 1187),[1] since, although revisions of the Gerard translation and retranslations of parts of the work began to circulate in the sixteenth century (see Chapter 5), the twelfth-century Latin text was the original basis of Western understanding of Avicenna's book. Furthermore, as we shall see, various of the later revised Latin versions retained much of Gerard's work. Given

---

[1] The list of translations attributed to Gerard by his pupils is most readily available, in English translation, in *A Source Book in Medieval Science*, ed. Edward Grant (Cambridge, 1974); for the *Canon* see p. 38, item 63. The text of the list is edited in Karl Sudhoff, "Die Kurze Vita und das Verzeichnis der Arbeiten Gerhards von Cremona," *Archiv für Geschichte der Medizin* 14 (1923), 73–82. Since the translations are so numerous, it seems likely that some of them were done under Gerard's supervision rather than by Gerard himself. I cite the Gerard version of the *Canon* from Avicenna, *Liber Canonis* (Venice, 1507; facsimile, Hildesheim, 1964). There is no modern critical edition of Gerard's Latin translation (the only complete one) or any other Latin version of the *Canon*. Studies of the Latin manuscript tradition and its relation to the original by Danielle Jacquart and by Ilona Opelt are in progress.

the length, complexity, and technical nature of the *Canon*, the translation attributed to Gerard of Cremona is a remarkable accomplishment. Certainly the long history of the use of this version attests that by and large Gerard or his pupils managed to produce a generally understandable rendering of Avicenna's opus. Nonetheless, even though comprehensive studies of the translation have yet to appear, various scholars in the sixteenth century and the twentieth have pointed out that it is characterized by a high proportion of both errors and obscurely rendered passages. It also retains numerous transliterated Arabic words, especially for names of plants and minerals in the pharmacological sections and for anatomical terms.[2] But whatever its merits or defects, the Gerard translation was the means whereby the *Canon* reached all its readers in western European medical schools up until the early sixteenth century, and a good many of them thereafter.

Considered as an encyclopedia of Greco-Arabic medicine, the *Canon* is in many respects distinguished by comprehensiveness and good organization. Praise of Avicenna's work for these qualities became, indeed, a commonplace among Latin commentators. As G. B. Da Monte put it, Avicenna was moved to write the *Canon* when he saw that "neither among the Greeks nor among the Arabs was there any single, complete, continuous book that taught the art of medicine," the Hippocratic writings being enigmatic and obscure, Galen extremely prolix, and Rasis confusing.[3] Elsewhere, the same author asserted that Avicenna "intended to reduce all the monuments of medical art scattered at large in various works of Galen into one, as it were, corpus. . . . Indeed, he collected much dispersed information into appropriate and defined places and arranged it in sequence."[4] One may certainly agree

---

[2] See Guy Beaujouan, "Fautes et obscurités dans les traductions médicales du Moyen Age," *Revue de synthèse*, 3rd series, 89 (1968), 143–52; and Hakim Abdul Hameed, "Gerard's Latin Translation of Ibn Sīna's *Al-Qanun*," *Studies in Islam* 8 (1971), 1–7; Ilona Opelt, "Zur Übersetzungstechnik des Gerhard von Cremona," *Glotta* 38 (1960), 135–70, a study of Gerard's translation of Aristotle's *De caelo* from an Arabic intermediary version, finds, however, that Gerard was often closer to the spirit of the Arabic than to that of the Greek original. For Renaissance opinions of Gerard's translation, see Part III, below.

[3] "Cum igitur videret Avicenna, neque apud Graecos, neque Arabes haberi ullum librum, qui integram, et continuatam, doceret artem medicinae . . . ," Da Monte, comm. *Canon* 1.1 (Venice, 1554) fol. 2ʳ. On Da Monte and this commentary, see Chapter 6, below.

[4] "Atque hac ego occasione Avicennam commotum crediderim, virum inter Arabas omnes acerrimi ingenii, ut omnia Galeni in medica arte monumenta sparsim in variis libris disseminata, in unum veluti corpus redigeret. . . . Verum, dum ille multa hinc inde dispersa in certas, propriasque sedes colligit, et seriatim disponit," G. B. Da Monte, preface, *Galeni opera ex sexta Juntarum editione* (Venice, 1586), sig. [A8ᵛ].

that the *Canon* is comprehensive. Few aspects of traditional Greek and Arabic medicine are left untouched in its five books, which together amount to about a million words in length. However, the *Canon* is at least as much a collection of essentially separate and distinct manuals and reference works as it is an architectonic *summa* of medicine. Moreover, while individual sections are as a rule clearly organized and succinctly expressed, the overall arrangement is somewhat confusing and involves a certain amount of overlapping. The reader turns with gratitude to the lengthy analytic table of contents found in the early printed editions of Gerard's translation immediately after Avicenna's preface to the whole work and before each of its subsequent books.

Book 1 is divided into four main parts, or fen, to use the term adapted from the Arabic by the Latin translator. It opens with the statement of principles and handbook of physiology. The second fen of Book 1 classifies varieties, efficient causes, and symptoms of disease. Diseases are divided primarily into those caused by imbalance of the four elementary qualities of hot, wet, cold, and dry in the body, those caused by faulty composition, or conformation of bodily parts, and those caused by *solutio continuitatis* or *continui*, which may be rendered, more or less, as trauma. The efficient causes of disease are categorized as either connected with environment, regimen, and psychology (among them are included the factors embraced in the traditional scheme of the "non naturals"—air, food, and drink; repletion and inanition; motion and rest; sleep and waking; and passions of the soul)[5] or as due to any of a wide range of individual physical events, some of which (for example, pain and swelling) the modern reader might be inclined to consider symptoms rather than causes. The section on symptomology both lists an array of individual signs of imbalance of complexion, of *solutio continuitatis*, of obstruction, and so on, and reviews the standard means of diagnosis by pulse and urine. The third fen of Book 1 concerns the conservation of health: separate sections on pediatric, adult, and geriatric regimen are followed by regimes for the delicate and complexionally imbalanced, and for travelers. The fourth and final fen of Book 1 deals with principles of therapy and forms of treatment appropriate for different conditions. Therapies discussed include emetic, cathartic, sedative, and other medications, bleeding, cauterization, blistering, and enemas.

Book 2 is on the subject of medicinal simples; most of it is given over

[5] See Saul Jarcho, "Galen's Six Non-Naturals: A Bibliographic Note and Translation," *Bulletin of the History of Medicine* 44 (1970), 370–77; Jerome J. Bylebyl, "Galen on the Non-Natural Causes of Variation of the Pulse," *Bull. Hist. Med.* 45 (1971), 482–85; Peter H. Niebyl, "The Non-Naturals," *Bull. Hist. Med.* 45 (1971), 486–92.

to a list—arranged more or less in Latin alphabetical order, presumably by the translator—of individual substances, their properties, and the conditions for which they are supposedly remedies. In his third book, Avicenna provided twenty-one fen on ailments peculiar to each major organ of the body—arranged from head to toe—and their treatment. Most of the sections are preceded by one or two chapters on the anatomy and aspects of the physiology of the organ in question. Book 4 surveys diseases and injuries that either affect the whole body or may occur in any part of it, and their treatment; of its seven fen, the most notable is probably the first, on fevers, which provided a famous and influential account of the subject. The remaining fen of Book 4 concern the concept of crisis or critical days in illness; tumors and pustules; *solutio continuitatis* in the form of wounds, bruises, sprains, and ulcers; dislocations and fractures; poisons of mineral, vegetable, and animal origins (including animal bites and stings); and skin conditions. The fifth and final book of the *Canon* is an *antidotarium*, or manual on the preparation of compound medicines.

If one wishes to use the *Canon* as a reference tool, the arrangement of material just summarized works well for some subjects, but a good deal less well for others. A reader who is primarily interested in disease, for example, finds a sequence of more or less self-contained treatises offering complementary information. He or she can begin with classification, efficient causes, and symptoms of disease in general in Book 1, Fen 2, and proceed to the survey arranged by varieties of treatment in Book 1, Fen 4. Then, moving from the general to the particular, there is the account of diseases affecting different parts of the body in Book 3 and of diseases affecting the body as a whole in Book 4. Yet the division of the material into separate sections, and the provision of the analytical table of contents, means that anyone who is interested only in one particular topic—*lepra*, say, or diseases of the eyes—can easily turn to a few chapters on that subject alone.

The results are also fairly satisfactory if one considers the material available to a reader primarily interested in therapy. There is a self-contained survey of treatment methods (1.4) and a dictionary of medicinal simples (2); much discussion of treatments appropriate for disease of particular bodily parts is found in Book 3, and of ills affecting the entire body in Book 4; Book 5 provides guidance for compounding medicines. The arrangement has the merit of making it possible to approach the subject of therapy from a variety of different standpoints. One can, for example, relatively easily find an answer to any of the following questions: When and in what conditions is bleeding an appropriate treatment? What are the medicinal powers of cinnamon? What treatments are recommended for deafness? For various kinds of fevers? How is theriac compounded? However, although no systematic survey has been attempted for present purposes, it is clear that consistency throughout the whole, whether in terms of therapeutic recommendations or of properties attributed to substances, is not always achieved.[6]

Least satisfactory, in some respects, is the arrangement of the physiological and anatomical material. Principles of physiology and the anatomy of bones, muscles, nerves, veins, and arteries are discussed in the first fen of Book 1; but the accounts of the anatomy and some further discussion of the physiology of other major organs (brain, lungs, heart, digestive and reproductive organs, for example) are scattered through the opening chapters of the twenty-one fen of Book 3. This separation, which is the result both of Avicenna's division of medicine into theory and practice and of the classification of bodily parts that he adopted, was, as we shall see, further accentuated by the curricula and practices of medieval university faculties of medicine. But in order to understand both the basis for Avicenna's treatment of physiology and anatomy and the principles underlying the organization of the *Canon* as a whole, it is necessary to turn to the content of the first fen of Book 1.

The easiest way to describe *Canon* 1.1 is as a manual of Galenic physiology, although such a description is slightly misleading because the work also contains other elements of considerable importance. Furthermore, although the subject matter of the treatise is primarily physiological, the discipline with which it is concerned is not coterminous with even the loosest and most general modern definition of the science of physiology. Instead, Fen 1, along with other parts of Book 1, deals with the theoretical part of medicine, a subject that embraced the definition of medicine and of its place among the arts and sciences, and the fundamental principles of medical learning. *Canon* 1.1 is subdivided into six *doctrinae*, the last four of which are mainly physiological in content. The first two sections concern the definition, subdivisions, and subject of medicine and the theory of the elements, the last being considered to provide the basis in physical science for physiological theory.

The first section (*doctrina*) of Fen 1 opens with a definition of medicine: "Medicine is the science by which we learn the various states of the human body, when in health and when not in health, whereby

---

[6] Commentators noted some of the inconsistencies. See, e.g., Dino del Garbo (d. 1327), *Chirurgia* (a commentary on sections of *Canon* 4), *Quaestio* 38, cited in Siraisi, *Alderotti*, p. 407.

health is conserved and whereby it is restored, after being lost."[7] Medicine is thus presented from the outset as a science in the Aristotelian sense of a body of knowledge derived by demonstrative reasoning from true premises,[8] but a science with a practical purpose. Implicit in the definition is the repudiation of any notion that medicine is merely a practical art, technology, or craft.[9] Avicenna next asserts that medicine is divided into theory and practice, rebutting the counterclaim that any true science must of necessity be entirely theoretical with the example of philosophy, also, in his view, divided into theoretical and practical parts. Furthermore, it is not the theoretical part of medicine alone that is categorized as *scientia*; the practical part is also *scientia*, since it too involves formally organized knowledge, in this case the knowledge of how the tasks of healing should be carried out.

The subject of medical science, we learn in the following chapter,[10] is the human body, insofar as it is subject to health and sickness. Since complete knowledge only comes with knowledge of causes, the physician must know the causes of health and sickness, these being classified in the Aristotelian manner into material, efficient, formal, and final causes. The subject of Fen 1 is announced to be the material, formal, and final causes of the human body as it is subject to health and sickness (efficient causes Avicenna identified with external factors affecting the body and discussed, as already noted, in Book 1, Fen 2). The *medicus*, who must also know regimen, symptoms, and medications, should investigate these causes by sense and anatomy, but he should take the fundamentals of physical science (for example, that the elements exist and are four in number) from natural philosophy without himself engaging in natural philosophical investigation.

The second *doctrina* of Fen 1, on the elements,[11] is an admirable illustration of this last principle, since it provides a highly compressed account of those, and only those, parts of a mainly Aristotelian element theory necessary to establish the human body as an object in the physical world and to provide the foundations for an understanding of two central concepts of Greco-Arabic medical theory, namely humoral

---

[7] "Dico quod medicina est scientia qua humani corporis dispositiones noscuntur ex parte qua sanatur vel ab ea removetur ut habita sanitas conservetur et amissa recuperetur." *Canon* (Venice, 1507), fol. 1ʳ. The translation is that of O. Cameron Gruner modified by Michael R. McVaugh in Grant, *Source Book*, p. 715.

[8] See, e.g., *Posterior Analytics* 1.2, 71b15–72b4.

[9] Some influential medieval authors, both Arabic and Latin (e.g., Hugh of St. Victor), classified medicine as a "mechanical" art, or grouped it with such activities as hunting and cooking. See James A. Weisheipl, O.P., "Classification of the Sciences in Medieval Thought," *Mediaeval Studies* 27 (1965), 54–90.

[10] *Canon* 1.1.1.2 (Venice, 1507), fol. 1ʳ⁻ᵛ. [11] Ibid., 1.1.2, fols. 1ᵛ–2ʳ.

physiology and the idea of *complexio*, temperament, or *krasis* (that is, the balance of the elementary qualities of hot, wet, cold, and dry in living bodies). We read that the human body, like all other bodies, is compounded of the elements. The two heavy elements, earth and water, contribute chiefly to the formation of its members; and the two light elements, air and fire, contribute mostly to the generation of *spiritus* and motion of the members (although only the soul actually moves the members). In addition to learning the natural place and qualities of each element (earth in the center, cold and dry, and so on), the reader is also reminded that earth preserves shapes and forms; that water receives all shapes but does not preserve them, that air helps in rarefying and elevating substances; and fire assists in processes of maturation, mixing, and making subtle. When one recalls, for example, the notion frequently expressed by medieval authors that a good memory is due to the physical retention of images by relatively dry (that is, earthy) brain tissue,[12] or the frequency with which the heating of mixtures plays a part in medical recipes, the medical and physiological relevance of the latter information becomes readily apparent.

The first two *doctrina* of Fen 1 thus constitute an important statement about the nature of medical learning. The definition of medicine is broad enough to include the study of all aspects of physical function. The status of medicine as a science is defended. Moreover, the subject is placed in the context of Aristotelian natural philosophy, through insistence on medicine's scientific character, the application to it of the concept of the four causes, and the assertion that the fundamental physical principles on which medicine rests are drawn from natural philosophy. The human body studied by the physician exists as part of the sublunary world of Aristotelian physics and is subject to its laws. At the same time the independence of medicine as a discipline is safeguarded by the warning that the *medicus* should not, *qua medicus*, investigate issues in natural philosophy. The significance of these assertions was not to escape Avicenna's Latin commentators.

In addition, the second of the two introductory sections, that on the elements, fulfills a transitional function. While it continues the Aristotelian and philosophical themes of *Doctrina* 1, it also leads directly into the mainly Galenic and physiological material of the rest of the treatise. The topics surveyed in the last four subdivisions of Fen 1 are *complexio*

---

[12] For example, "illi qui habent complexionem cerebri in posteriori ventriculo siccam melius memorantur: sed illi qui habent humidam, male memorantur: quia impressio in re sicca firmius adheret quam in re molli." *Thaddei Florentini* [i.e., Taddeo Alderotti], *Expositiones . . .* (Venice, 1527), fol. 361ᵛ. The idea is a commonplace, and other examples, both ancient and medieval, could be cited.

or temperament, the humors or bodily fluids, the parts of the body, and the virtues and operations, which include sensation, motion, pulsation, and so on. These categories, together with the elements and *spiritus* (discussed by Avicenna along with the virtues and operations), constitute the ancient scheme of the things natural.[13] In composing Fen 1, Avicenna superimposed the Aristotelian scheme of the four causes upon the set of seven things natural, redefining the latter as a sequence that proceeded from the most remote to the most immediate material causes, and ended with the final causes of the human body. Thus *Doctrina* 1 informs the reader that the body's material causes are the elements (remote), the humors (somewhat remote), and the members and *spiritus* (immediate). The virtues and operations, which usually come last in the scheme of things natural, Avicenna regarded, appropriately enough, as the final or teleological causes of the human body. These definitions accounted for the things natural except *complexio*, which Avicenna proclaimed the body's formal cause.[14] He discussed *complexio* in its accustomed place in the sequence of things natural between the elements and the humors. This position, somewhat awkward in terms of his arrangement according to the four causes, had perhaps to be retained because of the presence of another implied progression in the traditional order of the first four of the things natural (elements, *complexio*, humors, members), namely an ascending hierarchy of perceptibility to sense.

Within this whole scheme, each section leads logically to its successor, and all major bodily functions are neatly fitted into the system. Having learned that the human body, like all other sublunary bodies, is fundamentally composed of the four elements, each with its pair of qualities, the reader proceeds next to *Doctrina* 3 on *complexio*. The balance of the elementary qualities produces, in plant and animal species, in human individuals, in parts of the body, and in medicinal compounds, the *complexio*, which Avicenna, as transmitted by Gerard, defined as itself a quality. Complexion, used in this special sense, is either balanced or unbalanced, temperate or intemperate; in reality, however, complexion never achieves perfect balance, although in man it can come very close. A given complexion can only be identified by comparison with one of a series of norms (such as with the ideal for the species or the individual). According to Avicenna, eight varieties of temperate and eight varieties of distemperate complexion can be identified in this way. Medicines, too, can only be described as, for example, temperate, hot, or cold, with regard to their effect on a particular body

---

[13] See n. 5, above.   [14] *Canon* 1.1.1.1 (Venice, 1507), fol. 1ʳ.

or kind of body. The same medicine may be hot in regard to a scorpion and cold in regard to a man, or hotter for Peter than it is for Paul.[15] Whereas the elements in the human body were conceived of as not individually or directly perceptible to sense, complexion was supposedly to some extent detectable by physical means; in human beings, the skin of the palm of the hand is the most temperate organ and hence serves as the measure of the complexion of the other parts of the body and the manifestation of the complexion of the body as a whole. As is apparent from the foregoing, all the organs and humors of the body were thought of as individually complexionate. Avicenna accordingly provided his readers with four lists of bodily parts, each list being arranged in descending order from the extreme of hotness, coldness, wetness, or dryness to the palm of the hand.[16]

Since complexion in human beings was considered both as a kind of individual constitution and as sex-linked and subject to change in scientifically predictable ways over time (as well as in response to climatic and other conditions), discussion of complexion necessarily involved consideration of growth and aging as well as sex differences. Avicenna devoted a chapter to these topics, in which he considered some of the implications of the doctrine that life involves a process of diminution of heat and moisture from infancy to old age and ultimately death. A long section of this chapter weighs the relative complexional heat of children and youths; the problem was of interest because the theory just mentioned implied that infants ought to be the hotter, but the vigor of youth seemed to suggest the contrary.[17]

Doctrina 4 defines the humors as liquids into which nutriment is converted. In addition to the four primary humors (blood, phlegm, red bile, and black bile), four secondary humors are identified. All are said to be found in both good and bad varieties. The good varieties of the primary humors are absorbed into and nourish the substance of the body; the bad are "superfluities," which are either excreted or damaging to the body if retained.[18] Thus, discussion of the humors and their role in the body's economy involves attention to digestion, nutrition, and excretion, processes treated in a chapter on the generation of the humors. Topics covered include the stages of digestion and functions of mastication, saliva, stomach, intestines, liver, kidneys, and bladder.[19]

The topic of the humors is succeeded in *Doctrina* 5 by that of the *membra*, or parts of the body, which are here described as generated by the

---

[15] Ibid., 1.1.3.1, fols. 2ʳ–3ʳ.   [16] Ibid., 1.1.3.2, fols. 3ʳ⁻ᵛ.
[17] Ibid., 1.1.3.3, fols. 3ᵛ–4ᵛ.   [18] Ibid., 1.1.4.1, fols. 4ᵛ–6ʳ.   [19] Ibid., 1.1.4.2, fols. 6ʳ⁻ᵛ.

humors and sustained by their nutritive activity. The introductory chapter of this section contains generalizations about the members paralleling those about the humors and complexions in the two preceding parts of the work;[20] it is, however, followed by five *summae* containing a total of seventy-six chapters on the anatomy of the bones, muscles, nerves, arteries, and veins.[21] Well over half of Fen 1, in fact, consists of these chapters on anatomy. However, as we shall see in the next chapter, the only part of *Doctrina* 5 normally taught in European universities was the introductory chapter, and this is all that will be considered here. It is mainly concerned with various ways of classifying bodily parts. The first distinction made is between *membra similia* or *simplicia* (for example, bones, cartilage, nerves, ligaments, arteries, and veins) and composite or instrumental members (for example, the hands or the face); it will be observed that this distinction is not quite the same as that between tissues and organs, which it is sometimes said to resemble. Brief definitions of the nature and function of the more important *membra similia* follow. It is, of course, only such members that are treated in the subsequent anatomical chapters; for an account of the chief composite members as such the reader has to turn to the introductory chapters of each section of Book 3.

The next classification of members is according to whether they receive or emit virtue: examples of members that both receive and emit (*suscipiens et tribuens*) are the brain and the liver; a member that receives and does not emit is the flesh; one that emits and does not receive is, according to some, the heart, although others disagree. This allusion to the difference between the teaching of Aristotle and that of Galen on the role of the heart leads, appropriately enough, to consideration of the Galenic doctrine of the three, or four, primary or principal members. The discussion divides the parts into principal members and members that serve the principal members. The former are heart, brain, liver, and testicles; the subsidiary organs of the heart are the arteries and lungs, those of the liver the stomach and veins, and so on. Again, the members may be divided into those in whose generation the paternal sperm played a larger part (all *membra similia* other than flesh and blood) and those generated primarily from the retained menstrual blood of the mother (flesh and blood); discussion of this distinction leads into a brief excursus on embryology. Members may also be classified as fibrous (*villosa*) or nonfibrous in composition, the *membra villosa* being the stomach, intestines, urinary bladder, and gall bladder.

Discussion of the principal members leads naturally to consideration

---

[20] Ibid., 1.1.5.1 fols. 7ʳ–8ᵛ.   [21] Ibid., 1.1.5, *summae* 1–5, fols. 8ᵛ–23ʳ.

of the virtues, or powers, associated with each of them. These were divided into "natural," "vital" and "animal" virtues, a classification ultimately connected with the philosophical concept of the threefold character of the soul. Hence, *Doctrina* 6, the concluding section of Fen 1, opens (after a brief introductory chapter) with an account of the natural virtues (or in other terminology, powers of the vegetative soul) associated with liver and testicles: growth, the ability to convert and assimilate nutriment, and reproduction.[22] Avicenna then proceeded to a description of the role of *spiritus* in preparing the body for the reception of the animal virtues (that is, the powers associated with the sensitive soul possessed by all animals, including humankind) of motion and sensation. *Spiritus* in the Galenic tradition here followed by Avicenna was a highly refined bodily substance formed in part from inspired air; in Avicenna's version it was first generated in the liver from the vaporous part of the humors (to which, presumably, inspired air had contributed) and then received a second generation in the heart. Pervading the entire body, *spiritus*, which manifests itself in pulsation, serves as the vehicle of *virtus vitalis*, which keeps life itself in being. Specialized functions attributed to *spiritus*—the refinement of animal spirits in the brain and the role of visual spirits in seeing—were also briefly mentioned by Avicenna.[23] The account of the animal virtues focuses mainly on the process whereby messages from the senses are received and interpreted in the brain. For the Latin Middle Ages and Renaissance, Avicenna was of course a leading authority on psychology, although his reputation in this field was chiefly based on his *De anima* rather than the *Canon*.[24] Nonetheless, in the latter work, too, he weighed the validity of such classifications of brain function as *sensus communis*, *phantasia*, and imaginative, cogitative, estimative, and rational powers (the last of these being associated with the rational soul and reserved for humankind alone).[25] Fen 1 finally concludes with a chapter in which it is pointed out that many of the body's actual operations require the cooperation of both natural and animal powers.[26]

As will have become apparent from the foregoing summary, the first

---

[22] Ibid., 1.1.6.2–3, fols. 23ʳ–24ʳ.

[23] Ibid., 1.1.6.4, fols. 24ʳ⁻ᵛ. In the Gerard version, this chapter is titled "De virtutibus animalibus," although more than half of it is devoted to discussion of *virtus vitalis* and *spiritus*.

[24] Avicenna's psychology is contained principally in his *De anima*, also known in Latin as *Sextus de naturalibus*; see *Avicenna Latinus. Liber De anima seu Sextus de naturalibus I-II-III*, ed. Simone Van Riet, with introduction by G. Verbeke (Louvain and Leiden, 1972). The work was translated into Latin between 1152 and 1166, and survives in about fifty Latin manuscripts (ibid., pp. *91–*106).

[25] *Canon* 1.1.6, *summa* 1, 5 (Venice, 1507), fols. 24ᵛ–25ʳ.   [26] Ibid., 1.1.6, fols. 25ʳ⁻ᵛ.

fen of Book 1 of the *Canon* is a compendium based almost entirely upon ancient Greek sources, chiefly Aristotle and Galen. Yet Avicenna's selection, organization, and interpretation of his material resulted in a work with a distinctive character of its own. Investigation of the relationship of Fen 1 to its sources is beyond the scope of the present work; however, consideration of the way in which a few somewhat arbitrarily chosen examples of Aristotelian and Galenic doctrines appear in Avicenna's treatise may serve to throw light upon the special characteristics and apparent goals of that work.

Avicenna was both physician and philosopher, although he distinguished quite sharply between the two roles. Repeatedly, he warned the readers of Fen 1 that the *medicus* should not himself investigate natural philosophy, but should rather accept the conclusions of experts in that field. However, information and ideas derived from philosophy in general and from Aristotle in particular in fact play quite a large part in Fen 1. The Aristotelian framework provided for the whole work in its opening sections has already been noted. In addition, Avicenna took every opportunity that offered itself to point out specific differences between the physiological and psychological views of Galen and his followers and those of Aristotle and his. The most important differences between Aristotle and Galen on the subject of physiology were those relating to the functions of heart and brain and to conception. Regarding heart and brain, Aristotle usually held the heart to be the primary organ of the whole body,[27] whereas the Galenists, as already noted, considered the heart only one of several primary organs (namely, heart, brain, and liver, a triad to which the testicles were often added as a fourth).[28] The differing doctrines had extensive ramifications in that they also entailed differing views on sensation and motion, the blood vessels, and other topics. As regards conception, Aristotle held that the active or formative principle was contributed entirely by the male,[29] whereas Galen maintained that both sexes contributed actively to the formation of the fetus and that females as well as males therefore emitted sperm.[30]

[27] See, e.g., *De partibus animalium* 3.4, 666a5–b1; 3.4–5, 667a34–b31.

[28] An aphoristic statement of Galen's views is found in the *Ars* (also known as the *Tegni*) or *Microtechne*; in the medieval Latin version it runs "Principales igitur sunt cor, cerebrum, epar, et testiculi. Ab illis vero exorta sunt et illis famulantur nervi et spinalis medulla cerebro, cordi vero arterie, vene epati, seminalia vasa testiculis." *Tegni Galieni* 2.28–29 in *Articella nuperrime impressa* (Lyon, 1515), fol. cxi[r]. Elaborations of the concept are, of course, worked out in *De usu partium* and other longer treatises of Galen.

[29] See *De generatione animalium* 1.19–20, 727b5–729a33, and 2.4, 738b20–739a26.

[30] *On the Usefulness of the Parts*, tr. Margaret T. May (Ithaca, N.Y., 1968), 14.6–11, II.628–46; *De Semine* and *De foetuum formatione*, ed. Kühn, 4:512–702. For discussion and

Hence, in the first general chapter on the members, Avicenna informed his readers, according to the version attributed to Gerard, that the brain was held to be the *principium* of sense absolutely by some (the Galenists), but only intermediately by others (the Aristotelians).[31] A little farther on, he remarked that

> . . . the *medici* differ from a great man among the philosophers. For this great man among the philosophers said that the heart is the member that gives out and does not receive. For it is the first root of all the virtues, and it gives to all the other members their virtues by which they are nourished and live and by which they know and move. But the *medici* and some of the first philosophers shared out these virtues among the members and they do not say that [the heart] gives out and does not take in. And the opinion of the philosopher is indeed more subtly proved and truer. But the opinion of the *medici* when it is attended to in the first place (*in primis*) is more obvious.[32]

Later in the same chapter, referring to the simile used by "he who gave truth (*verificavit*) to the wise," likening the male contribution in conception to rennet and the female contribution to that of the milk passively acted upon by rennet, Avicenna observed:

> This word is to no small, nay, to a large extent, contrary to the words of Galen. For it seems to him that both the power of coagulating and the power of being coagulated is in each of the two [that is, male and female] sperms. . . .[33]

---

comparison of the views of Aristotle and other ancient and medieval authors on conception, see Howard B. Adelmann, *Marcello Malpighi and the Evolution of Embryology* (Ithaca, N.Y., 1968), II.734–47; and Joseph Needham, *A History of Embryology*, pp. 31–74.

[31] *Canon* 1.1.5.1 (Venice, 1507), fol. 7ᵛ: "Sed cerebrum quidem prebet sensum secundum quosdam absolute et secundum quosdam non absolute."

[32] "De aliis vero duabus divisionis partibus in una earum medici a magno philosophorum diversificati sunt. Philosophorum namque magnus dixit quod membrum tribuens et non recipiens est cor. Ipsum nam est omnium virtututum prima radix et omnibus aliis membris suas tribuit virtutes quibus nutriuntur et vivunt et quibus comprehendunt et quibus movent. Medici autem et quidam primorum philosophorum has virtutes in membris partiti sunt et non dixerunt quod sit membrum tribuens et non suscipiens. Et philosophi quidem sermo cum subtiliter certificatur est veracior. Sed medicorum sermo in primis cum attenditur est magis manifestus." Ibid.

[33] "Hoc autem verbum non parum immo multum verbis Galeni est contrarium. Sibi namque videtur quod cuique duorum spermatum inest virtus coagulativa et virtus coagulationem suscipiens: et propter hoc non se prohibet quando dicat quod virtus coagulativa in masculis est fortior. Virtus coagulationem suscipiens est fortior in feminis." Ibid., fol. 8ʳ. For Aristotle's simile of the rennet and the milk, see *De generatione animalium* 1.20, 729a,11–14.

In several passages of *Doctrina* 6, on the virtues, Avicenna returned at some length to the topic of the differences between the physiology of Aristotle and that of Galen, explaining that their differences over heart and brain were reflected in varying accounts of the vital, animal, and natural powers (associated with heart, brain, and liver, respectively).[34] In one of these passages the *medicus* was instructed that though the Aristotelian view was correct, it was not his business in his capacity as *medicus* to investigate the issue, since whether or not a particular organ was or was not the *principium* of one of the powers made no difference from the standpoint of medical treatment.[35]

Doctrina 6 also warns of differences between philosophical and medical terminology. Galenic medical writers normally described motion and sense as animal, and growth and reproduction as natural, powers. Avicenna, as Gerard represented him, pointed out that "the philosophers when they say *anima* mean *anima terrena*, the perfection of the natural instrumental body. And they mean the *principium* of every power, that principle indeed from which motion and diverse operations come."[36] Hence, the powers of growth and reproduction termed natural by medical writers might be described as *animales* in philosophical texts, although on other occasions *animalis* might be used to refer to the power of comprehending and moving. Furthermore, the reader is also instructed that philosophers use the term natural for "every power (*virtus*) through which operation occurs in a body according to the diversity of its form,"[37] and this usage refers to a higher faculty than the powers of reproduction and growth designated by the medical term *virtus naturalis*. Finally, yet other passages in the same *doctrina* point out differences between philosophers and medical writers over the proper classification of the internal powers of the brain.[38]

In Fen 1, the various discussions of the relationship of philosophical and medical teachings carry a double message. On the one hand, the *medicus* is repeatedly warned off philosophizing. He is, in effect, told on a number of occasions that although the Aristotelian teaching is true,

---

[34] *Canon* 1.1.6, *summa* 1, 4 (Venice, 1507), fol. 24ᵛ.

[35] "Medicus autem cum conceditur ei membra hec prenominata istarum virtutum principia ex existere non curat in eo quod de esse medicationis considerat an ex aliis habeantur principiis, que sunt ipsis priora vel non, neque illud ex eis existit que philosophus non ei levia facit." Ibid., 1.1.6, *summa* 1, 1, fol. 23ʳ.

[36] "Philosophi autem cum animam dicunt animam terrenam dicere volunt perfectionem corporis naturalis instrumentalis. Et volunt dicere principium omnis virtutis ex qua metipsi motus perveniunt et operationes diverse." Ibid., 1.1.6, *summa* 1, 4, fol. 24ᵛ.

[37] "Et naturalem volunt dicere pro omni virtute ex qua operatio pervenit in suo corpore secundum huius forme diversitatem." Ibid.

[38] Ibid., fol. 25ʳ.

he should for all practical purposes follow Galen and not worry about the discrepancy. On the other, the reader gets a good many tantalizing glimpses of philosophical views, and hints are not lacking that the dual roles of philosopher and physician may be combined in one person. That Avicenna himself had functioned in both capacities was, of course, well known to medieval and Renaissance readers of the *Canon* in Latin.[39] Furthermore, in *Canon* 1.1 Avicenna referred readers of Fen 1 to his own philosophical writings;[40] and he drew attention to Galen's philosophical interests with the remark that if Galen is to be attacked for his views on the division of medicine "he ought not to be attacked insofar as he is a *medicus* but insofar as he is a philosopher."[41]

For the strictly physiological, as distinct from the natural philosophical, material in *Canon* 1.1, Galen is by far the most important source. Almost all the physiological concepts schematized and abbreviated in Avicenna's treatise can be found in Galen's works. Except for the instances noted above, in which Galen's views are weighed against those of Aristotle, to the ultimate advantage of the latter, the Latin text of *Canon* 1.1 contains few or no examples of clearly intentional divergence from Galen's teaching. Moreover, Galen is several times cited by name, and is always mentioned with respect, even in instances when Aristotle's opinions are preferred from the standpoint of philosophy. Yet the spirit and approach of Avicenna in *Canon* 1.1 seems very different from that of Galen.

Avicenna's apparent goal in writing *Canon* 1.1 was to present a highly compressed yet comprehensive account of the whole of physiological theory; the work teaches a set of principles that have been, to a very large extent, effectively abstracted from any context of experience. Unified organization, clarity (usually), and brevity are achieved, but at a certain cost. Lacking, for the most part, are illustrative examples, admissions of uncertainty or limited knowledge, indications of divergence of views among ancient physicians, or acknowledgment of the presence of inconsistencies within the body of Galen's writings. By contrast, Galen's major treatises embody, as a rule, a leisurely and dis-

---

[39] For the dissemination of Avicenna's philosophical writings in western Europe in the Middle Ages, see M. T. d'Alverny, "Avicenna Latinus," *Archives d'histoire doctrinale et littéraire du Moyen Age* 28 (1961), 281ff.; 29 (1962), 217–33; 30 (1963), 221–72; 31 (1964), 271–86; 32 (1965), 257–302; 33 (1966), 305–27; 34 (1967), 315–43; 35 (1968), 301–35; 36 (1969), 243–80; 37 (1970), 327–61; 39 (1972), 321–41 (these volumes also bear a separate numeration by *année*).

[40] For example, "Qualiter autem sermo in hoc certificetur invenitur in nostris libris qui sunt de sapientiis radicalibus." *Canon.*, 1.1.5.1 (Venice, 1507), fol. 8ʳ.

[41] "Non debet aggredi inquantum est medicus: sed inquantum est philosophus." Ibid., 1.1.1.1, fol. 1ᵛ.

cursive investigation of a particular aspect of a unified science of medicine that is not sharply divided into theory and practice. Moreover, in Galen's writings physiological theory is generally interwoven into a context rich in detailed anatomical description, records of personal experience and observation, and, often, polemic against the holders of different scientific views. Without undertaking any detailed investigation of the way in which Avicenna used his Galenic sources (or the form in which these reached him), we may illustrate some of the ways in which the teaching of Galen is transformed by its presentation in the Latin text of *Canon* 1.1 by means of a comparison of a few passages therein with sections of three works of Galen that *Canon* 1.1 to some extent parallels in subject matter—namely, *De complexionibus* (*De temperamentis*), *De naturalibus facultatibus*, and *De usu partium*.[42]

Let us take our first example from the treatment of the subject of *complexio*. Most of the main ideas expressed in *Doctrina* 3 of *Canon* 1.1 can also be found in Books 1 and 2 of Galen's *De complexionibus*. Among the themes present in Galen's work that are also treated in *Canon* 1.1 are the relation of complexion to the elementary qualities;[43] the notion that the physician considers complexion not as a balance of weight (*ad pondus*) but *ad justitiam*, in terms of appropriateness for the species, individual, etc., under consideration;[44] the idea that complexion can only be expressed in relative terms and that the point of reference must always be specified;[45] the related idea that a given complexion may be cold in regard to one point of reference and hot in regard to another;[46] the assertion that man is the most temperate of all complex-

---

[42] I have used *Burgundio of Pisa's Translation of Galen's Peri Kraseon "De complexionibus,"* ed. R. J. Durling. *Galenus Latinus*, vol. 1 (Berlin and New York, 1976), since this presents Galen's work in a form in which it was available to early readers of the *Canon* in Latin. *De usu partium* was not available to Latin readers until the early fourteenth century; I have used the edition of the text by G. Helmreich (Leipzig, 1907; reprint, Amsterdam, 1968), and Galen, *On the Usefulness of the Parts of the Body*, tr. M. T. May (Ithaca, N.Y., 1968). *De naturalibus facultatibus* was consulted in Galen, *On the Natural Faculties*, ed. and tr. A. J. Brock, Loeb Classical Library (reprint ed., Cambridge, Mass., and London, 1979). The relevance of these three treatises to the subject matter of *Canon* 1.1 was long ago noted by Benedetto Rinio; they are by far the most frequently cited works among the marginal references provided in his edition of the Latin text of the *Canon* first published Venice, 1555 (see Chapter 5). It should be stressed once again that these treatises are not necessarily the only or a direct source of the related ideas in *Canon* 1.1; my intention is merely to illustrate some of the characteristics of the latter work.

[43] *De complexionibus*, ed. Durling, 1.1, p. 3.

[44] "Tale autem aliquid et iustitiam esse dicimus, non pondere et mensura id quod equale, sed decente et secundum dignitatem scrutantem." Ibid., 1.6, p. 30.

[45] Ibid., 1.5, pp. 23–24 and elsewhere.

[46] Ibid.

ionate beings and that the skin of the hand is the most temperate part of man;[47] and discussions of the different complexions of various ages[48] and sexes,[49] of the inhabitants of different regions,[50] and of the individual organs of the human body.[51]

De complexionibus 1, however, also contains extensive passages of exposition of differing views and polemic against them that have no parallel in *Canon* 1.1.3; futhermore, Book 3 of *De complexionibus* is devoted to detailed exposition of the complexion of various medicinal substances and the therapeutic applications of complexion theory, topics excluded from *Canon* 1.1. But the characteristic that most significantly distinguishes Galen's treatment from Avicenna's handling of some of the same material is the inclusion throughout Book 2 of *De complexionibus* of lengthy descriptions of the physical manifestations of different kinds of complexion. In Galen's treatise, the whole subject is closely related to anatomical experience, to observation of the patient, and to medical care; in Avicenna's, summary of the topic is explained by means of clearly stated but abstract and apparently arbitrarily determined rules, and examples are deliberately deferred until later in the *Canon*.[52] Thus, Galen's remarks on the complexion of the various organs relate the complexional characteristics of each part to its physical characteristics and especially to its consistency; the flesh of the heart is drier than that of the spleen, kidneys, and liver because it is harder.[53] The reader is urged to find out for himself that the heat of the heart is greater than that of any other organ by thrusting his fingers into an incision in the chest of a living animal.[54] By contrast, *Canon* 1.1's neatly schematized and readily memorable lists of organs in descending order of dryness and heat provide essentially the same information as that given by Galen—and a few gaps are filled in—but supporting references to physical experience are absent. In general, in Galen's much more than in Avicenna's account one is constantly reminded that complexion, and secondary characteristics dependent thereon, are to a significant extent accessible to sense.

Nowhere is this contrast more evident, perhaps, than in the treatment of the issue of whether the complexion of children or youths is hotter. In *Canon* 1.1, in one of the relatively few places in that treatise where a diversity of opinion among ancient physicians is acknowledged, otherwise unidentified *medici antiqui* are described as having

---

[47] Ibid., 1.9, pp. 42–43; 2.1, p. 51.   [48] Ibid., 2.2, pp. 53–57.   [49] Ibid., 2.4, p. 73.

[50] Ibid., 2.5, pp. 80–81.   [51] Ibid., 1.9, pp. 46–48.

[52] "Tu autem in libro 3° et 4° cuiusque xvi complexionum exemplum invenies." *Canon* 1.1.3.1 (Venice, 1507), fol. 3ʳ.

[53] *De complexionibus*, ed. Durling, 2.3, pp. 68–69.   [54] Ibid., p. 69.

been divided on the issue. Galen is said to have dissented from both views, and to have maintained that the heat of children and youths was *in radice* equal, but that the heat of children was greater in quantity and that of youths greater in quality. The rest of the passage is devoted to an explanation of Galen's supposed views, which turns on the two assertions: it is impossible to increase innate heat, and humidity declines throughout life. Thus, the heat of youths is conserved by less humidity than that of infants; they are at a stage of life in which the humidity is sufficient to preserve heat at a level that is qualitatively high, but not of such quantity as to permit further augmentation of the body in the form of growth.[55]

Turning to the Galenic account as presented in *De complexionibus*,[56] one is immediately struck by the much less abstract character of most of the discussion. Galen pointed out that the physician's evaluation of actual (as distinct from potential) complexional heat depended on touch, which with the aid of memory was indeed a satisfactory way of detecting changes in the heat of a single individual. However, if different individuals or whole categories of individuals were to be compared, then it was essential to compare like with like in regard to as many characteristics and conditions as possible—body type, diet, environment, and so on.[57] These remarks, interesting for the adumbration of the idea of controlled observation of numerous exemplars, find no echo in the Latin *Canon* 1.1.3. Moreover, Galen's conclusion in *De complexionibus* was firmly rooted in his clinical experience; he stated that having touched the bodies of numerous children and adolescents, he found it impossible to assert on the basis of the sense of touch that either group was simply and unequivocally hotter than the other.[58] However, the perspiration (a manifestation of heat, evidently) of children, was, owing to their greater humidity, greater in quantity, and that of adolescents more acrid in quality. This difference is because children have more innate heat, but the heat of adolescents is drier. Comparing this chapter with the passage in the *Canon*, one notes that the latter, characteristically, elaborates on Galen's conclusion, but does not contain those of his supporting arguments that depend upon clinical experience and sense perception. (*Canon* 1.1.3.3 does, however, also explain a few perceptible characteristics of small children in complexional terms.)

One more illustration of the way in which Avicenna handled Galenic material may be drawn from his treatment of the topic of digestion and

---

[55] *Canon* 1.1.3.3 (Venice, 1507), fols. 3ᵛ-4ʳ.
[56] *De complexionibus*, ed. Durling, 2.2, pp. 56–67.   [57] Ibid., pp. 62–63.   [58] Ibid., p. 64.

the digestive organs. We have seen that in *Canon* 1.1 there is a short narrative of the digestive process as a whole in the chapter on the generation of the humors (1.1.4.2); to this must be added the description of the coats of the stomach and intestines in the section on *membra villosa* in the general chapter on the members (1.1.5.1), and the account of the four nutritive powers (attractive, retentive, digestive, and expulsive) in the third chapter of *Doctrina* 6. Among the most important Galenic accounts of this part of physiology are Books 4 and 5 of *De usu partium* on the digestive organs and digestive process, and the lengthy discussion of nutritive power in *De naturalibus facultatibus*.

In its main outline, the brief summary of digestion in Avicenna's chapter on the generation of the humors is fairly similar to the much longer account presented by Galen in *De usu partium* and with parts of the account in *De naturalibus facultatibus*. Missing from Avicenna's highly compressed version are, however, both the emphasis on functional teleology and the richness of detail characteristic of *De usu partium* and the context of polemic against Erasistratus and his followers found in *De naturalibus facultatibus*. It is really only the opening generalities of *De usu partium* 4.1–4 that are paralleled in *Canon* 1.1.4.1. Any attempt at more detailed description of the individual digestive organs and their functions, similar to that occupying the remainder of Books 4 and 5 of Galen's work, is postponed in the *Canon* until scattered chapters of Book 3. Furthermore, even in passages that do closely parallel one another in Galen's account and in the *Canon*, Avicenna's version is greatly simplified. In some instances, the process of simplification, and the stripping away or deemphasis of the metaphors freely used by Galen to clarify his descriptions and render them more vivid, resulted in a presentation of Galenic ideas in the *Canon* in a form that was simultaneously both cryptic and perhaps more literal than Galen intended. One example will suffice. In both *De usu partium* and *De naturalibus facultatibus* Galen compared the concoction of the chyle in the liver to the fermentation of wine. In the former work, he said:

> Let us, then, compare the chyle to wine just pressed from the grapes and poured into casks, and still working, settling, fermenting, and bubbling with innate heat. The heavy, earthy part of its residues, which I think is called the dregs, is sinking to the bottom of the vessels and the other, light, airy part floats. This latter part is called the flower and forms on the top of light wines in particular, whereas the dregs are more abundant in heavy wines. In making this comparison, think of the chyle sent up from the stomach to the liver as bubbling and fermenting like new wine from the

heat of the viscus and beginning to change into useful blood; consider too that in this effervescence the thick, muddy residue is being carried downward and the fine, thin residue is coming to the top and floating on the surface of the blood.[59]

In *De naturalibus facultatibus* the same idea is presented as follows:

What else, then, remains but to explain clearly what it is that happens in the generation of the humors, according to the belief and demonstration of the Ancients? This will be more clearly understood from a comparison. Imagine then some new wine which has been not long ago pressed from the grape, and which is fermenting and undergoing alteration through the agency of its continued heat. Imagine next two residual substances produced during this process of alteration, the one tending to be light and air-like and the other to be heavy and more of the nature of earth; of these the one, as I understand, they call the flower and the other the lees. Now you may correctly compare yellow bile to the first of these, and black bile to the latter. . . .[60]

In the *Canon* the presentation of its idea runs as follows:

In every concoction of this sort there is to be found foam and sediment. . . . The foam is red [yellow] bile; and the sediment is melancholy [black bile].[61]

Avicenna's drastic condensation of Galenic material is accompanied on occasion not only by oversimplification, as in the instance just noted, but also by inconsistency, the latter sometimes merely echoing Galen's own. Thus, in the account of the *membra villosa* in the Gerard version of *Canon* 1.1, the urinary bladder is said in passing to have a single tunic; but in the account of the bladder's anatomy in Book 3 it is described as having two tunics.[62] This discrepancy presumably stems from the fact that Galen had assigned the bladder one tunic in *De usu partium* and in one passage of *De naturalibus facultatibus*, but in a second

[59] *De usu partium*, tr. May, 4.3, 1:205–6 (ed. Helmreich, 1:197–98).

[60] *De naturalibus facultatibus*, tr. Brock, 2.9, pp. 208–9.

[61] "In omni autem decoctione que est huiusmodi est res que est sicut spuma et res que est sicut hypostasis, et res fortasse erit cum eis aut que ad adustionem pertinet si decoctio superflua fuerit aut res que non est bene cocta si decoctio fuerit minor quam debet. Spuma autem est colera rubea et hypostasis est melancholia." *Canon* 1.1.4.2 (Lyon, 1507), fol. 6[r].

[62] *Canon* 1.1.5.1, and 3.19.1.1 (Venice, 1507), fols. 8[r], 343[r].

passage of the latter work had given it two.[63] Moreover, while the details of Galen's—and Avicenna's own—experience were excised from *Canon* 1.1, certain concepts adumbrated in Galen's works in *Canon* 1.1 were elaborated to the point where they may be regarded as original contributions. A case of this kind that has been the subject of modern scholarly attention is Avicenna's development of the concept of so-called radical moisture as an explanation of the process of aging.[64] It must be emphasized, however, that the focus in the physiological sections of *Canon* 1.1 upon the systematic presentation and explanation of principles, at the expense of detail and supporting evidence, is unquestionably part of the deliberate strategy of that treatise; other parts of the *Canon* are rich in material pertaining to the experience of the physician and the treatment of patients.

Avicenna was neither the first nor the earliest available in Latin among authors who had written in Arabic to produce a schematic general summary of Greco-Arabic medicine structured around a division into theory and practice. The collection of brief medical opinions attributed to Joannitius and known as the *Isagoge* begins with the assertion that medicine is divided into theoretical and practical branches and proceeds to a consideration of the naturals, the nonnaturals, and the things against nature (that is, diseases).[65] Avicenna has been shown to have drawn some of his material from the medical encyclopedia of Rasis (d. 925); another predecessor and possible partial source of the *Canon* was the survey of medicine written by Haly Abbas (d. 994).[66] As compared with these other works, the *Canon* offers a fuller and more intellectually demanding account of its subject matter than the highly abbreviated *Isagoge*, and its organization is somewhat easier to grasp than that of the work of Rasis. The work of Haly Abbas is fully

[63] Compare *De usu partium* 5.11 (ed. Helmreich, 1:282, tr. May, 1:267) and *De naturalibus facultatibus* 3.11 (tr. Brock, p. 280), with ibid., 1.13 (Brock, p. 50).

[64] See Thomas S. Hall, "Life, Death and the Radical Moisture: A Study of Thematic Patterns in Medical Theory," *Clio medica* 6 (1971), 3–23; and Michael McVaugh, "The 'humidum radicale' in Thirteenth-Century Medicine," *Traditio* 30 (1974), 259–83.

[65] The *Isagoge* became available in Latin before the end of the eleventh century; it was one of the earliest texts to be incorporated into the teaching *corpus* known as the *articella* (see Chapter 3) and was widely disseminated in the twelfth and thirteenth centuries. Joannitius is usually identified with Hunain ibn Ishaq (ninth century).

[66] The relationship between the *Canon* and the work of Rasis is discussed in A. Z. Iskandar, *A Catalogue of Arabic Manuscripts on Medicine and Science in the Wellcome Historical Medical Library* (London, 1967), pp. 2, 29–32. The work of Haly Abbas was the basis of the *Pantegni* of Constantinus Africanus (d. 1087), and was also translated in the twelfth century by Stephen of Antioch. I have consulted Haly Abbas, *Liber totius medicine* (Lyon, 1523).

comparable to the *Canon* in scope and sophistication as well as structure. It is divided into ten books on theory and ten books on practice, of which the first four books on theory roughly parallel *Canon* 1.1 in content. In organization, the *Liber totius medicinae* is in at least one respect superior to the *Canon*: Haly's entire account of physiology and anatomy is presented as a coherent unit in his opening books, whereas in the *Canon*, as we have seen, the treatment of internal organs is excluded from the physiological and anatomical material in Book 1, Fen 1. Like *Canon* 1.1, of which it may well have been one of the sources, the *Liber totius medicinae* contains lengthy passages summarizing Galenic concepts. But the Aristotelian element, which plays so marked a part in *Canon* 1.1 seems not to be found in the corresponding parts of the Latin version of Haly's work. It was precisely Avicenna's philosophical interests that gave *Canon* 1.1 its distinctive cast. In *Canon* 1.1, as in Avicenna's philosophical writings, elements of diverse origin were drawn together. It seems likely that, indeed, Avicenna's well-known readiness to incorporate both Aristotelian and Neoplatonic elements into his philosophical system stimulated his interest in considering the relationship between Aristotelian and Galenic thought, which also contained Platonic elements.[67]

Such, in barest outline, was the *Canon* as translated by Gerard of Cremona or his associates. The scope and organization of the work, the mass of practical information it contained, the author's summaries of Galenic thought (inadequate though these might sometimes be in detail), and the philosophical context in which Avicenna succeeded in placing medicine while preserving its independence as a distinct science—all initially secured for the *Canon* a place of honor in medieval western European medicine. Let us begin to trace its history in the West.

[67] See Philip De Lacey, "Galen's Platonism," *American Journal of Philology* 93 (1972), 27–39.

PART II

The *Canon* in the Schools

3

The *Canon* in the Medieval Universities and the Humanist Attack on Avicenna

By the 1520s, when the period with which this study is principally concerned opens, the *Canon* in its twelfth-century Latin translation was both a venerable part of a centuries-old tradition of medical teaching and a book that had been for a generation the object of attacks ranging from reasoned criticism to vitriolic abuse. In broad outline, the history of these developments is well known. Despite the availability of the Latin translation by 1187 at latest, significant awareness of the *Canon* in the West seems to have begun in the second quarter of the thirteenth century. By the latter part of that century, the work was routinely studied and much prized in the major centers of medical learning, and the production of a body of commentary—to which a number of the best-known learned physicians of the thirteenth to fifteenth centuries contributed—had begun. Meanwhile, criticisms of Arabo-Latin scholastic medicine, already expressed by Petrarch in the mid-fourteenth century, began in the late fifteenth century to be articulated by humanists within the medical community and to be especially concentrated upon Avicenna and the *Canon*. Nonetheless, much remains to be learned about the reception and uses of the *Canon* in the High Middle Ages. A full account of the work's place in the thought and culture of medieval Europe must await the completion of comprehensive studies of the manuscript tradition of the *Canon* and its commentaries and of the content of the commentary literature. The purpose of the following summary is merely to call attention to a few of the most salient features of the history of the *Canon* in the medieval West and of the shaping of the Latin commentary tradition.

Over the course of the late eleventh through the early fourteenth century, in medicine as in other branches of learning, the heritage of Latin antiquity was significantly enlarged by the translation of numerous texts of Greek and Arabic origin. These may be broadly classified into works of Greek origin translated directly from the Greek, works of Greek origin translated from Arabic versions, and works of Arabic origin that were largely based on Greek medical teaching.[1] Medical works of Arabic origin reached the West through two main channels, namely the translations of Constantinus Africanus of Monte Cassino, and those of the Toledan school of the twelfth century. Of these, only the Constantinian translations penetrated the Salernitan schools in the period in which Salerno was still at its height as a center of medical culture. But although Constantinus was appreciative of Arabic medical encyclopedism, as his famous *Pantegni*, a free rendering of Haly Abbas, shows, he did not undertake the task of translating the *Canon*.[2] Hence, the Salernitan teaching of the twelfth and early thirteenth centuries as reflected, for example, in the collections of Salernitan questions edited by Brian Lawn, shows almost no identifiable use of Avicenna.[3] The introduction of the *Canon* instead took place as part of the general dissemination of the corpus of scientific and philosophical works translated by the Toledo school. Toledo appears not to have been especially famed as a center of medical learning, but the medical component in the body of scientific texts translated there is considerable. For example, the Arabo-Latin translations attributed to Gerard of Cremona by his pupils include, besides the *Canon*, nine treatises by Galen and a major work of Rasis.[4]

Perhaps the earliest Latin work to incorporate whole passages drawn from the *Canon* is the *Anatomia vivorum* formerly ascribed to Ricardus Anglicus, which has been dated between 1210 and 1240, with the greatest probability attaching to about 1225. Since a relationship has been demonstrated between this work and parts of the later *De animalibus* of Albertus Magnus, written in the early 1260s, the consequent sugges-

---

[1] For the medieval Latin Hippocratic corpus, see Pearl Kibre, *Hippocrates Latinus: Repertorium of Hippocratic Writings in the Latin Middle Ages* (New York, 1985). For Dioscorides, see John M. Riddle, "Dioscorides," *CTC*, 4:1–143. The Galenic material in the older guide of Herman Diels, *Die Handschriften der antiken Aerzte* (Berlin, 1905–1907; reprint, Leipzig, 1970), is supplemented by Richard J. Durling, "Corrigenda and Addenda to Diels' Galenica. I. Codices Vaticani," *Traditio* 23 (1967), 461–76, and "II. Codices miscellanei," *Traditio* 37 (1981), 373–81. For an overview of the reception of Arabic medicine in the West, see Heinrich Schipperges, *Die Assimilation der arabischen Medizin durch das lateinische Mittelalter. Sudhoffs Archiv für Geschichte der Medizin und der Naturwissenschaften*, Beiheft 3 (Wiesbaden, 1964).

[2] Ibid., p. 54.

[3] Only one allusion to Avicenna is identified by the editor in *The Prose Salernitan Questions*, ed. Brian Lawn (London, 1979); see question B 256, pp. 124–125, and note on p. 124. The manuscript in which this question occurs is written in an English scholar's hand of about 1200 (p. ix).

[4] On the translation of medical works from the Arabic at Toledo, see Schipperges, *Die Assimilation*, pp. 95–103. The important *Chirurgia* of Albucasis was also translated at Toledo, perhaps by Gerard (Schipperges, *Die Assimilation*, p. 95).

tion that the *Anatomia vivorum* may have been composed in a Dominican house in Paris or Germany appears plausible.[5] Albertus himself, according to the editors of his works on animals, knew and used the *Canon*, independently of any use he may also have made of the *Anatomia vivorum*.[6] Although some of his knowledge of Avicenna's anatomy and physiology may have come via Avicenna's compendium *De animalibus*, in addition to, or instead of, the *Canon*, Albertus' use of Avicenna's pharmacology shows that he was definitely familiar with Book 2 of the latter work.[7] Another friar who probably drew on the *Canon* at a relatively early date (although here, too, the simultaneous or alternative use of Avicenna's *De animalibus* is a possibility) was the Franciscan encyclopedist Bartholomaeus Anglicus; his *De proprietatibus rerum*, probably composed in Paris between 1230 and 1250, contains several citations of Avicenna in Book 4 on the human body.[8] And around 1250, the canon of Amiens and physician and surgeon Richard de Fournival listed all five books of the *Canon* in the section of his library devoted to "lucrative sciences," that is, medicine and law.[9]

[5] George Corner, *Anatomical Texts of the Earlier Middle Ages* (Washington, D.C., 1927), pp. 38–44. However, Corner notes (p. 41) that Karl Sudhoff considered the *Anatomia vivorum* to be an early work of the Bolognese school. On the dating of *De animalibus*, see James A. Weisheipl, O.P., "The Life and Works of St. Albert the Great," in *Albertus Magnus and the Sciences: Commemorative Essays, 1980*, ed. James A. Weisheipl, O.P. (Toronto, 1980), p. 38.

[6] See, esp. Albertus Magnus, *Opera omnia*, ed. B. Geyer, vol. 12 (Cologne, 1955); *Quaestiones de animalibus*, ed. Ephrem Filthaut, O.P. pp. 323–24 (index of authors cited). In this collection of questions, Albertus cited Avicenna a number of times by name, but omitted to identify any particular work; the editor has identified the passages in question, distinguishing allusions to the *Canon* from those to other treatises by Avicenna. For discussion of Albertus' knowledge and use of medical writings, see also Nancy G. Siraisi, "The Medical Learning of Albertus Magnus," in Weisheipl, *Albertus Magnus and the Sciences*, pp. 390–404.

[7] Avicenna's compendium based on the Aristotelian works on animals was translated by Michael Scot before 1232. In Books 9 and 12–15 it deals with human anatomy and physiology. The work is printed in Avicenna (Ibn Sina,† 1037), *Opera philosophica Venise, 1508* (facsimile, Louvain, 1961), fols. 29ʳ–64ʳ (second set of foliation). For Albertus' use in his work on plants of Avicenna's pharmacology, see Jerry Stannard, "Albertus Magnus and Medieval Herbalism," *Albertus Magnus and the Sciences*, p. 370.

[8] See Bartholomaeus Anglicus, *On the Properties of Soul and Body*, ed. R. James Long (Toronto, 1979), pp. 82, 85, 94, 97. The date and place are suggested by the editor, pp. 4–5.

[9] See E. Seidler, "Die Medizin in der 'Biblionomia' des Richard de Fournival," *Sudhoffs Archiv für Geschichte der Medizin und der Naturwissenschaften* 51 (1967), 44–54. After Fournival's death in 1260, his books passed to Gerard of Abbeville; after the latter's death in 1272, to the Sorbonne; see Richard H. Rouse, "The Early Library of the Sorbonne," *Scriptorium* 21 (1967), 42–71, 227–251, and idem, "Manuscripts Belonging to Richard de Fournival," *Revue d'histoire des textes* 3 (1973), 253–67. Fournival was the son of one of

Hence, by the middle of the thirteenth century, the *Canon* was both recognized as a work indispensable for the learned medical or surgical practitioner, and also sufficiently well known to be used as a reference tool by encyclopedic writers on natural philosophy whose own learning was not primarily medical. And the *Canon* continued to be used in contexts other than the developing university medical faculties that are henceforth our main subject. Thus, it was drawn on by Vincent of Beauvais in the thirteenth century and Henry of Langenstein in the fourteenth.[10] Furthermore, the presence of the *Canon* in monastic libraries presumably attests to its usefulness both as a general work of reference and for the infirmarian. For example, probably in the late thirteenth century the rather large collection of medical books in the library of Christchurch Priory, Canterbury, was enriched by the addition of two volumes containing parts of the *Canon* acquired from Robert of Cornwall, an up-to-date *medicus* who also donated works of Taddeo Alderotti; nearby, St. Augustine's Abbey possessed five volumes of parts of the *Canon*, some of which seem to have been acquired in the late thirteenth or early fourteenth century.[11] Taddeo Alderotti himself willed his four-volume copy of the *Canon* to the Franciscan friars of Bologna.[12]

Moreover, the use of the *Canon* by secular professional medical men was not always exclusively in an academic context. The frequency with which copies of all or part of it were included in the personal libraries of prosperous university-trained practitioners in the fifteenth—and doubtless also the preceding—century is to be explained not as evidence of the fondness of these men for souvenirs of their student days, but by the *Canon's* reputation as a handy reference work for the practicing physician.[13] This reputation, which Matteo Corti was at pains to

---

the physicians of Philip Augustus and received papal permission to practice surgery, despite his position as chancellor of the cathedral chapter of Amiens, in 1246; see *Li Bestiaires d'Amours di maistre Richart de Fornival e Li response du Bestiaire*, ed. Cesare Segre (Milan and Naples, 1957), p. xxix.

[10] *Vincenti . . . Bellovacensis Speculum quadruplex, naturale, doctrinale, morale, historiale* (Douai, 1624), frequently draws on Avicenna for the books on plants (10–14) and on the human body (28); specific citations of the *Canon* occur, e.g., at 13:107, col. 1013, and 28:9, col. 1998. See also Nicholas H. Steneck, *Science and Creation in the Middle Ages: Henry of Langenstein (d. 1397) on Genesis* (Notre Dame and London, 1976), p. 144.

[11] M. R. James, *The Ancient Libraries of Canterbury and Dover* (Cambridge, 1903), p. 138, nos. 1706, 1707, 1712; pp. 332–33, nos. 1177–81. Regarding the date and identity of the donor of nos. 1177–80, see pp. lxxv–lxxvii.

[12] See his will, edited in Mauro Sarti and Mauro Fattorini, *De claris archigymnasii bononiensis professoribus a saeculo XI usque ad saeculum XIV*, ed. Carlo Albicini and Carlo Malagola, 2 vols. (Bologna, 1888–96), 2:227.

[13] For example, Giovanni Marco da Rimini (d. 1474), who also owned a large collec-

undermine in the 1530s (see Chapter 6), still survived at the very end of the sixteenth century, when Peter Kirsten's teachers at Leipzig told him that anyone who wanted to be a good practitioner had to be a good "Avicennista."[14] Furthermore, it seems likely that parts of the work (for example, Book 2 on simples, and Book 4, Part 1, on fevers) may have been used as manuals of practice by literate *medici* who were not university graduates. Some of the Latin collections of excerpts, maxims, or *flores* from the *Canon*, which apparently began to be compiled before the end of the thirteenth century, may also have been used outside the schools.[15]

Other traces of an influence of the *Canon* outside the universities may be seen in citations of Avicenna in vernacular medical treatises as well as in the existence of vernacular medical compendia purportedly based on Avicenna's work.[16] For example, a French treatise of which at least two copies survive (both in Italian libraries) claims to be "Avicen en romance." It is a little work on regimen that urges on the reader self-help and self-medication.[17] A complete study might reveal its actual re-

tion of Hippocratic and Galenic as well as modern Latin medical works; see Gerhard Baader, "Die Bibliothek des Giovanni Marco da Rimini: Eine Quelle zur medizinischen Bildung im Humanismus," *Studia codicologica*, ed. Kurt Treu, Texte und Untersuchungen zur Geschichte der Altchristlichen Literatur, 124 (Berlin, 1977), pp. 43–97. For other similar examples, see Bindo de Vecchi, "I libri di un medico umanista fiorentino del sec. XV," *La bibliofilia* 34 (1932), 293–301; Giuseppe Biadego, "Medici Veronesi e una libreria medica del sec. XIV," *Atti del R. Istituto Veneto di Scienze, Lettere ed Arti* 75 (1915–1916), 565–85; Léon Dorez, "Recherches sur la bibliothèque de Pier di Leone Leoni, médecin de Laurent de Médicis," *Revue des bibliothèques* 7 (1897), 81–106.

[14] "Praeceptores meos, haec et similia proferre judicia: Qui medicus bonus fieri vult practicus bonus necesse sit Avicennista." *Petri Kirsteni . . . Grammatices arabicae, Liber I. Sive orthographia et prosoda arabica* (Breslau [1608]), p. 3. On Kirsten and his work on the *Canon*, see Chapter 5, below.

[15] For example, Paris, Bibliothèque Nationale, MS lat. 7046 (TK 705), 13c, fols. 1ʳ–48ʳ, inc. "Medicina est scientia"; other examples, which I have not seen, are listed in TK 227, 695, 860, 1307. The wide range of formal education, social status, and intellectual interests in the medieval and Renaissance medical community has been delineated by various recent authors, notably Katharine Park, *Doctors and Medicine in Early Renaissance Florence* (Princeton, 1985).

[16] Two examples of vernacular excerpts from Avicenna, neither of which I have seen, are listed in P. Pansier, "Catalogue des manuscrits médicaux de France. IIIᵐᵉ partie. Manuscrits français," [Sudhoff's] *Archiv für Geschichte der Medizin* 2 (1908–1909), 388, namely, Paris, Bibliothèque de l'Arsenal, no. 2895, fols. 252 and 284, and no. 8216, both fifteenth century. I owe to Linda Voigts the information that Avicenna's views on synochal fevers are discussed in a Middle English *practica* written for a London barber surgeon before 1413 and contained in Cambridge, Gonville and Caius, MS 176/97.

[17] Florence, Biblioteca Medicea Laurenziana, Ashburnham MS 1260, 13–14c, 39 fols., inc. "Ici commence l'Avicen en romance"; Venice, Biblioteca Marciana, MSS Francesi, Appendice 10, no. 262, fols. 1–91, inc. "Dieu qui par sa grant poissance"; fol. 91ᵛ "Ce

lation, if any, to the *Canon*. Another vernacular treatise compiled in Italian in 1478 also claims to be based on Avicenna.[18]

Finally, the *Canon* played a major role in medieval Jewish medical culture. Nathan ha-Meati translated all five books of the *Canon* into Hebrew in 1279, and Zerahia ben Isaac ben Shealtiel Gracian also independently translated Books 1 and 2 into Hebrew during the thirteenth century. Nathan's translation was subsequently revised by Joseph ben Joshua ha-Lorki in about 1400. One hundred and eleven complete or partial manuscripts of these versions survive, most of them of Spanish or Italian provenance.[19] Thus, the most extensive use of the *Canon* outside the universities in western Europe during the Middle Ages was unquestionably by Jewish physicians (as one might expect, given that Jews were excluded from universities, the possessors of a learned medical culture, and in contact with the Arabic world). Nonetheless, the influence of the *Canon* on Western medical thought was chiefly exercised through the adoption of parts of the work as university textbooks.

During the thirteenth century, the study of medicine, like other branches of learning, was profoundly affected by the rise of university organization, the development of scholastic methodology in pedagogy and scientific inquiry, and the reception of Aristotelian natural philosophy. In turn, the teaching of medicine in public *studia generalia* fostered the emergence of medicine as a secular learned profession, so that in the case of medicine the content, the structure, and the uses of learning were all affected by these developments.[20] As already noted, the *Canon* of Avicenna had become available in the West at about the same

---

fuist l'avicenne en roumans" (I am grateful to John B. Friedman for drawing my attention to this manuscript and lending me a microfilm).

[18] Uppsala University Library, uncatalogued Waller 653 D:3, a. 1478, 67 fols., inc. "Questo sie uno fioreto trato de Avicena." I know of this manuscript through the kindness of Per-Gunnar Ottosson, and have seen only a photocopy of the first four and the last folios. Also Jole Agrimi, review of Michele Savonarola, *Libreto de tute le cosse che se manzano*, ed. J. Nystedt, in *Aevum* 2, Anno 58 (1984), 360, notes that some vernacular treatises on diet were based on part of the *Canon*.

[19] Benjamin Richler, "Manuscripts of Avicenna's Kanon in Hebrew Translation: A Revised and Up-to-date List," *Koroth* 8 (1982), 145*–168*; Richler's list greatly enlarges that earlier provided by Steinschneider.

[20] See Vern L. Bullough, *The Development of Medicine as a Profession: The Contribution of the Medieval University to Modern Medicine* (Basel and New York, 1966); Pearl Kibre, "Arts and Medicine in the Universities of the Later Middle Ages," in *Les universités à la fin du Moyen Age*, ed. Jacques Paquet and Jozef Ijsewijn (Louvain, 1978), pp. 213–27; Paul Oskar Kristeller, "Philosophy and Medicine in Medieval and Renaissance Italy," in *Organism, Medicine, and Metaphysics*, ed. S. F. Spicker (Dordrecht, 1978), pp. 29–36; and Siraisi, *Alderotti*.

time as several other major encyclopedic treatments of medicine or surgery of Arab origin and a number of important longer treatises of Galen. In the late twelfth century, too, the well-designed and widely studied core curriculum of short Hippocratic, Galenic, and other texts known as the *ars medicinae* or *articella* began to take shape.

The *Canon,* then, was only one of many medical works, most of them to a greater or lesser extent fundamentally Hippocratic and/or Galenic in content, which would from the beginning play a role in the teaching of the faculties of medicine in the universities. Hence, the *Canon* was studied alongside, not instead of, translations of Greek medical texts; at both Bologna and Montpellier, for example, in the years around 1300 leading medical masters expounded a rather substantial corpus of Galen's treatises. The high reputation achieved by the author of the *Canon* in the university milieu was doubtless chiefly owing to the suitability of various parts of his work as textbooks for teaching different branches of the medical curriculum, although Avicenna's status as a philosopher and the attention he gave to differences between Aristotle and Galen must also have served to enhance the value of the *Canon* in the eyes of physicians in the environment of the thirteenth-century universities.[21]

The actual process whereby the *Canon* entered university curricula is somewhat obscure, owing to the relatively late date of most of the university or doctoral college statutes mentioning the work. Nonetheless, some information can be gleaned about its reception at the main centers of university medical learning, namely Paris, Montpellier, and Bologna and other north Italian *studia.* The earliest list of medical books used at Paris is attributed to Alexander Neckam, who studied there from after 1175 until before 1195. As might be expected, it makes no mention of the *Canon.*[22] That work seems also to have been unknown

[21] Regarding the *articella,* see Paul Oskar Kristeller, "Bartholomaeus, Musandinus and Maurus of Salerno and Other Early Commentators on the 'Articella' with a Tentative List of Texts and Manuscripts," *Italia medioevale e umanistica* 19 (1976), 57–87. For Galenic works studied at Bologna and Montpellier, respectively, see Siraisi, *Alderotti,* pp. 100–7; and Luis Garcia Ballester, "Arnau de Vilanova (c. 1240–1311) y la reforma de los estudios médicos en Montpellier (1309): El Hipócrates latino y la introducción de nuevo Galeno," *Dynamis* 2 (1982), 97–158.

[22] See Charles H. Haskins, *Studies in the History of Mediaeval Science,* 2nd ed. (Cambridge, 1927), pp. 356–76. Medicine does not seem to have been a major subject at Paris until about the mid-thirteenth century; thereafter although fewer medical authors were associated with Paris than with Montpellier, the number of physicians known to have received their training in Paris consistently exceeds those similarly identified with Montpellier, sometimes by a large margin, until the end of the fifteenth century; see Danielle

to Gilles of Corbeil, the author of versified treatises on pulses and urines and on symptomology, whose training was Salernitan but who subsequently came to Paris, where he both taught and served as physician to King Philip II (1180–1223).[23] Precisely when the *Canon* entered the official curriculum at Paris is unclear, but it could presumably have been used to fulfill the requirement in the first officially issued list of books for medical study at the *studium* of Paris (1270–74) that candidates for a license in medicine must have read "one book on *theorica* and one book on *practica*."[24]

On the basis of manuscript evidence, Danielle Jacquart has established that the study of the *Canon* began at Paris between about 1230 and 1258.[25] Her dating appears to be confirmed by the content of Roger Bacon's *De erroribus medicorum*, which presumably refers to conditions at Paris and may, according to its modern editor, have been composed ca. 1250–60. Bacon's acidulous criticisms of the "vulgus Latinorum medicorum" contain several allusions to their insufficient knowledge of Avicenna's work on medicaments; on the other hand, they are also accused of overreliance on Avicenna's inadequate division of diseases. Doubtless, too, Bacon's complaints about the excesses of the current vogue for medical disputation may refer to habits fostered by the use of *Canon* 1.1.[26] The most prominent northern French medical author of the second half of the thirteenth century, Jean de St. Amand (d. before 1307), who may have taught at Paris and whose works were no doubt known there, drew heavily upon the *Canon* for his *Areolae*, a

---

Jacquart, *Le milieu médical en France du XIIᵉ au XVᵉ siècle* (Geneva, 1981), p. 365, Table 4:1, and p. 390, Table 28.

[23] See, e.g., *Egidii Corboliensis Viaticus de signis et symptomatibus aegritudinum*, ed. V. Rose (Leipzig, 1907). The main influences on Gilles' work appear to have been Salernitan. On his career and writings, see Ernest Wickersheimer, *Dictionnaire biographique des médecins en France au Moyen Age* (Paris, 1936), 1:196–97, and its *Supplément*, ed. Danielle Jacquart (Geneva, 1979), pp. 90–91.

[24] *Chartularium universitatis Parisiensis*, ed. H. Denifle and E. Chatelain (Paris, 1889), 1:517, no. 453. Of course, the requirement could also have been fulfilled by the study of other works, notably that of Haly Abbas. On the curriculum at Paris, see Vern L. Bullough, "The Medieval Medical University at Paris," *Bull. Hist. Med.* 31 (1957), 197–211.

[25] Danielle Jacquart, "La réception du *Canon* d'Avicenne: Comparaison entre Montpellier et Paris au XIIIᵉ et XIVᵉ siècles," *Actes du 110ᵉ Congrès national des sociétés savantes, Montpellier, 1984, section d'histoire des sciences et des techniques II. Histoire de l'école médicale de Montpellier* (Paris, 1985), pp. 69–77.

[26] *Opera hactenus inedita Rogeri Baconi*, ed. A. G. Little and E. Withington (Oxford, 1928), 9:150–79, esp. pp. 150–156, 162. The dating is suggested by the editors (p. xxviii). My supposition that Bacon's contacts with book-learned physicians were chiefly at Paris is based only on the fact that Paris was a more important center of medical learning than Oxford by the mid-thirteenth century.

pharmacological compendium. In addition, one of the earliest commentaries on *Canon* 4.1 (fevers) is attributed to this author.[27] Finally, although the work of an Italian and chiefly influential in Italy, the celebrated *Conciliator* of Pietro d'Abano, which is replete with references to Avicenna, is strongly influenced by Avicenna's philosophical as well as his medical teaching, and in part uses the same structural pattern of the *Canon*, was supposedly completed at Paris in 1303 and is certainly in large part the fruit of Pietro's studies there.[28]

At Montpellier, too, the study of the *Canon* in the medical schools seems to have begun in the middle years of the thirteenth century. It has been demonstrated that the first Montpellier medical author to make extensive use of the work was Cardinalis, who was already a master in the faculty of medicine in 1240 and who died about 1293.[29] Avicenna is among the authors prescribed for study in the papal bull of 1309 establishing a medical curriculum for Montpellier, but the portions of the *Canon* are not specified, and the substitution of other works is expressly permitted.[30] However, statutes of 1340 specify detailed instructions for the study of various parts of the *Canon* in three separate courses, two obligatory and one optional. Furthermore, the amount of time actually devoted to Avicenna seems to have increased in later centuries.[31]

[27] Citations of Books 2, 3, 4, and 5 of the *Canon* are numerous, and there are a few of Book 1, in *Die Areolae des Johannes de Sancto Amando (13. Jahrhunderts)*, ed. Julius Leopold Pagel (Berlin, 1893). The *Areolae* is part of a larger compendium and is also known under other titles; on this and on Jean's career, see Wickersheimer *Dictionnaire*, 2:476–77, and its *Supplément*, ed. Jacquart, pp. 179–80. The commentary on *Canon* 4.1 is found in Vienna, National-Bibliothek, MS 2426, 14c, fols. 92ʳ–123ᵛ; I have not seen this manuscript and cite it from TK 361.

[28] *Conciliator* (Venice, 1565; facsimile, Padua, 1985) (there are a number of early editions); on this work, parts of which seem to have been added after 1303, and Pietro's studies at Paris, see Eugenia Paschetto, *Pietro d'Abano, medico e filosofo* (Florence, 1984). The *Conciliator*'s first section, like that of the *Canon*, follows the sequence of the six things natural; the rest of Pietro's work covers a good many of the same topics as the rest of *Canon* 1. However, as already noted, the *Canon* was certainly not the only possible source of this kind of organization.

[29] Garcia Ballester, "Arnau de Vilanova," pp. 101–4.

[30] *Cartulaire de l'Université de Montpellier* (Montpellier, 1890), 1:220.

[31] Ibid., pp. 347–48. See also L. Dulieu, "L'arabisme médical à Montpellier du XIIᵉ au XIVᵉ siècle," *Les cahiers de Tunisie* 3 (1955), 86–95, where the rather small number of commentaries on the *Canon* produced at Montpellier in the thirteenth and fourteenth centuries and the translation there of minor medical works of Avicenna (*De viribus cordis* by Arnald of Villanova and the *Cantica* by Armengaud Blaise) are discussed. The statutes of 1340 were in effect until 1543; see Ernest Wickersheimer, "La question du judéo-arabisme à Montpellier," *Monspeliensis Hippocrates* 6 (December 1959), 3–11, at p. 4. Roland Antonioli, *Rabelais et la médecine*, Études Rabelaisiennes, vol. 12 (Geneva, 1976),

In Italy, the study of the *Canon* seems to have been first undertaken by surgical writers associated with Bologna and Padua. Several references to Avicenna's description of and suggested treatments for the condition or conditions termed *cancer* are contained in Rolando da Parma's explication of the twelfth-century surgery by Roger. Rolando was active in Bologna; his treatise was probably written ca. 1230–40.[32] Much more extensive use of Avicenna was made by Bruno Longoburgo da Calabria in his *Cyrurgia magna,* finished at Padua in 1252. Bruno advertised his book in its preface as a compilation bringing together the wisdom of Galen, Avicenna, Rasis, Albucasis, and Haly Abbas, a claim that appears amply justified by the frequency with which these authors are mentioned in the body of the work.[33] Bologna was already a center of medical and surgical teaching, study, and practice in the first two decades of the thirteenth century, but as at Padua, the first indication of the existence of a formal organized student university and doctoral college of arts and medicine appears to date from the 1260s.[34] Thus, although the composition of Latin books on surgery is presumably in itself an indication of didactic intent, and although, as is well known, the Italian universities later offered degrees in surgery as well as medicine, there is no evidence that either Rolando or Bruno was engaged in public teaching of surgery in a university setting.

The *Canon* may, however, have been used in medical, as distinct from surgical, teaching and study in the *studium* of Siena before 1250. The most prolific medical writer associated with any northern or central Italian school in the middle years of the thirteenth century was Petrus Hispanus, the future Pope John XXI (d. 1276), who was the author of a widely used medical handbook, the *Thesaurus pauperum;* commen-

---

Travaux d'humanisme et de Renaissance, no. 143, p. 43, indicates that the proportion of time devoted to Avicenna rose beyond the statutory amount in the late fifteenth and early sixteenth century.

[32] *Libellus de Cyrurgia editus sive completus a magistro Rolando,* Book 3, chap. 27 in *Cyrurgia Guidonis de Cauliaco et Cyrurgia Bruni Theodorici Rolandi Rogerii Bertipalie Lanfranci* (Venice, 1498, Klebs, 494.1), fol. 157 [156]ᵛ. On the dating of Rolando's work and his association with Bologna, see C. H. Talbot, *Medicine in Medieval England* (London, 1967), p. 92.

[33] *Cyrurgia magna Bruni Longoburgensis,* in *Cyrurgia Guidonis* (Venice, 1498), fols. 83 [82]ʳ–102 [101]ʳ. The work opens: "Rogasti me iam est diu Andrea Vincentine venerabilis amice mi, quod tibi brevi et apto sermone in medicamine cyrurgie librum describerem collectum et excerptum ex dictis glorioxisimi Galieni, Avicenne, Almansoris, Albucasis et Alyabatis. . . ." Talbot regards the introduction of this work at Bologna as marking a significant break with Salernitan tradition there; see Talbot, *Medicine in Medieval England,* p. 97.

[34] For a summary of the evidence, see Siraisi, *Alderotti,* chap. 1; and idem, *Arts and Sciences at Padua,* chap. 1.

taries on five of the *articella* works, on works of Isaac, and on the Aristotelian books on animals; and a set of celebrated and influential treatises on logic. Petrus most likely acquired his medical training at Paris before he came to Siena, where he was teaching in 1246; he was apparently still in the latter city in 1250 and perhaps remained there longer. His medical commentaries are presumably to be associated with the period in his life when he was teaching medicine rather than with the later stages of his career, when practice as a papal physician and ecclesiastical affairs took more of his attention.[35] In his commentary on the work on diets attributed to Isaac Judeus, Petrus frequently introduced citations of Avicenna.[36]

At Bologna, the *Canon* had certainly entered the curriculum well before the end of the thirteenth century, judging by the fact that Taddeo Alderotti produced commentaries—presumably based on his lectures—on several short sections.[37] The same is probably true of Padua, since the *Tractatus de conservatione sanitatis* of Zambonino da Gaza of Cremona, who was a regent master of medicine at Padua in 1262, contains citations of Avicenna.[38] At Salerno and Naples, however, statutory provisions of the late 1270s gave no place to the *Canon* in the formal curriculum (although, the work may have been studied there by that time).[39]

The *Canon* was frequently copied in its entirety and much studied as a reference work. However, both the commentary tradition as it developed from the late thirteenth century and academic statutes of the fourteenth and fifteenth centuries make it clear that the whole of the *Canon* was never prescribed as a textbook—the work's length alone would make such a requirement impossible. Instead, portions of the work were early isolated for use in teaching separate courses in *theoria*, *practica*, and probably surgery. While early statutes listing required

[35] On his studies and career as a professor of medicine, see Richard Stapper, *Papst Johannes XXI. Eine Monographie* (Münster i. W., 1898), pp. 4–26.

[36] See, e.g., *Omnia opera Ysaac* (Lyon, 1515), fol. xi^r.

[37] Taddeo commented on a chapter on things eaten and drunk from *Canon* 1.2, a chapter on *lepra* from *Canon* 4.3, and on *Canon* 4.2. A commentary on a few chapters of *Canon* 1.4 is doubtfully ascribed to him. For incipits, manuscripts (and in the case of the last an early edition), see Siraisi, *Alderotti*, pp. 416–417, 422, 425, 426.

[38] Padua, Biblioteca del Seminario Vescovile, MS 173, 14c, last twelve unnumbered folios. For discussion, see Siraisi, *Arts and Sciences*, p. 145; and Paolo Marangon "Il trattato 'De conservatione sanitatis' di Zambonino da Gazzo († dopo il 1298)," *Quaderni per la storia dell' Università di Padova* 8 (1975), 1–17, where two brief excerpts from the treatise are edited.

[39] Salvatore de Renzi, *Collectio Salernitana ossia Documenti inediti e trattati di medicina appartenenti alla scuola medica salernitana* (Naples, 1852), 1:360–62.

books do not necessarily make the distinction between *theoria* and *practica* explicit, the content of the works used in different courses, the currency given to the division by the language of the *Canon* itself,[40] and the appointment of professors of *practica* at Bologna from the early fourteenth century all suggest that this distinction was implicitly present in the organization of university medical teaching from an early date.[41] But as Tiziana Pesenti has pointed out, at Padua, at any rate, the separation of the two categories seems to have become sharper as time went on.[42] In the main, the goal in teaching *theoria* appears to have been to provide the student with an understanding of general philosophical and physiological principles; the goal in teaching *practica* was to convey specific information of proven medical usefulness, although this goal did not, of course, preclude discussion of the general principles on which particular conclusions or recommendations were based. The distinction between *theoria* and *practica*, considered as branches of the university curriculum in medicine, was not so much in subject matter as in context, in degree of direct relevance to treatment, and probably in the extent of presentation of concrete physical detail. Thus, for example, a discussion of the causes of fever in the context of an exposition of the doctrine of *complexio* would presumably rate as part of theory; yet, appropriately, a discussion of the causes of fever also forms the first part of a treatise by Taddeo Alderotti entitled *Practica de febribus*, which is essentially a work on treatment.[43] Moreover, works written to aid in the teaching of *practica* were not necessarily less academic or scholastic than those on theory; what ties them to *practica* is not any particular pedagogical or investigative methodology, but their concern with anatomical, pathological, or therapeutic factual detail.

The widest use made of the *Canon* was probably in teaching *practica*. Sections of the work commonly used for this purpose at various times and places included Part 4 of Book 1, Book 3, and parts of Book 4. For example, the very detailed curriculum in *medicina*, including numerous

---

[40] Explication of the proper understanding of the division is the main theme of the opening chapter of the *Canon*.

[41] Mondino de' Liuzzi received a public salary as a professor of *practica* in 1324; see Elia Colini-Baldeschi, "Per la biografia di Cecco d'Ascoli," *Rivista delle biblioteche e degli archivi* 22 (1921), 71, document no. 2.

[42] Tiziana Pesenti, "Generi e pubblico della letteratura medica padovana nel Tre- e Quattrocento," in *Università e società nei secoli XII–XVI*, Atti del nono Convegno Internazionale di studio tenuto a Pistoia nei giorni 20–25 settembre 1979 (Bologna, 1983), pp. 531–32.

[43] For manuscripts, see TK 1288. I have consulted Padua, Biblioteca Universitaria, MS al numero provvisorio 202, 14c, fols. 107^r–115^r, inc. "Quoniam nihil melius ad veritatis indagationem."

Galenic works, found in the statutes of the student University of Arts and Medicine of Bologna issued in 1405, provides for the study of *Canon* 1 (omitting some sections of Fen 1–3) in three years out of a four-year cycle of courses.[44] Both the Montpellier statutes of 1340 and the Paduan statutes of 1465 prescribe the whole of Book 1, the latter as part of the instruction to be given by *theorici*.[45] Yet it is clear that Part 4 of Book 1 (on general therapy) was by the early fourteenth century treated as a text in *practica*, just as it is in later university documents;[46] this is apparent from the title of Dino del Garbo's highly academic commentary on *Canon* 1.4, namely *Dilucidatorium totius practice medicine*.[47] Dino's exposition appears to be the earliest example of a long tradition of separate commentary on this part of the work. Also required by the Bologna statutes of 1405 for *medicina* was the study of *Canon* 4.1–2, dealing with fevers and other diseases of the whole organism, and *Canones secundi Avicenne*, presumably meaning Book 2 on simples.[48] Here, as at Montpellier in 1340, where *Canon* 4.1–2 was also prescribed,[49] we must assume that we are dealing with texts thought of as useful for *practica*. As is the case with *Canon* 1.4, the designation of *Canon* 4, especially 4.1, as a text in *practica* is frequent at a later date.[50]

In addition to providing for the study of practically oriented parts of the *Canon* under the rubric *medicina*, the Bologna statute of 1405 also provided for a separate course of study called *practica*. This was to consist in its entirety of a four-year cycle of lectures on *Canon* 3: parts of the body with their anatomy, physiology, and diseases, arranged from head to toe. Judging from the content of the sections specified, the first year was devoted to the head and brain; the second to the lungs, heart,

[44] Carlo Malagola, ed., *Statuti delle Università e dei Collegi dello Studio bolognese* (Bologna, 1888), pp. 274–276.

[45] See n. 31, above, and *Statuta dominorum artistarum achademiae patavinae* (Padua, n.d. [ca. 1529]; Hain 15015, where it is erroneously dated ca. 1496; microfilm at Columbia University, N.Y., supplied by courtesy of William H. Scheide), Book 2, no. 16, fol. 24ᵛ: "Ordinarii theorici primo anno legere teneantur totum primum canonis." The Paduan statutes were issued in 1465 and revised in 1495.

[46] *Canon* 1.4 was regularly the subject of lectures on *practica* at Bologna from 1589 until 1716, and doubtless before; see Umberto Dallari, ed., *I rotuli dei lettori legisti e artisti dello studio bolognese dal 1384 al 1799*, 4 vols. (Bologna, 1888–1924), vols. 2 and 3.

[47] *Dyni Florentini super quarta fen primi Avicenne preclarissima commentaria: que Dilucidatorium totius practice generalis medicinalis scientie nuncupatur* (Venice, 1514).

[48] Malagola, *Statuti*, p. 276. [49] *Cartulaire*, 1:347.

[50] "The topic of fevers was an important part of university courses in practical medicine. The prescribed text was usually the first *fen* of the fourth book of Avicenna's *Canon*." Lonie, "Fever Pathology," p. 20. The *rotuli* of Padua and Bologna in this period frequently provide for lectures *de febribus*, without specifying the textbook.

and thoracic cavity; the third to the liver, stomach, and intestines; and the fourth to the urinary and reproductive systems.[51] This statute partially parallels the Montpellier provision of 1340 that additional, optional, books to be read should include *Canon* 4.3–4 and selections from *Canon* 3. Surgical teaching in the Italian universities also drew upon practically oriented portions of the *Canon*; evidence for the use of parts of *Canon* 4 as a textbook of surgery is provided by the interest of thirteenth-century north Italian surgical writers in Avicenna, alluded to above, and also by Dino del Garbo's *Chirurgia*, an academic commentary on *Canon* 4.3–5.[52] That the *Canon* was regarded by some as useful for anatomical teaching is indicated by some disparaging remarks of Berengario da Carpi, writing in 1521.[53]

If the number of commentaries is any guide, the most highly valued of all the parts of the *Canon* used in teaching *practica* was Book 4, especially its first section on fevers. At least eighteen Latin commentaries on *Canon* 4.1 were written before 1500;[54] no doubt more could be identified. The earliest known Latin commentary on a part of the *Canon* is, as already noted, on this section; it is also the subject of one of the latest printings of any medieval Latin commentary on the work, namely that by Giovanni Arcolano (Arculanus, Herculanus, d. 1458), reissued at Padua in 1685.[55] By contrast, Thorndike and Kibre list only seven commentaries on *Canon* 1.4 written before 1500. Commentaries on the whole of Book 3 are few (perhaps none, since Gentile da Foligno's, which covers most of the book, appears not to be complete); however, the various subdivisions of this part of the *Canon* gave rise to fairly numerous commentaries by different authors on separate short sections. Despite the requirement for the study of *Canones secundi Avicenne* in the Bologna statute of 1405, there appear to be few extant commentaries on *Canon* 2. *Canon* 5, the antidotarium, appears to have been relatively little studied in the schools, and to have attracted commentary only from the indefatigable Gentile da Foligno.[56]

---

[51] Malagola, *Statuti*, pp. 276–77.

[52] *Expositio super 3ª et 4ª fen Avicenne et super parte quinte* (Ferrara, 1489, Hain *6166), a work generally known as Dino's *Chirurgia*.

[53] Regarding Berengario da Carpi's dissatisfaction with the *Canon* as an anatomical text, see Roger French, "Berengario da Carpi and the Use of Commentary in Anatomical Teaching," in *The Medical Renaissance of the Sixteenth Century*, ed. A. Wear, R. K. French, and I. M. Lonie (Cambridge, 1985), pp. 42–74.

[54] On the basis of TK.

[55] *De febribus Joannis Arculani in Avicennae IV Canonis Fen primam dilucida atque optima expositio* (Padua, 1685). Arcolano taught at the University of Pavia.

[56] For some editions of Gentile's commentaries on Books 3 and 5, see Appendix 1; the manuscripts of his commentary on Book 3 listed in TK appear all to be on various subsections, not the whole book. Commentaries on Book 2 include those of Gentile da Fo-

Book 1 alone, and no other part of the *Canon*, emerged as a textbook
for the teaching of medical *theoria*. It was early adapted for this role by
selective omission. Of its four parts, or fen, it seems likely as we have
just seen that *Canon* 1.4 early migrated to *practica*. Moreover, in pre-
scribing this book, the Bologna statutes of 1405 indicate omissions
from Fen 1 and 2, and require only five chapters of Fen 3.[57] The insignificant position accorded to *Canon* 1.3 in medieval university education in medical theory is further indicated by deficiency of commentary. Not only are independently surviving commentaries on this
section alone rare, but some major commentators on Book 1 excluded
Fen 3 from consideration. Thus, for example, Giacomo da Forlì and
Ugo Benzi both expounded *Canon* 1.1–2, omitting the third fen[58] (Ugo
also wrote a separate commentary on *Canon* 1.4).[59] The portions of the
Canon used in teaching medical theory were therefore usually drawn
from the first two fen of Book 1; of these two sections, it was the first
that was primarily valued as a compendium of basic principles. Hence
the practice of writing separate commentaries on *Canon* 1.1 was not, as
one might be tempted to suppose, a later innovation introduced at a
time when the role of Avicenna in medical education was diminishing
in importance, but can be traced back to the earliest beginning of Latin
commentary on the *Canon*. The oldest Latin commentary on any part
of Book 1 appears to be a set of lectures taken down by Alberto of Bologna from Antonio da Parma, probably at Bologna between 1310 and
1323; these *recollectiones* are on *Canon* 1.1 alone.[60]

---

ligno (see TK 231) and Dino del Garbo's *Expositio Dini super canones generales de virtutibus
medicinarum simplicium secundi Canonis Avicenne*, printed with his *Dilucidatorium* (Venice,
1514) (TK 1438). On Gentile's education, teaching career at Siena and Perugia, practice
and intellectual influence in Padua, and death of the plague in 1348, see Siraisi, *Alderotti*,
p. xxi; Carl C. Schlam, "Graduation Speeches of Gentile da Foligno," *Mediaeval Studies*
40 (1978), 96–119; and Fausto Bonora and George Kern, "Does Anyone Really Know
the Life of Gentile da Foligno?" *Medicina ne' secoli* 9 (1972), 29–53.

[57] Malagola, *Statuti*, pp. 274–276.

[58] See *Jacobi Foroliviensis medici singularis expositio et quaestiones in primum Canonem
Avicennae* (Venice, 1547) and *Expositio Ugonis Senensis super primo Canonis Avicennae cum
questionibus eiusdem* (Venice, 1498, Klebs 998.2). Both works include Fen 2 as well as Fen
1 of Book 1. On Giacomo da Forlì's biography, see Paolo Sambin, "Su Giacomo della
Torre († 1414)," *Quaderni per la storia dell' Università di Padova* 1 (1968), 15–47; for Ugo's
biography see n. 59. On their intellectual characteristics, see Graziella Federici Vescovini,
"Medicina e filosofia a Padova tra XIV e XV secolo: Jacopo da Forlì e Ugo Benzi da
Siena (1380–1430)," in her *"Arti" e filosofia nel secolo XIV: Studi sulla tradizione aristotelica
e i "moderni"* (Florence, 1983), pp. 231–78.

[59] For manuscripts and editions, see Dean P. Lockwood, *Ugo Benzi: Medieval Philosopher and Physician, 1376–1439* (Chicago, 1951), pp. 198–205, 395.

[60] Biblioteca Apostolica Vaticana, MS Vat. lat. 4452, fols. 1ʳ–47ᵛ, inc. "[I]n primis deo
gratias. Intentio Avicenne in hoc libro."

Nor was Fen 1 taught in its entirety. As noted in the last chapter, the fifth part of this fen, on the parts of the body (*Doctrina de membris*) contains an introductory chapter followed by subsections on bones, muscles, nerves, arteries, and veins—a total of fifty-six chapters, which together provide quite a substantial short account of aspects of Galenic anatomy. It was the subject of at least one separate commentary, which survives in a fifteenth-century manuscript.[61] Yet the major commentaries on Fen 1 written in the Italian schools simply omit all but the introductory chapter of the anatomical section. This is true of the commentary of Antonio da Parma in the early fourteenth century, of that of Gentile da Foligno in the mid-fourteenth century, and of that of Giacomo da Forlì in the early fifteenth century. Gentile da Foligno remarked of this practice at the end of his comments on the general introductory chapter: "We next proceed to the chapter on the virtues, following the common error. For the science of anatomy ought to be taught first to beginners, just as letters of the alphabet are taught to anyone who must learn and read."[62] That the omission of the anatomy was standard practice is confirmed by the Bologna statutes of 1405, which specify that this portion of Fen 1 is to be passed over.[63]

One is immediately struck by the fact that at Bologna the practice of omitting commentary on the anatomical portions of Fen 1 seems to have emerged in the very years in which the teaching of anatomy as a distinct branch of medical study was becoming established in the curriculum. Antonio da Parma was a contemporary and probably a colleague at Bologna of Mondino de' Liuzzi (d. 1326), author of a celebrated work on anatomical demonstration by dissection of a human subject.[64] According to Gui de Chauliac, Mondino and his pupil and successor Niccolò Bertruccio (Gui's own teacher) habitually instructed

---

[61] Paris, Bibliothèque Nationale, MS lat. 6936, fols. 1ʳ–148ʳ, inc. "Determinatio de membris generaliter in capitulo precedenti." I have not seen this manuscript and cite it from TK 405.

[62] "Nos deinceps procedamus ad capitulum de virtutibus sequendo communem errorem. Nam scientia anathomie deberet primo doceri introducendis sicut doceatur littere alfabeti debenti discere et legere," *Primus Avicenne Canon cum argutissima Gentilis expositione* (Pavia, 1510), fol. 54ᵛ. Compare Giacomo da Forlì, comm. *Canon* 1.1 (Venice, 1547), fol. 51v: "Et sic explicit hoc capitulum huius quintae doctrinae primae Fen primi Canonis Avicennae. Nunc sequuntur quinque summae huius quintae doctrinae, quas summas Jacobus iste Foroliviensis non curavit exponere."

[63] Malagola, *Statuti*, pp. 274–76.

[64] Antonio's connection with Bologna has been disputed, but his lectures on *Canon* 1.1 were taken down "per me Albertum Bononiensem" (MS Vat. lat. 4452, fol. 47ᵛ). For a summary of Mondino's career at Bologna, and of the evidence as regards his influence on anatomical teaching there, see Siraisi, *Alderotti,* pp. 66–69, 110–14, and bibliography there cited.

their students in this way.[65] While it is thus tempting to connect the exclusion of Avicenna's anatomy from the general course on medical principles with the emergence of a separate place for anatomy in the curriculum, I know of no evidence for the conscious or purposive connection of the two developments by those responsible for them. It seems likely, however, that the exclusion of anatomy from lectures on Fen 1 reflects a consensus of opinion (although evidently one not shared by Gentile da Foligno) that concrete physical detail of the kind contained in the omitted chapters more properly belonged to the study of *practica* than that of general principles. Certainly, Fen 1 without the anatomical section is a handy short textbook of medical philosophy and physiology. In this form, it is easy to comprehend its being alternated, as it was at Padua for so long, with the Galenic *Ars*, or *Microtechne*.

Although Latin commentary on the various parts of the *Canon* began to appear in the late thirteenth century, the major expositions were mostly the products of a period extending from the early fourteenth to about the mid-fifteenth century. The few commentaries, mostly brief, that were composed before 1300 appear to have had little lasting influence; and the composition of major commentaries seems to have tapered off after about 1450. All Latin commentaries were probably in some way or another linked with academic medical instruction in the university setting, although the nature and directness of the connection varied. Thus, Jacques Despars (d. 1458) began ten years of preparatory work for his commentary on *Canon* 1, 3, and 4.1 after leaving the position of regent master of medicine at the University of Paris, which he held from 1411 until 1419; his commentary was actually written in the years 1432 and 1453 at Cambrai and his native Tournai, where he held ecclesiastical benefices.[66] This commentary is therefore certainly not simply a redaction of lectures the author had given in various courses on different parts of the *Canon* at Paris; nonetheless, the choice of sections on which to comment suggests that the original inspiration of the commentary may have been connected with his university teaching.

An author who seems to have set out to produce a complete commentary that would transcend the limitations of academic curricula was Gentile da Foligno, apparently the only Latin writer to expound all five books. Nonetheless, Gentile's commentary (or commentaries) shows abundant evidence of classroom origin. More commonly, separate commentaries on major subdivisions of the *Canon* were probably

---

[65] Gui de Chauliac, *Chirurgia* (Venice, 1498), fols. 5r-v.

[66] Danielle Jacquart, "Le regard d'un médecin sur son temps: Jacques Despars (1380?–1458)," *Bibliothèque de l'Ecole des Chartes* 138 (1980), 35–86, at pp. 35–38.

the fruit of a single course of lectures on a portion of the text prescribed as part of a formal curriculum. Thus, Dino del Garbo began his commentary on *Canon* 1.4 while lecturing at Bologna, although he polished it up by subsequent editing, including a dedication to his patron King Robert of Sicily.[67]

Yet other, briefer, commentaries reflected the practice of isolating for discussion very small segments of the work (a chapter or so) that dealt with theoretical or practical problems of some importance. As examples, one might mention Taddeo Alderotti's exposition of three chapters on *lepra*,[68] and the same author's disquisition on the problems regarding specific and substantial form raised by a chapter "on things eaten and drunk";[69] Alberto de Zanchariis' treatment of the section on *lepra*;[70] and the expositions of Mondino de' Liuzzi, Tommaso del Garbo (d. 1370), and Giacomo da Forlì of Avicenna's treatment of the generation of the embryo.[71] The latter section no doubt attracted commentary both because of the existence of philosophical debates about such topics as the nature of *virtus formativa* and the animation of the fetus and because the account of mammalian conception is a major point of difference between Aristotle and Galen. Medical masters seem to have exercised fairly free choice of subject matter for these short commentaries or lectures. The format was flexible, and Books 1, 3, and 4 of the *Canon* were a treasure trove of topics. Some of these short pieces can be found both as separate manuscript items and incorporated into a longer commentary on a whole book of the *Canon*. For example, this is the case with a number of Gentile da Foligno's expositions of various fen of Book 3—although in this case it may be that they were first collected by the early printers. It is not always possible to tell whether one is dealing with a passage excerpted from a long commentary or an originally independent item that was subsequently incorporated or planned for incorporation into a longer work. The short commentaries

[67] For Gentile's commentaries, see Appendix 1. Dino, *Dilucidatorium*, fol. 2ʳ, and comm. *Canon* 2, fol. 1ʳ (both Venice, 1514).

[68] Florence, Biblioteca Medicea Laurenziana, MS Ashburnham 217 (149) fols. 91ᵛ–93ʳ; Biblioteca Apostolica Vaticana, MS Palat. lat. 1240, fols. 100ᵛ–102ʳ.

[69] Biblioteca Apostolica Vaticana, MS Palat. lat. 1246, fols. 78ᵛ–97ᵛ.

[70] Paris, Bibliothèque Nationale, MS lat. 7148, fols. 24ʳ–44ᵛ. Inc. "Lepra est infirmitas mala etc. medice laboranti." I have not seen this manuscript and owe the reference to Luke Demaitre. Alberto, who became a professor of medicine at Bologna, was a pupil of both Mondino de' Liuzzi and Antonio da Parma.

[71] Mondino's commentary is found in Biblioteca Apostolica Vaticana, MS. reg. lat. 2000, fols. 1–23ʳ. Those of Tommaso and Giacomo are printed in *Expositio Jacobi supra capitulum Avicenne De generatione embrionis* (Venice, 1502).

are as a rule complete in themselves and cannot properly be described as fragmentary.

Although the full extent of the body of commentary produced before 1500 on the various portions of the *Canon* cannot be mapped before the completion of a comprehensive study of the manuscript tradition, it appears that individual commentaries, long or short, usually survive in relatively few copies, and that only a few authors succeeded in producing commentaries on Avicenna with lasting reputation in the schools. The first certainly seems to be true of the only major commentary or set of commentaries for which the manuscript tradition has been thoroughly examined in a published study by a modern scholar. Jacquart's list of the manuscripts of Jacques Despars' commentary includes a single set of codices containing the whole work and a number of copies of the various subdivisions (some of which together form partial sets). Among the separate copies of subdivisions, the expositions of *Canon* 1.1 and 1.4 survive in the largest number, with five copies each. Thus, while the total number of manuscripts of all parts of Jacques Despars' work on Avicenna amounts to thirty-nine, the maximum number of copies of any single section is six. Yet Despars was an exceptionally celebrated and influential commentator of enduring repute, as is demonstrated by the fact that all of the twenty-nine dated manuscripts of sections of his commentary were copied after his death and that excerpts were printed in several early editions.[72] Indeed, it seems likely that where commentaries on medical works lectured on in the schools are concerned, any multiplication of copies, even if limited, indicates that commentator or commentary was held in special esteem. Over the centuries, the great majority of expositions of the *Canon* were doubtless classroom lectures intended for no wider audience than the teacher's own students; many such lectures must have left either no written trace at all, or existed in written form only in the master's own copy. Potentially somewhat longer-lasting and wider influence is suggested in those cases where a copy in the shape of *recollectiones* or a *reportatio* was taken down by a scholar among the master's auditors. But only masters of some distinction might expect copies of their work to be further multiplied, either in their lifetime or posthumously.

The most celebrated fourteenth- and fifteenth-century Latin commentators on the *Canon*—Dino del Garbo, Gentile da Foligno, Giacomo da Forlì, Ugo Benzi, Giovanni Arcolano, and Jacques Despars—

---

[72] Jacquart, "Le regard d'un médecin," pp. 39–43. Of the manuscripts listed by Jacquart only one is included in TK (see TK 423), a fact indicative of the scope of the Latin manuscript tradition of the *Canon* and its commentaries that remains to be investigated.

have already been mentioned in the course of this chapter. To their names should perhaps be added those of Antonio da Parma, Tommaso del Garbo, Marsiglio di Santa Sofia (d. 1405),[73] Giovanni Matteo Ferrari da Grado (d. 1472)[74] and Biagio Astario (d. 1504),[75] although the range of *Canon* commentary in the latter group was more restricted and some of them left expositions that did not attract the attention of early printers. This list does not, of course, include the authors of important works that were to a significant extent based on the *Canon* in content, arrangement, or both, but did not take the shape of formal commentaries; for example, the *Chirurgia* of Leonardo da Bertipaglia (d. after 1448), which is described as "recollecte habite super quarto Avicenne," the *Conciliator* of Pietro d'Abano, and the *Summa medicinalis* of Tommaso del Garbo.[76] One may note again that the provenance of all these authors, with the solitary though important exception of the Frenchman Jacques Despars, lies in the north Italian universities. It seems safe to say that in the fourteenth and fifteenth centuries the practice of commentary on the *Canon* was most flourishing and most diverse in the schools of northern Italy. This productivity made local reputations and

[73] Marsiglio produced expositions of *Canon* 1.1 (TK 713) and *Canon* 1.2 (TK 414) and collections of recipes from *Canon* 1.4 (TK 1544) and *Canon* 4.1 (TK 189). Of these, only the works on *Canon* 1.2 and *Canon* 1.4 appear to have been printed. On Marsiglio's career at Padua, see Andrea Gloria, ed., *Monumenti della Università di Padova (1318–1405)* (Padua, 1888), 1:390-95.

[74] G. M. Ferrari da Grado produced an exposition of *Canon* 1.2 printed in the first volume of the five-volume edition of the *Canon* (Venice, 1523), and one of *Canon* 3.22, printed in the third volume of the three-volume edition of *Canon* 3 (Venice, ca. 1505), and in the second volume of the two-volume edition of *Canon* 3 (Venice, 1522); for details of these editions, see Appendix 1. On his career, see H. M. Ferrari da Grado, *Une chaire de médecine au XVᵉ siècle: un professeur à l'Université de Pavie de 1432 à 1472* (Paris, 1899).

[75] Biagio Astario taught at Pavia and died in 1504. His work on fevers, based on *Canon* 1.4, is perhaps a compendium rather than a commentary. See *Blasii Astarii de curis febrium libellus utilis*, bound with *Marci Gatinarie de curis egritudinum particularium* (Venice, 1521). There are a number of other editions.

[76] Printed in *Cyrurgia Guidonis* (Venice, 1498; see n. 32, above); inc., fol. 233ʳ: "He sunt recollecte habite super quarto Avicenne ab egregio et singulari doctore Magistro Leonardo Bertipalia." Lynn Thorndike remarked that this work seemed "less a commentary upon the text of Avicenna than a collection of recipes . . . cures, unguents, and plasters." Lynn Thorndike, "The Manuscript Text of the Cyrurgia of Leonard of Bertipaglia," *Isis* 8 (1926), 268. Thorndike also noticed rather wide divergence between the manuscripts and the printed text of this work. On Leonardo's career, see Tiziana Pesenti Marangon, " 'Professores chirurgie,' 'medici ciroici' e 'barbitonsores' a Padova nell'età di Leonardo Buffi da Bertipaglia († dopo il 1448)," *Quaderni per la storia dell'Università di Padova* 11 (1978), 1-38. I have consulted Tommaso del Garbo's *Summa* in the edition of Venice, 1506.

ensured a local supply of manuscripts, factors that help to explain the frequency with which such commentaries were selected for publication, and their influence extended and perpetuated, by Renaissance Italian printers.

The contributions of these various interpreters of Avicenna differed not only in regard to the portions of the work commented on but also, obviously, according to their individual interests. Many of the themes they took up are not necessarily peculiar to the exposition of the *Canon* but can also be traced in other medical and philosophical literature of the same period. In general, Latin scholastic medical commentary is characterized by the use of dialectic and especially of the question method in discussing scientific problems; by the discussion of certain standard questions or topics such as, for example, the differences between Aristotle and Galen on the subject of heart and brain or of conception; by some degree of readiness to introduce philosophical and general scientific issues into works on medical theory; and by an even-handed respect for most ancient and Arabic authors and a desire to reconcile their divergent views wherever possible.[77] In the case of the fourteenth- and fifteenth-century commentaries on the *Canon*, we may add respect for Avicenna as an independent authority and a willingness to place his views on a par with those of Galen when the two differed or appeared to differ. In the case of commentaries of Italian provenance, another important goal appears to have been to acquaint the reader with the views of leading professors in the Italian schools from the time of Taddeo Alderotti to that of the writer. Thus, Gentile da Foligno referred repeatedly to the opinions of *Canon* 1.1 of Antonio da Parma, and Giacomo da Forlì frequently cited those of Dinus and Mundinus (presumably Dino del Garbo and Mondino de' Liuzzi), as well as those of Gentile himself. Commentary was for these authors both a vehicle of current debate and a means of transmitting the views of the most celebrated doctors of the Italian medical schools to another generation.

Beyond these few generalizations, no summary of the content of these usually lengthy and diffuse works will be attempted here. For present purposes, it may be sufficient to emphasize once again not only the broad usefulness attributed to different parts of Avicenna's *Canon* for various branches of medical training, but also the fact that in the fourteenth and fifteenth centuries the production of commentaries on

---

[77] The characteristics of scholastic medical commentary are discussed and extensively illustrated in Per-Gunnar Ottosson, *Scholastic Medicine and Philosophy: A Study of Commentaries on Galen's Tegni (ca. 1300–1450)* (Naples, 1984).

Avicenna's work served to enhance the reputation, among their contemporaries and immediate successors, of men who were numbered
among the most distinguished masters of the Italian medical schools.
In particular, the names Dino del Garbo, Gentile da Foligno, Giacomo
da Forlì, and Ugo Benzi crop up over and over again in biographical
collections listing exceptionally celebrated physicians.[78] In several accounts, the distinction of these men is linked in a very specific and explicit way to the writing of commentaries and/or to Avicenna. Thus,
Filippo Villani noted as one of the chief accomplishments of Dino del
Garbo that his commentaries on the *Canon* immediately became and
remained valued university textbooks;[79] half a century later Michele
Savonarola said the same of the *lecturae, quaestiones,* and *commenta* of
Marsiglio di Santa Sofia and Giacomo da Forlì.[80] For Benedetto Accolti, as already noted, Gentile, Marsiglio, Giacomo, and Ugo were
"philosophers" worthy to be placed alongside Avicenna, Averroes,
and Thomas Aquinas.[81]

While the commentators who have just been discussed belong
mostly to the fourteenth and first half of the fifteenth centuries, their
expositions of the *Canon* probably achieved widest circulation between
the 1470s and the 1520s, when Venetian and other north Italian presses
issued and reissued numerous editions of fourteenth- and fifteenth-century medical texts. During that period, with the exception of the expositions of Book 1 by Antonio da Parma and Marsiglio di Santa Sofia,
all of the fourteenth- and fifteenth-century commentaries mentioned
so far in this chapter were printed, many of them several times. We
may take the single, but doubtless not uncharacteristic, example of
Ugo Benzi, chosen because the printing history of his works has already been the subject of thorough investigation by a modern scholar;
between 1478 and 1524, Ugo's commentary on *Canon* 1.1–2 appeared
in five editions; his commentary on *Canon* 1.4 (general therapy) was
printed eleven, perhaps twelve, times; and his commentary on *Canon*
4.1 (fevers) five times. Thereafter, apart from excerpts included in
Lockwood's study, none of Ugo's Latin commentaries was ever
printed again.[82] In the same approximately fifty-year period centering
on 1500, the lectures on the *Canon* of contemporary teachers seem to

---

[78] See Siraisi, "Physician's Task."

[79] Villani, *Liber de . . . famosis civibus,* p. 27.

[80] Michele Savonarola, *Libellus de magnificis ornamentis regie civitatis Padue,* ed. A. Se-
garizzi, in *Rerum italicarum scriptores,* n.s. 24, p. 15 (Città di Castello, 1902), pp. 36–37.

[81] Accolti, *Dialogus de praestantia virorum sui aevi,* printed with Villani, *Liber de . . . famosis civibus,* pp. 122–123.

[82] Lockwood, *Benzi,* pp. 382–98.

have been less frequently regarded as worth disseminating by means of print.[83] In short, one contribution of the printing industry was to provide sixteenth-century readers with excellent opportunities for access to a substantial body of commentary on the *Canon* produced by a handful of celebrated authors whose names were synonymous with the early fame of north Italian university medicine, but whose achievements had already receded into the fairly distant past.

Editions of scholastic commentaries on the *Canon* hence appeared in greatest numbers in precisely the period in which medical learning was becoming permeated by a humanistic insistence on the superiority of the direct study of ancient Greek authors either in the original language or in modern translation and, in some instances, on the need for a fresh and systematic confrontation of ancient teaching and modern experience. The goals of medical humanism were already defined in the late fifteenth century; the new Latin translations of Galen and other medical writers from the Greek, so prized by humanist physicians even though many of the texts had been available in medieval Latin versions for centuries, multiplied between 1500 and 1531; and the long and eagerly awaited first printed edition of Galen's collected *Opera* in Greek issued from the Aldine press in 1525.[84] However one may rate the actual importance of medical humanism for the development of medicine, there can be no doubt that those involved perceived themselves as introducing or advocating changes of profound significance.[85] Very few phy-

[83] There are, of course, exceptions to this generalization, e.g. the work of Pietro Antonio Rustico, *Qui atrocem horres pestem pestilentemque times febrem* (Pavia, 1521), and the commentary of Leonardo Legio on *Canon* 3.1.1.29 (Venice, 1523) (for both, see Appendix 2); but these are minor works, not cited by later authors. No doubt, too, the difficulties of the universities of Bologna and Padua in the disturbed times of the early sixteenth century reduced the output, not just the preservation, of academic discourses of all kinds.

[84] Studies include Richard J. Durling, "A Chronological Census of Renaissance Editions and Translations of Galen," *Journal of the Warburg and Courtauld Institutes* 24 (1961), 230–305, and "Linacre and Medical Humanism," in *Linacre Studies: Essays on the Life and Work of Thomas Linacre, ca. 1460–1524,* ed. Francis Maddison, Margaret Pelling, and Charles Webster (Oxford, 1977), pp. 77–106; Vivian Nutton, "John Caius and the Linacre Tradition," *Medical History* 23 (1979), 373–89, and "Medicine in the Age of Montaigne," in *Montaigne and His Age,* ed. K. Cameron (Exeter, 1981), pp. 15–25, 163–70; see also Temkin, *Galenism,* pp. 125–74.

[85] Much new light is thrown on the goals and accomplishments of sixteenth-century medical humanism and Galenism by Vivian Nutton, "John Caius and the Eton Galen: Medical Philology in the Renaissance," *Medizinhistorisches Journal* 20 (1985), 227–52. See also Walter Pagel, "Medical Humanism—A Historical Necessity in the Era of the Renaissance," in *Linacre Studies,* pp. 375–86; and for the impact of humanism on different specific aspects of medicine, *Humanismus und Medizin,* ed. Rudolf Schmitz and Gundolf Keil (Weinheim, 1984).

sicians shared the levels of linguistic and philological interest and accomplishment of leading medical humanists such as, say, Leoniceno, Linacre, or Caius; moreover, some, as we shall see, reacted vigorously against the explicit or implied repudiation of medicine's recent past. Nonetheless, by the 1520s there could have been few academically educated physicians who remained wholly unaware of or unaffected by the humanist climate of opinion, and the influence of the movement remained widespread throughout the century. And as is well known, the rhetoric of medical humanism frequently incorporated a strong vein of denigration of the Arabs and their Latin scholastic interpreters.

The origins of the attack on the Arabs by physicians are of course primarily to be sought in the general influence of the literary and philological humanism of the fifteenth century. However, scattered and occasional criticism of the influence of Arabic authors in medical teaching can be traced back to the thirteenth century. The earliest manifestations of such criticisms belong to the history of strictures on medicine and physicians emanating from outside the medical profession and usually based on accusations of intellectual arrogance, ineffectiveness, and/or excessive concern for the things of this world.[86] We have already noted Roger Bacon's complaints that the *medici* of his day relied too heavily on Avicenna's classification of diseases and expended too much energy on disputation irrelevant to the task of healing. In the next century, Petrarch grounded his much paraded hostility to medicine in part on a disdain for "Arab lies," for as he explained to his correspondent, the physician Giovanni Dondi, "I hate the whole race."[87] As one might expect, Petrarch's dislike of Arabic medical advice, like his similar attitude toward scholastic natural philosophy, seems more to have been inspired by religious, moral, and literary than by scientific

---

[86] The history of medieval attitudes toward and concerns about medicine up to the early thirteenth century is well summarized in Jole Agrimi and Chiara Crisciani, *Medicina del corpo e medicina dell'anima: Note sul sapere del medico fino all'inizio del secolo XIII* (Milan, 1978); see also Darrel W. Amundsen, "History of Medical Ethics: Medieval Europe: Fourth to Sixteenth Century," in *The Encyclopedia of Bioethics* (New York and London, 1978), 3:938–51. It seems likely that the change to the pursuit of medical learning in the university setting that took place in the thirteenth century in itself served to engender new themes in the criticism of medicine.

[87] *De rebus senilibus liber XII* in his *Opera* (Basel, 1554; facsimile, Ridgewood, N.J., 1965), 2:1001, 1007–9; esp. p. 1009: "Unum antequam desinam te obsecro, ut ab omni consilio mearum rerum, tui isti Arabes arceantur, atque exulent, odi genus universum." On the relationship between Petrarch's criticisms and later attacks on the role of the Arabs in medicine, see Gerhard Baader, "Medizinisches Reformdenken und Arabismus im Deutschland des 16. Jahrhunderts," *Sudhoffs Archiv für Geschichte der Medizin und der Naturwissenschaften* 63 (1979), 270.

considerations. Similar views were not necessarily an integral part of various other evaluations of medicine by fourteenth- and fifteenth-century literary humanists. For example, Coluccio Salutati, who was strongly critical of many aspects of the medicine of his day, referred to Avicenna approvingly as a "remarkable man who brought great light to medicine."[88] Moreover, as already noted, the leading scholastic commentators on the *Canon* were on the whole kindly treated by their humanist contemporaries.

Among those professionally concerned with medicine, there was an early awareness of the defects of some of the Arabo-Latin translations, particularly as regards the nomenclature of substances used in pharmacology. Dietlinde Goltz has pointed out that Latin manuscripts of the *Canon* and other medical works of Arabic origin copied in the thirteenth and fourteenth centuries frequently contain glossaries giving Latin equivalents for some transliterated Arabic technical terms, and that in the concluding portions of his commentary on *Canon* 5 (the *antidotarium*) Gentile da Foligno recorded his inability to find the meanings of various of Gerard of Cremona's transliterations. More generally, the desire to clarify a technical terminology derived from three different languages was doubtless a principal motivating force behind the whole development of medieval medical lexicography, of which the *Clavis sanationis*, or *Synonima*, of Simone of Genoa (fl. ca. 1290) is a leading example.[89] Moreover, skepticism about the value of Avicenna's own medical teaching (not just of the Latin translation) was forcefully expressed by Arnald of Villanova, the leading medical professor of late thirteenth-century Montpellier.[90]

Although important themes in the attack on the Arabs in medicine were thus prefigured earlier, the criticisms launched in the late fifteenth and early sixteenth centuries were more sweeping in nature and scope

---

[88] "Digestor et ordinator egregius Avicenna . . . vir plane mirabilis et qui lumen maximum attulerit medicinae." Coluccio Salutati, *De nobilitate legum et medicinae. De Verecundia*, ed. E. Garin (Florence, 1947), p. 70.

[89] Dietlinde Goltz, *Studien zur Geschichte der Mineralnamen in Pharmazie, Chemie und Medizin von den Anfängen bis Paracelsus, Sudhoffs Archiv für Geschichte der Medizin und der Naturwissenschaften*, Beiheft 14 (Wiesbaden, 1972), pp. 321–24, 328–30. See also Loren C. Mackinney, "Medieval Medical Dictionaries and Glossaries," in *Medieval and Historiographical Essays in Honor of James Westfall Thompson*, ed. J. L. Cate and E. N. Anderson (Chicago, 1938), pp. 240–68.

[90] "Ubi ad sensum mostravimus solidam veritatem Galieni non fuisse intellectam ab Avicena qui in medicina maiorem partem medicorum latinorum infatuat." Quoted in editors' introduction to *Commentum supra tractatum Galeni De malicia complexionis diverse*, ed. Luis Garcia Ballester and Eustaquio Sanchez Salor, in *Arnaldi de Villanova Opera medica omnia*, vol. 15 (Barcelona, 1985), p. 34.

and more powerful in their impact than anything that had gone before. Specific criticism of the *Canon* and its Latin commentators in this period must be understood as part of a broadly based attack on the Arabs in general, which aroused controversies in university faculties of medicine throughout Europe and generated a fairly large literature. Recent studies have charted the progress of these arguments not only in Italian humanist circles, but also in the schools of Montpellier, Paris, Tübingen and elsewhere in Germany, and Alcalá and elsewhere in Spain.[91] Moreover, the attack on the Arabs was intimately linked not only to humanistic enthusiasm for Greek medical texts, but to the interest, both philological and practical, in the development of botany and botanical nomenclature and the purification of pharmacology, and was thus intertwined with other major concerns of medical innovators of the period. Yet because segments of the *Canon* played a prominent part in university curricula, and because the sections on simples and the composition of remedies in Avicenna's work were both lengthy and notably problematical, in medical circles criticism of the Arabs frequently tended to focus on Avicenna.[92] Without attempting any detailed analysis of these developments, we may simply note their broad chronology and a few of the main themes of criticism.

Although controversy over the issue of the Arabs in medicine probably reached its height in the late 1520s and early 1530s in France and Germany, criticism of Avicenna was already an important ingredient in the medical teaching of Nicolò Leoniceno at the University of Ferrara in the last decade of the fifteenth century. Leoniceno's once celebrated treatise *De Plinii et plurium aliorum medicorum in medicina erroribus*, first published in 1492, aroused controversy chiefly because of its author's willingness to attribute defects to Pliny's own teaching rather than to errors introduced in the process of transmission.[93] However,

---

[91] In addition to the general articles mentioned in n. 84, above, see Felix Klein-Francke, *Die klassische Antike in der Tradition des Islam* (Darmstadt, 1980), pp. 17–43; Heinrich Schipperges, *Ideologie und Historiographie des Arabismus*, Sudhoffs Archiv für Geschichte der Medizin und der Naturwissenschaften, Beiheft 1 (Wiesbaden, 1961), pp. 6–26; Goltz, *Studien*, pp. 334–48; for Germany, Baader, "Medizinisches Reformdenken"; for Spain, Luis Garcia Ballester, "The Circulation and Use of Medical Manuscripts in Arabic in Sixteenth-Century Spain," *Journal for the History of Arabic Science* 3 (1979), 183–99, esp. pp. 186–89; for Montpellier, Antonioli, *Rabelais*, pp. 40–50.

[92] In turn, Klein-Franke *Die klassische Antike*, p. 19 , points to the role of medical humanism in stimulating criticisms of Arabo-Latin translations of philosophical works (e.g., Vives' attack on Averroes and his Latin translators in *De causis corruptarum artium*, 5.3, in his *Opera* [Valencia, 1782–90], 6:191–98).

[93] I have consulted this treatise in Leoniceno's *Opuscula* (Basel, 1532), in which its four books occupy fols. 1r–61v. On this work, and the fairly widespread debate over it in hu-

the work also contains more than twenty chapters dedicated to exposing specific errors by Avicenna and his "recent interpreters." Usually
the accusations turn on the allegation that Avicenna has misunderstood
or confused Greek botanical and anatomical terminology; however,
several chapters also accuse him of providing erroneous terminology
for processes of digestion.[94] Leoniceno's chief disciple, Giovanni Manardo, who also taught at Ferrara, broadened the attack in his collection
of "medical epistles" first published in 1521 and widely disseminated
in several subsequent enlarged editions. In addition to discussing specific errors by Avicenna, Manardo characterized the *Canon* in general
as filled with "a dense cloud and infinite chaos of obscurities." Furthermore, he laid stress on the idea that medieval translations were in
general unreliable, and pointed out that Avicenna's work was itself a
pastiche based on the writings of other Greek and Arabic medical authors.[95]

Nor was Ferrara the only center of anti-Arab polemic in Italy. Denigration of Avicenna was the central theme of a collection of treatises
published in 1533 under the title *Little Works of the New Florentine Academy and against the Neoteric Physicians Who, Neglecting the Discipline of
Galen, Cultivate the Barbarians.*[96] The author of the first of these trea-

---

manist, medical, and botanical circles, see Charles G. Nauert, Jr., "Humanists, Scientists, and Pliny: Changing Approaches to a Classical Author," *American Historical Review*
84 (1979), 72–85. On Leoniceno's intellectual position in general, see Daniela Mugnai
Carrara, "Profilo di Nicolò Leoniceno," *Interpres* 2 (1978), 169–212.

[94] A few examples of Leoniceno's chapter headings, chosen more or less at random
(numbered by book and chapter), are: 1.18, "Error Avicennae ac Serapionis, in herba
Isatide, quam Nile Arabice nominarunt"; 1.29, "Error Avicennae, multas herbas figura
et natura diversas uno capite confundentis"; 3.8, "Error novi expositoris Avicennae, in
herba tinctorum citrina, quam Avicenna sic nominat"; 3.25, "Error Avicennae seu potius eius expositorum, non recte gutturis partes enumerantium."

[95] I have consulted *Joannis Manardi . . . in Galeni doctrina et Arabum censura celeberrimi et
optime meriti epistolarum medicinalium libros XX* (Basel, 1540). See 1.1, p. 1: "In cuius tamen libro [the *Canon*] praeter densam caliginem, infinitum esse ambagum chaos"; 2.1,
p. 13, for faults of older translations; 3.4, p. 37, for the derivative nature of Avicenna's
work. The criticisms of Avicenna are also found in the much briefer first edition of 1521.
Manardo's medical epistles were also printed at Paris, 1528; Basel, 1535; and Venice,
1542. Many more instances of his criticisms of Avicenna could be cited; however, it
should not be assumed that he, or others, who had a generally critical stance toward the
Arabs, necessarily opposed them automatically on every issue. For example, the hotly
debated question of the identity and safety of *scamonea* cut across party lines, pitting Manardo against another noted critic of the Arabs, Symphorien Champier; see Brian P. Copenhaver, *Symphorien Champier and the Reception of the Occultist Tradition in Renaissance
France* (The Hague, Paris, New York, 1978), p. 77.

[96] *Novae Academiae Florentinae opuscula adversus Avicennam et medicos neotericos qui, Galeni disciplina neglecta, barbaros colunt* (Venice, 1533). The so-called academy seems to have

tises, a dialogue entitled *Barbaromastix*, was apparently Bassiano Landi, who in 1551 became first ordinary professor of medical theory at Padua.[97] Under the cloak of anonymity, the young Landi expressed the hope that "whole volumes about Avicenna's errors will issue from our Academy."[98] He also characterized the famous Italian commentators on the *Canon* as men of great ingenuity who had been misled by following the bad leadership of the Arabs.[99] In this dialogue specific criticism of Avicenna largely focuses on errors and confusions in botanical and pharmacological terminology and is placed in the context of a plea for the direct study of plants in nature as well as of ancient authorities. Pietro Francesco Paolo and Leonardo Giacchini, the authors of the other two treatises, described themselves as "Galenic physicians" and practiced in Florence and Pisa, respectively. Paolo's treatise refutes as erroneous Avicenna's teaching regarding the administration of therapeutic phlebotomy, and Giacchini's criticizes the pharmacology of Avicenna and Mesue.[100]

North of the Alps, criticism of Avicenna appeared in print at Paris in 1513; the preface to Guillaume Cop's translation of Galen's *De locis affectis* asserts that the unintelligibility of the older translations of Hippocrates and Galen has induced students to turn to the *Canon*, where they find not, as is claimed, light and order, but rather darkness and chaos.[101] A few years later, Pierre Brissot followed with a tract refuting Avicenna's views on bloodletting, in which he referred to the latter's "tyranny" over the schools.[102]

The anti-Arabism of Leonhart Fuchs and other medical and botanical

---

been an informal grouping of medical teachers who perceived themselves as modern and Galenist; among their models was Matteo Corti (see Chapter 6, below); see Nutton, "John Caius and the Eton Galen," p. 245. Their efforts attracted the attention and approval of Leonhart Fuchs, who was immediately informed of the publication of their *Opuscula* by a correspondent in Italy; see Fuchs' *Paradoxorum medicinae libri tres* (Basel, 1535), fol. B[v]. My attention was drawn to this passage by Vivian Nutton.

[97] See Bartolo Bertolaso, "Ricerche d'archivio su alcuni aspetti dell'insegnamento medico presso la Università di Padova nel Cinque- e Seicento," *Acta Medicae historiae patavina* 6 (1959–60), 23.

[98] "Spero ut ex nostra Academia de Avicennae erratis iusta volumina prodeant." *Barbaromastix*, fol. 10[v].

[99] Ibid., fol. 9[v].

[100] It would seem likely that Paolo was aware of Brissot's treatise on the same subject, published a few years earlier (see n. 102, below).

[101] *Galeni de affectorum locorum notitia libri sex Gulielmo Copo . . . interprete* (Paris [1513]), fol. 3[r].

[102] Pierre Brissot, *Apologetica disceptatio, qua docetur per quae loca sanguis mitti debeat in viscerum inflammationibus* (Paris, 1525; reprint, Brussels, 1973), sig. i 3[v]. The treatise was published posthumously, as Brissot died in 1522.

innovators in Germany has recently been analyzed by Gerhard Baader and will not be further examined here. Opposition to the Arabs among German physicians was by 1530 sufficiently widespread to stimulate Lorenz Fries to publish his *Defensio medicorum principis Avicennae ad Germaniae medicos.*[103] Fuchs himself participated vigorously in the controversy over the Arabs in the early 1530s, and made Tübingen, where he taught from 1534, a center of anti-Arabism. For example, his *Paradoxorum medicinae libri tres,* first published in 1535, consists of a series of detailed attacks on Avicenna and other Arabic authors on a host of specific issues regarding medicinal simples, causes of diseases, and anatomy. The preface of this work reaches new levels of anti-Arab polemic with the assertion that the Arabs, having taken all their materials from the Greeks, like harpies defiled all they touched.[104]

Montpellier also had a leading opponent of the Arabs in the person of Symphorien Champier, who in 1533 produced a defense of the Greeks against the errors of the Arabs and a reply to Lorenz Fries.[105] It has several times been pointed out that in so doing Champier reversed his own earlier acceptance of Arab authors as medical authorities. Yet his was no sudden conversion, but rather a gradual evolution of thought of which the direction was not always maintained.[106] Although, no doubt, Champier's various shifts in position on the subject of the Arabs were in part dictated by the rhetorical strategies and specific issues of the different disputes in which he became involved, his various writings on the subject provide insight into the development of one man's views over almost the entire period when the role of the Arabs was a central issue in debates over the reform of medicine. Champier was exposed to Italian humanist influences early in his career, perhaps while still a student in Paris in the 1490s; in particular, as

[103] Strasbourg, 1530. Regarding this work, see Ernest Wickersheimer, "Laurent Fries et la querelle de l'arabisme en médecine (1530)," *Les cahiers de Tunisie* 9 (1955), 96–103. See also Baader, "Medizinisches Reformdenken."

[104] *Paradoxa,* preface *ad studiosos,* sig. [A6ʳ], Fuchs remarked: "Arabes quotquot fuerunt, nihil aliud studuerunt quam . . . sequi alienis atque adeo furtivis vestirent plumis. Id quod sane tolerandum erat, ni suo foedissimo contactu, harpyiae ritu, omnia contaminassent."

[105] On Champier as a critic of the Arabs in medicine, see Antonioli, *Rabelais,* pp. 46, 104–13; Copenhaver, *Champier,* pp. 66–81; and for the controversy stimulated by these works, Ernest Wickersheimer, "Die 'Apologetica epistola pro defensione Arabum medicorum' von Bernhard Unger aus Tübingen (1533)," *Sudhoffs Archiv für Geschichte der Medizin und Naturwissenschaften* 38 (1954), 322–28.

[106] Antonioli, *Rabelais,* p. 46; Baader, "Medizinisches Reformdenken," pp. 276–77, both note Champier's apparent change of heart. The various strands in his thought are well delineated by Copenhaver, *Champier.*

is now well known, he was strongly influenced by the thought of Marsilio Ficino.[107] He also became an admirer of the work of Leoniceno and Manardo, although his own criticism of Avicenna and other Arabic authors clearly has independent elements.[108] About 1506, Champier published a brief bio-bibliographical history of medicine. Avicenna appeared in a category devoted to the founders of medicine and royal personages who had practiced medicine, and was described as "a man of most outstanding genius and certainly the most distinguished of all."[109] However, the passage further stressed that Avicenna had been a Moslem and warned the reader of the spiritual and moral dangers of Islam.

By 1515, at the latest, although Champier clearly still attached some value to Arabic contributions to medicine, he found it desirable to distinguish them from those of the Greeks. He published a topically arranged *Practica* in which each condition discussed was accorded three chapters: one giving the views of the Greek authorities, one those of the Arabs, and one the remedies recommended by recent authors.[110] In 1518, Champier published annotations to Arcolano's commentary on *Canon* 4.1, thus presumably indicating his belief at that time that an older scholastic exposition could remain useful if revised. The revision was dedicated to Pietro Antonio Rustico, a professor at Pavia with whom Champier was shortly to collaborate on another project involving the *Canon*, and Matteo Corti, one of the principal advocates of medical reform in Italy, who in the course of his career taught at Pavia, Pisa, and Padua.[111]

In 1522, Champier collaborated with Rustico in the publication of a new edition of the *Canon* in which the prefatory matter included both strongly hostile remarks about Islam and a denunciation of Avicenna's philosophical and moral opinions and also a list of scientific issues on which Avicenna erred by differing from Galen and Dioscorides (see Chapter 5). In 1528, Champier announced that his *Symphonia Galeni ad Hippocratem, Cornelii Celsi ad Avicennam* had been written "lest Avi-

[107] Ibid.

[108] Champier's repeated denunciations of the religion of Islam introduce a theme not common in other medical works of the period.

[109] *De medicine claris scriptoribus in quinque partitus tractatus* [Lyon, ca. 1506], fol. xv[r]: "[Avicenna] Eminentissimi ingenii vir omnium certe clarissimus."

[110] *Practica nova in medicina aggregatoris lugdunensis domini Symphoriani Champerii* (Lyon, 1517). The first edition of this work appeared between 1509 and 1515. See Durling, *Catalogue*, no. 937.

[111] *Joannis Herculani Veronensis expositio perutilis in primam fen quarti canonis Avicenne una cum adnotamentis prestantissimi viri domini Symphoriani Champerii* (Lyon, 1518). Letter of dedication on fol. 1[v]. On Corti, see Chapter 6.

cenna and Averroes, that impious apostate, deceive Christian physicians through inane and barbarous philosophy."[112] In the same work, he also stressed the stylistic barbarism of Avicenna, making no distinction between the original and the Latin translation. In another treatise published the same year, he went so far as to pronounce a curse on the doctors of Padua, Salerno, Pavia, and Montpellier who allowed their schools to be occupied by "Arabs, Persians, Indians, and Mahometans" in a way pernicious for men and calamitous for good letters.[113]

Yet in some respects Champier's *Officina apothecariorum*, published in 1532, seems to reflect a return to a more moderate stand, with its assertion that, despite the turpitude of Islam and their clumsy language, the Arabs had made a few useful contributions to medicine and were not to be rejected out of hand. Of them, Avicenna was the noblest.[114] In the same work, Champier included a list of celebrated physicians in which relatively recent Latin writers are classified into *sophistae* (scholastics) and *atticissantes* (humanists). To the first class, are assigned such major fourteenth- and fifteenth-century commentators on the *Canon* as Giacomo da Forlì and Ugo Benzi; to the second, Cop, Leoniceno, Manardo, Fuchs, and so on.[115] The same idea is taken up in Champier's *Castigationes seu emendationes pharmacopolarum*, where the reader learns that there are three sects in medicine—Greek, Arabic, and Latin—the Arabs being merely compilers from books, while the Greeks knew nature and the art of medicine firsthand. Among the Latins, the *neoterici* are subdivided into *Latini*, who follow Hippocrates and Galen (again, Leoniceno, Cop, Fuchs, etc.), and *barbari*, including Gentile da Foligno and Jacques Despars.[116] Apart from their polemic value, the publication of such lists must surely have helped to foster an understanding of medicine's history that stressed the idea of distance between the leading medical writers of the fourteenth and early fifteenth centuries and their late fifteenth- and early sixteenth-century successors.

What was subsequently to become the most celebrated of all early sixteenth-century repudiations of Avicenna was quite different from the evaluations that have just been described and could have had little

---

[112] "Hanc Symphoniam scripsi, ne Avicenna et Averhous ille impius apostata Christianos medicos per inanem ac barbaram philosophiam decipiant." *Symphonia Galeni ad Hippocratem, Cornelii Celsi ad Avicennam, una cum sectis antiquorum medicorum ac recentium, a D. Symphoriano Campegio . . . composita* [Lyon, ca. 1528], p. 5.

[113] *Clysteriorum campi contra Arabum opinionem, pro Galeni sententia* ([Lyon, ca. 1528]; bound with the foregoing item), p. 26.

[114] *Officina apothecariorum . . . D. Symphoriani Campegii* (Lyon, 1532), fol. 2ᵛ.

[115] Ibid., fols. 3ᵛ–4ʳ.

[116] Bound with the preceding item, separately foliated; fols. 8ʳ–9ʳ.

or no impact on them. Whether or not Paracelsus actually burned the *Canon* in the St. John's Day bonfire at Basel in 1527, he certainly voiced his hostility to both Avicenna and Galen often enough.[117] Yet Paracelsus used these names as symbols for the whole system of school- and book-learned medicine—a system he wished to reject in its entirety— whereas the authors discussed here were engaged in debate within the academic medical community. It would seem likely that an intellectual climate in which hostility to the Arabs had become a shibboleth of modernism in medicine may have played a part in stimulating Paracelsus' more sweeping attack on tradition, but that is a supposition that takes us beyond the scope of this book.

Several salient features emerge from the series of attacks by academic medical writers on Avicenna and the Arabs. First, the criticisms put forward in the works just reviewed and other similar productions were evidently disseminated and discussed throughout the European medical community. Without taking up the question of lines of influence, it is clear that the leading opponents and defenders of the Arabs in widely separated centers were mutually aware of one another's work, and that their ideas circulated through personal contacts and correspondence as well as by means of print. Therefore, the absence of Padua and Bologna from the list of major centers of production of polemical treatises specifically directed against the Arabs and their Latin expositors does not mean that the controversy passed those universities by. (Political disruption sharply reduced all forms of academic output at Padua for almost a decade, 1509–17, when the controversy was running high.) On the contrary, by 1522 Leoniceno was able to claim that he had more supporters than opponents at Padua.[118] Hence one must assume some degree of familiarity with the attacks on the Arabs on the part of any Latin author translating, revising, editing, commenting upon, or otherwise discussing the *Canon* after at latest the early 1530s.

Second, although the approach of medical humanists to the Arabs certainly included its share of purely rhetorical and polemical elements, the grounds on which the *Canon* was criticized were for the most part

---

[117] The story is based on a passage in Paracelsus' *Paragranum* (in his *Schriften*, ed. Karl Sudhoff [Munich, 1924], 8:58); Sudhoff denied that Paracelsus was referring to the *Canon* in this passage, but Pagel accepted the identification on the basis of independent contemporary witness; see Walter Pagel, *Paracelsus: An Introduction to Philosophical Medicine of the Era of the Renaissance* (Basel and New York, 1958), pp. 20–22. Whatever the case, the *Paragranum* and its various prefaces (*Schriften*, 8:33–125, 131–221), like Paracelsus' other medical writings, contain numerous animadversions on Avicenna. The *Paragranum* was written 1529–30, but first published in 1565.

[118] Bylebyl, "School of Padua;" p. 345.

both practical and highly specific. The emphasis was primarily on evaluating the extent of the actual usefulness of the *Canon* for contemporary practitioners. Although the defenders of the *Canon* accused its at-
tackers of excessive concern for literary elegance rather than
substance,[119] such in fact seldom seems to have been the case. Moreover, Champier's suspicion of the taint of Islam was not echoed by
other authors. Instead, Leoniceno, Brissot, Fuchs, and Champier himself, as well as others, expended considerable effort in identifying particular instances in which Avicenna's supposed misunderstanding of a
text of Greek origin or the obscurities of Gerard of Cremona's Arabo-
Latin technical terminology produced confusions and errors that led to
an imprecise understanding of Galenic physiology and anatomy and to
mistakes in therapy and the identification of pharmacological substances. It was indeed the pharmacological portions of the *Canon* that
were the chief focus of critical attention, doubtless, as already suggested, both because these were the parts in which the Latin translation
was least comprehensible, and because of the growing general interest
among early sixteenth-century physicians in medical botany and pharmacology. The other main themes present, the ascription of general
unreliability to medieval translations and of purely derivative medical
teaching to Avicenna, were as a rule less emphasized and treated in less
detail. Little attention was paid by these authors to the question of the
usefulness of the *Canon* to students as a general guide to the basic principles of Galenic medicine and physiology. It is hard to evaluate the
rhetorical element in one other very frequent complaint, namely that
the teaching of Avicenna dominated or tyrannized the medical schools.
Yet there may be grounds for such complaints so far as late fourteenth-
and fifteenth-century medical curricula were concerned. After a century and a half of translating activity, the production of translations of
Greek medical works fell off in the early fourteenth century, and was
not resumed until the late fifteenth. And at the end of the thirteenth
century and beginning of the fourteenth, at Montpellier and Bologna,
commentaries were written on more than a dozen works of Galen,[120]
most of which do not appear to have inspired commentary (or at any
rate none that has survived) between about 1350 and 1500.

Third, criticism of the *Canon* was almost always closely linked not
just to denigration of the fourteenth- and fifteenth-century commentators, but also to an emphasis on the differences separating their med-

[119] See, for example, Fries, *Defensio* (1530), a2ᵛ–a3ʳ.
[120] For these developments at Bologna, see Siraisi, *Alderotti*, pp. 100–103; for Montpellier, Arnald of Villanova, *Opera*, 15:15–37.

ical teaching from that of their humanist critics, an emphasis sufficiently exaggerated to obscure real and important continuities. For
physicians trained in the northern Italian schools, acceptance of the humanist critique of Avicenna involved if not the outright repudiation of
their most distinguished local predecessors, then certainly the ability to
place them at a distance.

Thus, by the second or third decade of the sixteenth century, the accessibility of Greek medical works in the original and in numerous new
or modernized translations, rhetorical polemics against the Arabs in
general, the identification of specific errors or mistranslations in the
Canon especially as regards pharmacology, and the dimininishing reputation of earlier Latin scholastic commentators all argued against continued reliance on Avicenna. These arguments were genuinely persuasive and their force was widely recognized; yet they did not prevail.
The *Canon* survived in numerous university medical curricula, continued to be taught seriously in many universities, including leading centers of medical education, and continued to be consulted by practitioners. Academic, administrative, and professional tradition; the convenience of parts of the *Canon* for introductory teaching of Galenic
physiology and pathology; and the belief that the Arabs had added to
the store of remedies bequeathed by the Greeks—all these played a part
in ensuring this result. More fundamentally, philosophical eclecticism
and confidence in the power of humanist philology to recapture the
core of ancient wisdom made it difficult or impossible for most sixteenth-century intellectuals to jettison any traditionally authoritative
text with links to Greek antiquity. A much more common goal was to
purify, to reinterpret, to integrate. Thus, in the case of the *Canon*, the
introduction of philological humanism into medicine, which engendered the attack on the Arabs, also served to engender a reactive body
of opinion, which held that the cause of sound medical teaching would
be better served if the *Canon*, instead of being scorned, was supplied
with an improved Latin text and a modern body of commentary, both
of which would clarify Avicenna's relationship to Galen and confirm
or enlarge the practical usefulness of the work. Let us now turn from
Avicenna's critics to those who continued to find a use for his book.

4

The *Canon* in Italian Medical
Education after 1500

When the sixteenth century opened, the *Canon* was a ubiqui-
tous feature of the medical curricula of European universities. By the middle years of the century, humanist critics of
the Arabs had succeeded in either ending or limiting its use in some
places. For example, the statutes of the University of Tübingen, drawn
up in 1538, perhaps with the participation of Leonhart Fuchs, contain a
programmatic statement critical of the study of the Arabs;[1] in the
1550s, new statutes at several German universities—Heidelberg, Ingoldstadt, and Freiburg—increased emphasis on the Greeks at the expense of the Arabs, although in the 1570s the last two reverted to a
more traditional curriculum, which gave significant place to Avicenna
and Rasis.[2] In Spain, where innovations in medical teaching spread rapidly in this period, teaching based on the *Canon* was abolished at the
University of Alcalá de Henares, a noted center of Spanish humanism,
in 1565.[3] And the statutes that John Caius drew up for the London College of Physicians in 1563 confirmed the college's practice of examining students only on Galenic texts.[4] At Montpellier, although the place
of Avicenna in the medical curriculum was formally reasserted in 1550,
courses based on the *Canon* seem virtually to have disappeared after
1545, at any rate for the rest of the sixteenth century. Instead, courses
were offered with some frequency on the encyclopedic work of Paulus
Aegineta, which resembled the *Canon* in being for the most part a derivative compendium based on Galen. But Paulus' work, which ignored physiological theory, contained a noted section on surgery and

---

[1] *Urkunden zur Geschichte Universität Tübingen aus den Jahren 1476 bis 1550* (Tübingen,
1877), pp. 311–12; and for discussion, Gerhard Fichtner, "Padova e Tübingen: La formazione medica nei secoli XVI e XVII," *Acta medicae historiae patavina* 19 (1972–73), 43–
62.

[2] Nutton, "John Caius," p. 377.

[3] Luis Garcia Ballester, *Historia social de la medicina en la España de los siglos XIII al XVI.*
I. *La minoría musulmán y morisca* (Madrid, 1976), p. 89. On medicine in Spain during this
period, see further Luis S. Granjel, *Historia general de la medicina española.* II. *La medicina
española renacentista* (Salamanca, 1980), esp. pp. 153–93.

[4] Nutton, "John Caius," p. 377.

was the work of an author who had written in Greek—both features to recommend it to sixteenth-century medical *moderni*.[5]

However, the victory of the humanists was far from complete. In northern Europe, not only did the *Canon* retain at least a formal place in many university curricula, but statutes or directives specifically mandating its continued use were issued: for example, at Jena in 1591 (where *Canon* 1.1 and 4.1 were to be read alongside a range of Hippocratic and Galenic texts), at Würzburg in 1610, at Ingoldstadt in 1611, and at Louvain in 1617.[6] Furthermore, although few actual sets of lectures based on the *Canon* written after 1520 in universities north of the Alps appear to have survived (which suggests that university statutes were often honored in the breach), evidence of continued use of Avicenna by physicians is easy to find. Thus, the University of Paris, which had the largest medical faculty in sixteenth-century Europe, was in the 1520s and 1530s "the centre of the industry of editing and translating the classics of Greek medicine, especially Galen."[7] One might suppose that, despite the survival of highly traditional curricular arrangements until the French Revolution,[8] the *Canon* would be effectively ignored by the sixteenth-century Parisian Hippocratics and Galenists. No doubt this was the case as far as the use of portions of the *Canon* as textbooks for the systematic presentation of Galenic medicine was concerned. Thus, one of the most celebrated medical humanists and Galenists at Paris, Jacobus Sylvius (Jacques de la Böe, 1478–1555), made a deliberate effort to expunge any reliance on and almost all reference to Avicenna and other Arab authors from his expository works. Yet Gerhard Baader has shown that when it came to *materia medica* and their prescription, Sylvius, like other physicians of his day, was unable to detach himself from the Arabs or even their medieval Latin commentators.[9] Among Sylvius' colleagues, Jacques Houllier (d. 1562),

---

[5] Louis Dulieu, *La médecine à Montpellier*. II. *La Renaissance* (Avignon, 1979), pp. 141, 144–46, and tables on pp. 150, 152. On the Renaissance fortuna of Paul of Aegina, see Eugene F. Rice, "Paulus Aegineta," *CTC* 4:145–91.

[6] Heinz Goerke, "Die medizinische Fakultät von 1472 bis zur Gegenwart," in *Die Ludwig-Maximilians Universität in ihren Fakultäten* (Berlin, 1972), 1:191 (re Ingoldstadt); Ernst Giese and Benno von Hagen, *Geschichte der medizinischen Fakultät der Friedrich-Schiller-Universität Jena* (Jena, 1958), pp. 17–20; Franz X. von Wegele, *Geschichte der Universität Wirzburg* [sic] (Würzburg, 1882; reprint, 1969), vol. 2, *Urkundenbuch*, document 94, p. 249, medical statutes of 1610.

[7] Iain M. Lonie, "The 'Paris Hippocrates': Teaching and Research in Paris in the Second Half of the Sixteenth Century," in Wear et al., *Medical Renaissance*, pp. 155, 158.

[8] Charles Coury, "The Teaching of Medicine in France from the Beginning of the Seventeenth Century," in *The History of Medical Education*, ed. C. D. O'Malley (UCLA Forum in Medical Sciences, no. 12, Los Angeles, 1970), pp. 121–72.

[9] Gerhard Baader, "Jacques Dubois as a Practitioner," in Wear et al., *Medical Renaissance*, pp. 146–51. In his *De febribus*, a work on a subject often taught from *Canon* 4.1 in

whose *Omnia opera practica* were sufficiently useful to be reprinted more than a century after his death, and Vesalius' Galenist teacher at Paris, Guinter of Andernach (1505–1574), also noted appreciatively and made use of Arab contributions to pharmacology.[10]

Lyon was another major center of medical learning and activity in sixteenth-century France; there, the absence of a university was perhaps more than compensated for by the surgical education available at the Hôtel-Dieu, and the presence of an active college of physicians, and a flourishing medical publishing industry. At Lyon, Jacques Dalechamps, attending at the Hôtel-Dieu from 1552 until 1588, fostered the international dissemination and cultivation of Galenic and humanist ideals in medicine by means of his wide-ranging correspondence, and also pioneered the translation into French of Greek books on surgery and anatomy.[11] One of his principal achievements was his *Chirurgie françoise*, a translation of Book 6 of Paulus Aegineta's work, accompanied by his own commentary. And in the latter he drew frequently upon Abulcasis, and occasionally upon Avicenna; furthermore, he drew attention to his use of these authors on his title page.[12]

When one turns from France to the Low Countries and the German

---

the sixteenth century, Sylvius drew his readers' attention to his avoidance of Arab sources: "Hunc porro commentarium ex duobus rei medicae clarissimis luminibus, Hippocrate et Galeno eius interprete absolutissimo excerpere malui, quam ex Graecis aliis aut Arabibis, aut horum sectatoribus, quod in his quicquid est lectione aut imitatione dignunt, ex Hippocratis Galenique fontibus purissimus exhaustum est." *Iacobi Sylvii Ambiani medici et professoris regii parisiensis Opera medica* (Geneva, 1630), pt. 4, p. 312.

[10] "Vixerunt Graeci in media luce literarum. Extiterunt Arabes, et inde ductae familiae, iam desertis ac sepultis melioribus disciplinis, digna tamen luce aeternaque memoria nobis reliquerunt. E vivis fontibus Graecorum remedia primum petenda sunt, sed ita, ut nec Arabum rivos, nec posteritatis ingenia contemnamus. . . . Atque omnino hac parte perlustranda nobis naturae fertilitas, a qua omnis ubertas et quasi silva remediorum ducta primum est." Preface to *De materia chirurgia*, in *Iacobi Hollerii . . . Omnia opera practica* (Geneva, 1623), p. 156. On Houllier, see Lonie, "Paris Hippocratics," pp. 157–64, who notes on p. 159 Houllier's continued use of Arabic pharmacology. The numerous editions of Houllier's works include, according to *The National Union Catalog Pre-1956 Imprints*, 256:159, a reissue of this collection of his works on *practica*, Paris, 1674. According to Guinter, "Si enim Aristoteles multa ex Platone, Galenus ex Hippocrate, Dioscorides ex Democrate et aliis transcripserint, cur non mihi etiam nonnulla instituto idonea ex Graecis, Latinis, Arabibus, et Barbaris cuiuscunque linguae in hae nostra volumina traducere, veterum inventa augere, elaborare, et meliora quocunque modo reddere liceret?" *Ioannis Guintherii . . . De medicina veteri et nova . . . commentarii duo* (Basel, 1571), letter of dedication to Maximilian II, fol.★★★2r. On Guinter's career, see *Biogr. Lex.*, 2:878–89.

[11] On Dalechamps, and Lyon as a medical center, see Vivian Nutton, "Humanist Surgery," in Wear et al., *Medical Renaissance*, pp. 83, 85–87.

[12] Jaques Dalechamps, *Chirurgie françoise* (Lyon, 1570). According to the title page, the work includes "Les passages d'Aëce Grec, Cornelius Celsus Latin, Avicenne & Albucasis Arabes qui concernent la matiere traictee de Paul [of Aegina]." In fact, Dalechamps did not quote passages, but wove the opinions of the authors into his own commentary.

lands the picture is much the same. The prevailing mood of progressive medical men inside the universities in the middle years of the sixteenth century was one of enthusiasm for the Greeks, and only the Greeks. Yet as soon as one begins to look closely a number of signs that the *Canon* was still read and used, and to some extent still openly acknowledged and appreciated, appear. One may note the endeavors of Gilbert Fusch, or Fuchs, of Limburg (1504–67), who was sufficiently well known as a devotee of Avicenna to be memorialized for this attribute in Boissard and de Bry's collection of portraits and biographies of learned men.[13] The fruit of Fusch's dedication was a work, published at Lyon in 1541, in which he purported to show how Avicenna could be reconciled with Hippocrates and Galen and purged of errors. In his preface, Fusch acknowledged that Avicenna had made mistakes, but declared that he was nevertheless a glory not only of his own age, whenever that may have been, but also of the modern one.[14]

In 1550, Jacob Milich published at Wittenberg an oration on the life of Avicenna (whose birth he dated 1140) in which he declared that he had transmitted ancient medicine "more purely than any other of the Arab writers," and expressed the standard praises for the good organization of the *Canon* and the ease with which it could be consulted.[15] Johann Lange (1485–1565), physician to the Elector Palatine, urged that reformed university medical teaching include instruction in the Arabic language, on the grounds that a well-trained physician ought to know the Arabic names of herbs, and wrote a letter enthusiastically describing exotic *materia medica* (including cane sugar) that he had found available at Venice, and that he associated with Arab lands and Arab medical learning.[16] Lange, like many other sixteenth-century German

---

[13] *Bibliotheca sive thesaurus virtutis et gloriae in qua continentur illustrium eruditione et doctrina virorum effigies et vitae . . . per Ian. Iacobum Boissardum . . . incisae a Ioan. Theodor. de Bry*, pt. 4 (Frankfurt, 1631), pp. 198–201. Fusch's portrait is captioned with the verse "Quantum Asiae medicos hoc tollit et evehit aetas,/Ipse ego tantum Arabes teque Avicenna veho."

[14] "Quandoquidem Avicenna princeps fuit, rarum non sui tantum, sed etiam nostri seculi decus, et exemplum." [Gilbert Fusch], *Modus et ordo, quibus possint medicinae studiosi Avicennam, medicum Arabem, cum Hippocrate, Galeno, caeterisque medicis Graecis conciliare* (Lyon, 1541), p. 5.

[15] "Et quamquam plerique multas corruptelas arti admiscuerunt, tamen nemo ex omnibus Arabicis scriptoribus artem purius ipso Avicenna tradidit." *Oratio Jacobi Milichii doctoris artis medicae de Avicenna vita*, printed with his *Oratio de consideranda sympathia et antipathia* (Wittenberg, 1550), sig. b iiii[v].

[16] On Lange and his ideas about university reform, see Nutton, "Humanist Surgery," pp. 92–96. The epistle entitled *De exoticis medicamentis Arabum, sero a Graecis cognitis* is 1.64 in *Ioannis Langii Lembergii . . . Epistolarum medicinalium volumen tripartitum . . .* (Hanover, 1605), pp. 316–22. His plea for the teaching of Arabic is ibid., 3.6, p. 933.

physicians, had been trained and had his professional and scientific ideas formed in Italy.[17] And in Italy, as we shall see, Avicenna continued to play a prominent role in the curriculum of the most celebrated schools. Moreover, in the Low Countries and the German lands, manifestations of interest in the *Canon* continued well after 1600. In the seventeenth century, this interest took the form of several attempts, admittedly scattered and incomplete, to retranslate the text directly from the Arabic (see Chapter 5).

Doubtless many more examples could be adduced of continued use of Avicenna in northern Europe even at the height of the vogue for Greek medicine in the first half of the sixteenth century. The use of Avicenna is unlikely to have been less, and may have been more, widespread in the years around 1600, when the enthusiasm for the Greeks may have passed its peak, and when intellectual innovation of any kind perhaps began to appear increasingly threatening to religious or scientific conservatives, particularly in regions that were being retaken for the Catholic church.[18] Yet the overall impression left by various scattered references to Avicenna by northern medical authors, and from the way some of them used his work, is that the *Canon* was valued chiefly as a reference work for the practicing physician, and chiefly for its pharmacology and therapeutic recommendations.[19] Such authors seem seldom to have expressed positive views about the use of portions of the *Canon* as textbooks on which to base university lectures, or on which to depend for the systematic presentation of Galenic medical doctrine.

For a much more active tradition of university teaching based on the *Canon* after about the 1520s, one must turn to southern Europe, that is, to the Iberian peninsula and to Italy. From these regions, too, one can find expressions of appreciation for the *Canon* considered as a storehouse of Arab *materia medica*, or a handy guide to treatment. But it appears to have been almost exclusively in the south that the merits of the *Canon* as a text on which to base university lectures on medicine were highly enough regarded in the sixteenth and seventeenth centuries to give rise to numerous Latin editions for the use of professors and stu-

---

[17] Nutton, "Humanist Surgery," pp. 92–93.

[18] A valuable account of the nature of culture and learning in the re-Catholicized German-speaking imperial territories in the early seventeenth century is to be found in R.J.W. Evans, *The Making of the Habsburg Monarchy* (Oxford, 1979), pp. 311–80.

[19] Various works present *materia medica* from the *Canon* along with those of other authors. An example is *Medicinae tam simplices quam compositae . . . ex Hippocrate, Galeno, Avicenna, Aegineta, et aliis per Georgium Pictorium Villinganum, doctorem medicum, ordine sic alphabetico in unum conscriptae* (Basel, 1560).

dents and to engender the continued production of new lectures and commentaries specifically on portions of Avicenna's work.

In Spain, the approach to the *Canon* was influenced by the general openness to humanist interests and to the new anatomy that marked Spanish medicine for some years during the sixteenth century. The abandonment of teaching from the *Canon* at the University of Alcalá in the 1560s has already been mentioned. The early work of Francisco Vallés (1524–92), who taught at Alcalá de Henares from 1557, was marked by insistence upon the direct study of classical medical texts and by a marked interest in anatomy.[20] In his *Controversariarum medicarum et philosophicarum libri decem* (1556), which, like *Canon* 1, provided a general survey of medical theory, he arranged his topics in a nontraditional sequence and omitted some of the philosophical subject matter. In the same work, he condemned excessive reliance on dialectic in medicine, and criticized Avicenna for summarizing medical dogma without demonstration and requiring acceptance on the basis of faith rather than reason, and for postulating unnecessary and imaginary qualities of things.[21] But the *Canon* was affected positively as well as negatively by sixteenth-century Spanish endeavors to modernize the medical curriculum, as evidenced by the new (published in 1547–48) translation of and commentary on *Canon* 1.1 by Miguel Jeronimo Ledesma, professor of medicine at Valencia. This innovative edition, and its linguistic context, will be more fully discussed in Chapter 5.

In the long run, however, neither the abandonment of the *Canon* nor Ledesma's unusual effort to draw on local resources in the way of Arabic manuscripts and native Arabic speakers in order to get a better idea of the original nature of Avicenna's work was to prove characteristic of the Spanish universities. In the latter part of the sixteenth century, the religious and intellectual reaction against humanism and the repression of all aspects of Arabic language and culture combined to reinforce the most conservative and scholastic aspects of the medical curriculum.[22]

[20] See José Maria López Piñero, *Ciencia y técnica en la sociedad española de los siglos XVI y XVII* (Barcelona, 1979), pp. 344–47.

[21] *Controversarium medicarum et philosophicarum Francisci Valesii . . . editio tertia* (Frankfurt, 1590: I take the date of the first edition from López Piñero, *Ciencia,* p. 345). Preface to Book 1, p. 1: "Nam qui inter illos totam artem sibi proposuerunt pertractandam, ut Avicenna, aut omnia, aut pleraque, sine demonstratione tradunt, sive sine ratione haberi fidem postulantes."; 1.6, p. 17: "Sed multo probabilius, et Galeni doctrinae magis consonum est, non esse hanc qualitatem quam Avicenna dicit complexionem. Sed barbarorum hic semper fuit mos; supervacaneas quasdam et fictitas qualitates et proprietates singulis rebus imaginari, illustriorem se doctrinam ita reddere putantes."

[22] López Piñero, *Ciencia,* p. 351; Luis Garcia Ballester, *Los Moriscos y la medicina* (Barcelona, 1984), pp. 31–66.

Vallés' slightly younger contemporary Luis Mercado (1525–1611)—
like him, one of the leading Spanish medical writers of the age—already reflected such a trend.[23] (It should be noted that, although especially marked in Spain, neoscholasticism in medicine was by no means
peculiar to Spain; some evidence of the same tendency in parts of the
German lands has already been noted, and we shall see somewhat parallel developments in Italy.) Mercado, too, was a Galenist; but his
Opera omnia (1590) are wholly scholastic in organization and cite Avicenna frequently and uncritically.[24] After the turn of the century, some
commentaries on the *Canon* published in Spain were preoccupied with
issues that seemed at least as much metaphysical or even theological as
medical (regarding the content of these works, see Chapter 6). Thus,
for example, whatever the situation at Alcalá de Henares in its humanist heyday, before 1611 Dr. Pedro Garcia Carrero (later physician to
King Philip IV) was lecturing there on *Canon* 1.1 and before 1628 on
Canon 1.4 (see Appendix 2). One hopes the lectures on which the
printed *Disputationes medicae* he published in those years were presumably based were shorter than the printed versions; Garcia Carrero's
Disputationes on *Canon* 1.1 make up a tome that can only be described
as weighty, consisting, as it does, of 1398 folio-sized pages.

Moreover, at Salamanca, which was at the height of its reputation as
a center of medical education during the sixteenth and part of the seventeenth centuries, the *Canon* seems to have been taught actively and
seriously throughout the period, if one may judge by the survival of
seven lengthy sets of manuscript lectures on different parts of the
work, written by Salamanca medical professors between the 1540s and
the 1670s (see Appendix 2). The Salamanca curriculum provided the
model for the struggling and only intermittently existing medical faculties of various universities in Spain's New World colonies. An official report, drawn up in 1617, after consultation with learned men from
the universities of the mother country, on the difficulties of the young
University of Mexico, concluded that the main problem with the faculty of medicine was that the professors did not really lecture on, and
the students did not really study, the doctrines of Hippocrates, Galen,
and Avicenna. Instead, professors preferred to teach their own works
and the students, regrettably deficient in Latin, preferred to ask their
teachers straightforward questions about practice and get short an-
swers.[25] It is unclear whether the commission's report sufficed to cor-

---

[23] López Piñero, *Ciencia,* pp. 351–53.

[24] *Ludovici Mercati Operum tomus primus* (Frankfurt, 1620).

[25] Agueda Maria Rodriguez Cruz, O.P., *Historia de las Universidades Hispanoamericanas
periodo hispánico,* 2 vols. (Bogotá, 1973), pp. 12–24, 43, 48, 161, 196–98, 301, 315–16.

rect this in its view deplorable state of affairs. In Spain and its dependencies, as elsewhere in Europe, the final elimination of Avicenna from even a nominal place in medical curricula was a development of the eighteenth, not the seventeenth, century.[26]

Although serious attention to Avicenna as a text for university medical teaching after about the mid-sixteenth century tended to be more a feature of Catholic than of Protestant Europe, the situation in Italy was very different from that in Spain. Whereas the universities of sixteenth-century Spain were for a time receptive to new trends in medicine, those of Italy were among the main centers where such trends originated. Moreover, the major Italian centers of medical education, and particularly the University of Padua, attracted large numbers of foreign students (especially Germans), so that the influence of the form of medical education offered at Padua was very widely felt.[27] At the same time, the output from Italy of editions of the *Canon* and of new commentaries on it was a good deal larger than from the rest of Europe put together. (The same may well be true of notes, lectures, and commentaries left in manuscript, although here the accidents of survival evidently play so large a role that one hesitates to generalize.) Hence, the Italian schools offer both the largest body of material for a study of the influence of the *Canon* on Renaissance and early modern medical education, and the most striking examples of the interaction in the medical ideas of the period of humanist Galenism, scientific innovation, Aristotelian and eclectic natural philosophy, and Galenism in its medieval Arabo-Latin form.

However, judging by the output of material relating to the *Canon*, the importance accorded to the work was by no means uniform throughout the Italian universities. To some extent, the difference between institutions merely reflects differences in their sizes and general levels of academic productivity. Thus, to consider only three of the more prominent universities, the teaching staff in all faculties at Pisa in the late sixteenth century was less than half that of Bologna. Padua, apparently only slightly larger than Pisa in number of medical faculty,[28]

---

[26] See Michael E. Burke, *The Royal College of San Carlos: Surgery and Spanish Medical Reform in the Late Eighteenth Century* (Durham, N.C., 1977), pp. 43–65.

[27] See Bylebyl, "School of Padua," esp. pp. 335, 351; also E. Martellozzo Forin and E. Veronese, "Studenti e dottori tedeschi a Padova nei secoli XV e XVI," *Quaderni per la storia dell'Università di Padova* 4 (1971), 49–102.

[28] Charles B. Schmitt, "The Faculty of Arts at Pisa at the Time of Galileo," reprinted in his *Studies in Renaissance Philosophy and Science* (London, 1981), pp. 243–72 (original pagination), at p. 251. On the cultural and intellectual ambience of the University of Pisa in the sixteenth century, see also Paola Zambelli, "Scienza, filosofia, religione nella Toscana di Cosimo I," in *Florence and Venice: Comparisons and Relations*. II. *Cinquecento* (Flor-

enjoyed in the late sixteenth and early seventeenth centuries an out-standing reputation as a center of medical learning, a reputation that was both created by and fostered the contributions of its professors to all aspects of the subject. And Padua also had the advantage of prox-imity to a major center of the printing industry. But the output of ma-terial relating to the *Canon* was unquestionably also affected by varia-tions of emphasis in statutory curricula—which, although generally similar to one another, were by no means identical—and by the local intellectual climate.

Thus, the lack of material relating to *Canon* 1.1 by authors associated with Pisa is doubtless partially a result of the fact that at Pisa, unlike Padua and Bologna, *Canon* 1.1 was not part of the cycle of books on which ordinary (that is, senior) professors of medicine were required to teach. Instead, at Pisa this cycle consisted only of the Galenic *Ars* and Books 1 and 3 of the Hippocratic *Aphorisms*. The otherwise conserva-tive medical curriculum prescribed in the statutes that governed the University of Pisa from its revival in 1543 by Cosimo I of Tuscany un-til the eighteenth century found a place for *Canon* 1.1 only as part of the three-year cycle of texts assigned to extraordinary (that is, junior) pro-fessors of *theoria*.

One certainly cannot attribute to Cosimo I or his advisers any gen-eral determination to expel the Arabs from the medical schools; a glance at the curriculum in *practica*, which required both ordinary and extraordinary professors to lecture on *Canon* 4.1 (fevers) every three years, and furthermore drew the set books for the other two years of the cycle from the *Almansor* of Rasis, is sufficient to dispel any such no-tion.[29] Yet the minor position accorded *Canon* 1.1 and the early ap-pointments of some well-known antitraditionalists to the medical fac-ulty—even if these appointments were inspired more by a desire to

---

ence, 1980), pp. 3–52. Pisa in the late sixteenth century had five chairs in theoretical med-icine, two in practical medicine, one in botany, and one in anatomy and surgery (Schmitt, "Faculty of Arts," p. 252). The number of medical chairs at Padua varied from time to time over the course of the century, but in the 1590s comprised four chairs in *theoria*, six in *practica*, one in anatomy, and one in medicinal botany (simples), with two additional instructors in surgery (Bartolo Bertolaso, "Ricerche d'archivio su alcuni as-petti dell'insegnamento medico presso la Università di Padova nel Cinque- e Seicento," *Acta medicae historiae patavina* 6 [1959–60], 23–34).

[29] The statute is printed in F. Buonamici, "Sull'antico statuto della Università di Pisa: alcune preliminari notizie storiche," *Annali delle università toscane*, 30 (1911), the medical requirements appearing on p. 47. It should be noted that at Siena, too, *Canon* 1.1 was apparently taught only by extraordinary professors; see Alcide Garosi, *Siena nella storia della medicina, 1240–1555* (Florence, 1958), p. 237, where, however, the date of this pro-vision is not made clear.

secure famous professors for Pisa than by any special fondness for their views—certainly suggests an openness to the humanist and anti-Arabist intellectual climate of advanced medical circles in the 1540s. The faculty at Pisa in the 1540s and 1550s not only included, briefly, the anatomists Realdo Colombo and Gabriele Falloppia, but also Matteo Corti, Giovanni Argenterio, and Leonardo Giacchini.[30] Corti, near the end of his career when he came to Pisa for a few months shortly before his death, is best remembered for a commentary on the *Anatomia* of Mondino de' Luizzi largely dedicated to an attack on the author of that work (see Chapter 6). Argenterio had among contemporaries a reputation as a medical innovator and critic of received authorities, including Galen himself, almost equal to that of Fernel.[31] Leonardo Giacchini was, as already noted, one of the authors who had issued anti-Arabist medical treatises supposedly under the auspices of a "new Florentine academy." However, the contents of the large personal library owned by Giulio Angeli of Barga, ordinary professor of *theoria* at Pisa from 1577 to 1592, indicate that in the latter part of the century a good deal of the material actually taught, at any rate in *theoria*, was highly eclectic, and probably neither less nor more traditional than in other universities. Angeli's books included recent editions of classical medical authors and a wide selection of modern medical treatises, alongside the *Canon*, the works of the leading medical scholastics of the fourteenth and fifteenth centuries, including their commentaries on the *Canon*, and sixteenth century expositions of that work.[32]

Annual *rotuli* (announcements of courses and lecturers) and the series

[30] Angelo Fabroni, *Historiae academiae pisanae* (Pisa, 1792), 2:248–49, 254–57, 258–59; Giovan Battista Picotti, "Per la storia dell'Università di Pisa," in his *Scritti vari di storia pisana e toscana* (Pisa, 1968), p. 42; also Schmitt, "Faculty of Arts," pp. 250–51, who notes that the most distinguished personages tended not to stay at Pisa for very long. Of the medical figures, this is certainly true as regards Colombo (1546–48) and Falloppia (1548–51), and Corti and Giacchini died soon after arriving. However, Giovanni Argenterio (1543–55) and Girolamo Mercuriale (1592–1606), both renowned in their day, stayed at Pisa for respectable periods of time, although not for their entire careers. But Mercuriale, at any rate, was enticed to devote the last phase of his career to Pisa by an exceptionally handsome salary.

[31] See Lonie, "Fever Pathology," p. 36, citing the views of Laurent Joubert. On Argenterio, see *DBI* (Rome, 1960), 4:114–16.

[32] Giulio Angeli's list of the books contained in his personal library is reproduced in facsimile and transcribed in Laura Zampieri, *Un illustre medico umanista dello Studio pisano: Giulio Angeli* (Pisa, 1981), pp. 28–109. An idea of the eclecticism of Angeli's collection may be gained from the fact that he owned commentaries on the *Canon* by both the fourteenth-century author Dino del Garbo (p. 44) and Angeli's own contemporary A. M. Betti (p. 52)—together with the *opera* of both Galen and Hippocrates in Greek (p. 46). For Angeli's career, see ibid., pp. 9–10.

of surviving lecture notes of Giulio Angeli indicate that at Pisa the prescribed rotations of books for *theoria* and *practica* were adhered to in actuality, although apparently with the addition of lectures on other books and topics, throughout the sixteenth century.[33] Furthermore, from the late 1560s until 1605, Pisa also endowed a "supraordinary" chair of theoretical medicine, although at first it was only intermittently occupied. This chair appears to have functioned as a distinguished professorship, since for most of this period the fortunate occupant enjoyed an emolument about three times that of the highest-paid ordinary professor and ten times that of the highest-paid extraordinary professor. The *supraordinarius* also appears to have enjoyed somewhat more freedom to select the books on which he would lecture, judging from lectures on the *Physics*, *De anima*, and *De generatione animalium*, all somewhat unusual in a medical program, in the years 1583–85. When the famous Girolamo Mercuriale was *supraordinarius* from 1592 to 1605 he chose to lecture on Hippocrates: *De natura humana* (*De natura hominis*); the third, fifth, and seventh books of the *Aphorisms*; and the sixth book of the *Epidemics*.[34] Thus, at Pisa, the only lectures on *Canon* 1.1 appear to have been given by poorly paid *extraordinarii* in the early stages of generally undistinguished teaching careers that were seldom productive of written works of any kind. Hence it comes as no surprise to learn that apparently the only surviving commentary on *Canon* 1.1 by a professor at Pisa is a highly abbreviated and wholly routine exposition; it was written, probably early in his career, by Giuseppe della Papa (1649–1735), who late in life achieved modest success

[33] Angeli, a teacher whose degree of organization one can only envy, kept his lecture notes on the assigned texts in *theoria* in separate books, one for each year; those for the years 1578–88 are now Pisa, Biblioteca Universitaria, MSS 333–42. With the exception of 1585, which is missing, and 1584, when he taught on diseases of the head, these notebooks show that Angeli maintained the prescribed rotation of the *Ars*, *Aphorisms* 1, and *Aphorisms* 3 throughout the decade. Archivio di Stato, Pisa, Università G 77 contains sixteenth-century *rotuli* and administrative records (compiled in the eighteenth century by Angelo Fabroni for his history of the university), which, from 1565 to 1604, name texts as well as professors and their salaries (fols. 159^r–243^r), and also show substantial adherence to the statutes.

[34] On Mercuriale's lectures, see ibid., for 1596, 1599, 1600, 1602, 1604. The *supraordinarius* in 1583–85 was Andrea Camuzio, whose career and philosophical interests are described in Charles B. Schmitt, "Andreas Camutius on the Concord of Plato and Aristotle with Scripture," in *Neoplatonism and Christian Thought*, ed. Dominic J. O'Meara (Norfolk, Va., n.d.), pp. 178–84, 282–86. Giulio Angeli was also interested in the comparison of Plato and Aristotle if one may judge by the fact that he copied some notes from "Georgii Gemisti, qui et Plethonis dicitur, de iis quibus Aristotelis a Platone differt," into one of his notebooks (Pisa, Biblioteca Universitaria, MS 234, fols. 90^r–99^v). On Mercuriale, see *Biogr. Lex.* (Berlin, 1931), 4:171–72.

as a grand-ducal physician and the author of a few minor medical works.[35] For other portions of the *Canon* we seem to have no commentaries from Pisa, unless Argenterio's own work on fevers is to be ranked as such; as Iain Lonie has pointed out, although Argenterio deplored teaching by commentary, this work closely follows the organization of *Canon* 4.1.[36]

Yet in Italy, as in northern Europe, a formal curriculum that accorded the *Canon* a more prominent place than it held at Pisa was not in itself enough to guarantee the production of commentary where the local intellectual climate was sufficiently unfavorable. Thus, at Ferrara late fifteenth-century statutes of the University of Arts and Medicine provided for a program of lectures on various parts of the *Canon* that in its thoroughness and complexity recalls the statutes issued in 1405 by the University of Arts and Medicine at Bologna.[37] The extent to which the Ferrara statutes were actually observed over the course of the sixteenth century is, like their source, unclear. Throughout its heyday as a center of medical and humanistic studies in the later fifteenth and much of the sixteenth century, the small university of Ferrara was dominated by the Estensi court, by a board of Riformatori dello Studio responsive to the wishes of the court, and by leading faculty members who enjoyed the ducal favor and often filled court as well as professorial positions.[38] For a time, Ferrara acquired a European reputation as a center of medical learning largely as a result of the teaching of Leoniceno and Manardo, the propagators, as we have seen, of a strongly anti-Arabist brand of medical humanism. The dominant figure on the medical faculty in the middle years of the century, Antonio Musa Brasavola, a pupil of Leoniceno, was an exponent of innovative medicine who was especially noted for his work on pharmacological botany. Brasavola combined the roles of ducal physician and, from 1541 to 1555, first ordinary professor of *practica* (earning in the latter

---

[35] Venice, Biblioteca Marciana, MS lat. VII.23 (3491). A brief notice of Del Papa's career is included in *Nouvelle Biographie Générale* (Paris, 1862), 29:155.

[36] Lonie, "Fever Pathology," p. 20, n. 4.

[37] These undated late fifteenth-century statutes are printed in Ferrante Borsetti Ferranti Bolani, *Historia almi Ferrariae Gymnasii*, vol. 1 (Ferrara, 1735), with medical textbooks appearing in statute no. 57, p. 433. Borsetti believed these statutes to be of student origin.

[38] On the history of the *studium* of Ferrara during the Renaissance, see Adriano Franceschini, *Nuovi documenti relativi ai docenti dello studio di Ferrara nel secolo XVI*. Deputazione Provinciale Ferrarese di Storia Patria. Serie Monumenti, 6 (Ferrara, 1970); Alessandro Visconti, *La storia dell'Università di Ferrara* (Bologna, 1950), pp. 1–111; Giuseppe Pardi, *Lo studio di Ferrara nei secoli XV° e XVI° con documenti inediti* (Ferrara, 1903); Girolamo Secco Stuardo, "Lo studio di Ferrara a tutto il secolo XV," *Atti della Deputazione Ferrarese di Storia Patria* 6 (1894), 25–294.

capacity a higher salary than the first professor of *theoria*). Like his predecessors, he attracted and influenced a notable circle of pupils.[39]

At Ferrara, in addition to the usual lectureships on anatomy and simples introduced at a number of Italian universities in the course of the sixteenth century, a lectureship "on the works of Galen" was instituted in 1543, and another on the works of Hippocrates in Greek was added in 1562.[40] Alongside these chairs, lectures on *theoria* by senior professors continued to be given throughout the sixteenth century, although without attracting much attention.[41] And for medical *theoria* at least it seems likely that the *Canon* continued to serve as a textbook, since it was again assigned to the first ordinary professor of theory in 1611 (by which time the university had fallen under papal control), and once more in 1742.[42] But as long as the University of Ferrara remained vigorous, the faculty of which Leoniceno and Manardo had been the chief ornaments showed no interest in commenting on the *Canon*; only one exposition, dating from after 1600 and remaining in manuscript, can be even tentatively associated with Ferrara.[43]

The concentration at Padua, Pavia, and Bologna—the three major Italian universities of the period—of the active pursuit, and indeed renewal, in the sixteenth and early seventeenth centuries of the practice of writing commentaries on the *Canon* was clearly not due to any lesser vitality in those institutions as a whole. In particular, the importance in this period of Padua as a center of Aristotelian natural philosophy, Galenic and generally grecophile and humanistic medical learning, and botanical, anatomical, physiological, and clinical teaching and investigation scarcely requires further emphasis. Yet the frequent circulation of philosophical and medical faculty among the Italian universities suggests that Padua's uniqueness lay more in Europe-wide renown and in

[39] Franceschini, *Nuovi documenti*, pp. xv, 236, 240; Visconti, *Storia*, pp. 50–52, Pardi, *Studio*, p. 85.

[40] Franceschini, *Nuovi documenti*, pp. 247, 249, 250.

[41] From both the documents in Angelo Solerti, "Documenti riguardanti lo studio di Ferrara nei secoli XV e XVI conservati nell'Archivio Estense," *Atti della Deputazione Ferrarese di Storia Patria* 4 (1892), 5–51, and the lists of professors and salaries printed by Franceschini, *Nuovi documenti*, pp. 236–51, it is clear that lectures on *theoria* and *practica* continued to be given in addition to the lectures on the works of Galen and on Hippocrates in Greek. The chair on works of Galen disappears from the lists in 1573, and that on Hippocrates in Greek in 1594, but the lectures on *theoria* and *practica* continued.

[42] Visconti, *Storia,* pp. 110–11.

[43] Alessandro Ferri(?), comm. *Canon* 1.1, Modena, Biblioteca Estense MS Alpha U.7.19 (lat. 542). On fol. 1ʳ is the inscription Alexandri Ferri Regiensis/Ferrarie 1620 Patavii 1626. It is unclear from this whether Ferri was the author of the exposition or took it down from someone else's lectures. Nor is it clear whether the names of the cities and dates represent places where the lectures were delivered.

cultural, social, and political factors, and perhaps also in the possession of a larger critical mass of active scholars and scientific investigators and celebrated medical practitioners, than in any especially distinctive procedures or strains of thought.[44] However, local conditions that fostered special attention to the *Canon* at Padua certainly existed. Attention has, for example, been drawn to manifestations of interest in Avicenna as a philosopher in late fifteenth-century Paduan circles.[45] In a more practical vein, it was of course the Venetian presence in the Middle East that made possible the textual work of Ramusio and Alpago (see Chapter 5), and the Venetian printing industry that disseminated Alpago's revised edition of the *Canon*.

But at both Padua and Bologna, the most important factor contributing to the continued production of commentaries may simply have been that a larger medical faculty and the partial observance of curricular traditions of greater antiquity than those of the other institutions so far discussed multiplied the actual number of lectures on the *Canon*. In turn, this meant that a fair number of faculty members had a vested professional and economic interest in curricular conservatism. At Bologna in the late sixteenth and seventeenth centuries three ordinary professors and three or four extraordinary professors of *theoria* normally expounded *Canon* 1.1 as part of a three-year cycle of texts; a similar number of professors of *practica* taught *Canon* 1.4, and apparently *Canon* 4.1, as two parts of a three-year cycle.[46] At Padua, an essentially

---

[44] The bibliography on the intellectual life of Padua in the fifteenth, sixteenth, and early seventeenth centuries is, of course, very large. Recent overviews include, for philosophy and science in the fifteenth and early sixteenth centuries, *Scienza e filosofia all'Università di Padova nel Quattrocento*, ed. A. Poppi (Padua and Trieste, 1983); for medicine, Bylebyl, "School of Padua," pp. 335–70, and Giuseppe Ongaro, "La medicina nello Studio di Padova e nel Veneto," in *Storia della cultura veneta*, vol. 3, pt. 3 (Vicenza, 1981), 75–134; for philosophy and science, stressing the interaction between universities, Charles B. Schmitt, "Philosophy and Science in Sixteenth-Century Italian Universities," and idem, "Aristotelianism in the Veneto and the Origins of Modern Science: Some Considerations on the Problem of Continuity," both reprinted in his *The Aristotelian Tradition and Renaissance Universities* (London, 1984), pp. 104–23 and 297–336 (original pagination). A bibliography of Paduan university history is published serially in *Quaderni per la storia dell'Università di Padova*, vol. 1– (1968–).

[45] Marie Thérèse d'Alverny, "Avicenne et les médecins de Venise," in *Medioevo e Rinascimento: Studi in onore di Bruno Nardi* (Florence, [1955]), 1:178–97.

[46] See Dallari, *Rotuli*, vol. 2 (Bologna, 1889), which covers the period 1513–1660. One part of the cycle in *practica* is simply titled "De febribus," but the textbook was probably *Canon* 4.1. In addition, propositions from Avicenna were sometimes assigned as the subjects of the disputations whereby candidates competed for the annual "lectura universitatis" reserved for poor scholars in the late fifteenth and early sixteenth centuries. Heads of some of these disputations survive in ASB, Riformatori dello Studio, Dispute e ripetizioni di scolari per ottenere letture d'università, 1487–1527; see, e.g., no. 17, dated

similar arrangement prevailed as regards *Canon* 1.1 and 4.1;[47] *Canon* 1.4 seems not to have formed a regular part of the Paduan curriculum in this period,[48] but as we shall see, certain other chairs making use of portions of the *Canon* as a textbook were introduced at different times.

The presence of a course or courses of lectures on a given book in annual *rotuli*, and still less in university statutes, is not of course in itself a guarantee that the lectures in question were actually delivered, or if delivered were not either drastically truncated or unattended. Such possibilities are implied by the very existence of the regulations, common in one form or another to various Italian universities, that provided for the presence of lecturers and their progress through the as-

---

1487–88, where the subject is "textum Avicene in primo libro in secunda doctrina quae incipit *Elementa sunt corpora.*" I am grateful to Herbert Matsen for his kindness in drawing my attention to this collection. The lectureship is described in his "Students' 'Arts' Disputations at Bologna Around 1500, Illustrated from the Career of Alessandro Achillini (1463–1512)," *History of Education* 6 (1977), 169–181. On the general history of the University of Bologna in the Renaissance and early modern periods, see Luigi Simeoni, *Storia dell'Università di Bologna. II. L'età moderna* (Bologna, 1940).

The program at Pavia seems to have been similar in essentials: see Baldo Peroni, "La riforma dell'Università di Pavia nel Settecento," *Contributi alla storia dell'Università di Pavia pubblicati nell' XI centenario del Ateneo* (Pavia, 1925), pp. 121–22, and, more generally, Pietro Vaccari, *Storia della Università di Pavia*, 2nd ed. (Pavia, 1957), and [A. Corradi], *Memorie e documenti per la storia dell'Università di Pavia* (Pavia, 1878). According to *Statuti e ordinamenti della Università di Pavia dall'anno 1361 all'anno 1859* (Pavia, 1925), no early statutes of the University of Arts and Medicine survive (p. ix), and the statutes of the College of Doctors of Arts and Medicine (pp. 118–29, 130–43), do not mention books.

[47] See Bertolaso, "Ricerche d'archivio" (1959–60), pp. 23–25, 27–28, 30–31. Most of the *rotuli artistarum*—that is, annual lists of chairs, teachers, and textbooks in liberal arts, natural philosophy, and medicine—from Padua survive for the period 1430–1815. So far, only scattered examples have been published, although publication of the entire series is planned by the Istituto per la Storia dell'Università di Padova. Most of the *rotuli* for the period 1519–1740 are contained in Archivio Antico dell'Università di Padova, *filze* 651 and 242 (for the locations of the entire series, see A. Favaro, "Indice dei rotuli dello Studio di Padova," *Monografie storiche sullo Studio di Padova* [Venice, 1922], pp. 22–27); however, by no means all the *rotuli* provide the titles of textbooks. Those that do (e.g., in *filza* 651, those for 1579, fols. 283^r–84^v; 1583, fols. 292^r–94^v; 1584, fols. 301^r–2^r; 1585, fol. 304^{r-v}; 1586, fol. 308^{r-v}; 1589, fols. 311^r–12^r; 1590, fol. 317^{r-v}; 1592, fols. 329^r–30^r; 1603, fols. 374^r–75^v) make it clear that both ordinary and extraordinary professors of theory rotated *Canon* 1.1 with the *Aphorisms* and the *Ars*; the *ordinarii* and *extraordinarii* in *practica* rotated instruction *de febribus* (clearly using *Canon* 4.1 as a text, judging from the number of sixteenth-century Paduan commentaries and a remark to that effect of Vettor Trincavella opening his comm. *Canon* 4.1, 1553, in his *Opera* [Venice, 1599], vol. 3) with teaching on diseases affecting parts of the body from the head to the heart, and from the heart downward (probably using Rasis, *Almansor*, which was prescribed by name in 1583, and described as frequently used in teaching *practica* by Giambatista Da Monte, comm. *Canon* 1.2 [Venice, 1557], p. 8).

[48] To the regret of Da Monte (ibid.).

signed books to be checked at regular intervals.[49] Nonetheless, whatever may have been the practice in the later seventeenth century and thereafter,[50] or among earlier teachers whose lectures do not survive, sets of lectures on the *Canon* from the sixteenth and early seventeenth centuries do not appear notably truncated or cursory. A full academic year's course was usually supposed to amount to about eighty or ninety lectures.[51] To take a few rather randomly chosen examples from manuscripts, Matteo Corti left 63 lectures on *Canon* 1.1; Girolamo Capodivacca, 77 on *Canon* 4.1; and Bernardino Paterno's lectures on *Canon* 1.4 fill a volume of 277 leaves.[52] Furthermore, while it was rather common for a lecturer not to get through the whole of *Canon* 1.1, the treatment of individual topics and the length of individual lectures were usually quite full. For example, Giambatista Da Monte's exposition of *Canon* 1.1 in the printed version amounts to about 80 percent of the length accorded to the same portion of the work by that extremely prolix scholastic Gentile da Foligno.[53] It seems fair to assume from these surviving examples that during the sixteenth century a significant number of the prescribed lectures on Avicenna at Padua, Bologna, and Pavia were actually delivered and were not pro forma treatments.

At Padua, one result of these curricular arrangements was that, of nine holders of the first ordinary chair of medical theory between 1524 and 1624, four produced full-scale commentaries on *Canon* 1.1.[54] Thus,

[49] See Stefano de Rosa, "Studi dell'Università di Pisa, I, Alcune fonti inediti: diari, lettere e rapporti dei bidelli (1473–1700)," *History of Universities* 2 (1982), 97–125.

[50] It is, for example, clear from a report on the state of the university drawn up in 1741 by G. B. Morgagni and other faculty members that the teaching of the official curriculum had by that time become a formality (AAUP 507, fols. 89–108); complaints that all real teaching was conducted by means of private lessons were already heard in 1672 (AAUP 722, document of 26 February 1672). See further below.

[51] Administrative reforms at the University of Siena in 1589 included the stipulation that each professor must give at least ninety lectures in the academic year; see Danilo Marrara, *Lo studio di Siena nelle riforme del Granduca Ferdinando I (1589 e 1591)* (Milan, 1970), p. 22.

[52] Corti, comm. *Canon* 1.1, 1528(–29), Bologna, Biblioteca Comunale dell'Archiginnasio, MS A 922 (the commentary ends somewhere in *Doctrina* 4, on humors, and occupies the entire codex of 173 folios); Capodivacca, comm. *Canon* 4.1, Siena, Biblioteca Comunale, MS C IX 18, 1579–80, fols. 1ʳ–129ᵛ; Paterno, comm. *Canon* 1.4, Mantua, Biblioteca Comunale MS 83 (A.III.19), 1551, whole sections of which are only schematic outlines, especially toward the end (these lectures were probably delivered at Pavia, where Paterno taught for a time early in his career).

[53] Based on a very rough estimate and comparison of the number of words in Da Monte, comm. *Canon* 1.1 (Venice, 1557), and Gentile da Foligno, comm. *Canon* 1.1 (Pavia, 1510—for this edition see Appendix 1).

[54] Bertolaso, "Ricerche d'archivio" (1959–60), p. 23, lists the following names and

in the Paduan milieu, lecturing on the *Canon* was not an activity restricted to isolated or peripheral figures, or to those of especially conservative bent, but was a normal part of the output of leading professors who played a major part in the life of the school. Nor was the writing of commentaries on the *Canon*, at Padua or elsewhere, confined to those who taught *theoria*, arguably the branch of the curriculum least responsive to innovation either in methodology or content; commentaries on *Canon* 1.4 and 4.1 were the work of professors of *practica*, among them men of such contemporary renown as Vettor Trincavella and Girolamo Capodivacca.[55] In the course of the sixteenth century the entire traditional curriculum at Padua, especially in *theoria*, although not supplanted, seems to have been squeezed to one side by new topics, new materials, and new interests. But within the traditional parts of the curriculum, the teaching of the *Canon* was treated seriously and, as we shall see, was infiltrated by innovations in content and approach. However, the place of the *Canon* in the sixteenth-century Paduan curriculum was not determined by tradition and ancient statute alone, but was affected by various contemporary efforts at curricular reform that reveal a good deal about the actual uses of the work in university teaching.

Teaching the Canon at Padua, 1521–50

At Padua, the emergence of a new phase in the teaching of the *Canon* may conveniently be dated from the official endorsement given by the College of Philosophers and Physicians in 1521 to Andrea Alpago's emendations of the Latin text (on the content of Alpago's work, see

---

dates of appointment: 1524, Mathaeus de Curte; 1532, Benedictus Vict. de Faventia; 1539, Franciscus Cassianus; 1541, Pamphilius Monte; 1543, Johannes Bapt. de Monte; 1551, Bastianus Landus; 1563, Bernardinus Paternus; 1592, Horatius Augenius; 1611, Sanctorius Sanctorius. Of these, Corti, Da Monte, Paterno, and Santorio wrote commentaries on *Canon* 1.1.

[55] Trincavella held the first chair in *practica* at Padua from 1551 until his death in 1563. He was celebrated both as a practitioner and for his study of Greek medical texts. On his career and writings, see Bertolaso, "Ricerche d'archivio" (1959–60), *Biogr. Lex.*, 6:9–10, and Richard Palmer, "The Control of Plague in Venice and Northern Italy, 1348-1600," (Ph.D. diss., University of Kent at Canterbury, 1978), pp. 255–59; and Richard Palmer, *The Studio of Venice and Its Graduates in the Sixteenth Century* (Padua and Trieste, 1983), p. 19, correcting the death date given in *Biogr. Lex.* Girolamo Capodivacca held the second ordinary chair in medical *practica* at Padua from 1564 until his death in 1589; his reputation was based in part on his success in the treatment of venereal disease, and in part on his numerous published writings. On him, see Bertolaso, "Richerche d'archivio" (1959–60), p. 24; *DBI*, 18:649–51; and Palmer, "Control of Plague," pp. 242–54, recounting a singularly unsuccessful episode in his career.

Chapter 5). Before examining the implications of the decision itself, it may be useful to place it in the context of the general history of the university in the early sixteenth century and the function of the college therein.

When university organization of higher learning emerged at Padua in the thirteenth century, the *studium* was made up of a number of separate self-governing academic and professional corporations. These were student universities of law and of arts and medicine (the latter apparently in existence in the 1260s, although only gaining full recognition from the church, the universities of law, and the city government in the next century) and doctoral colleges of law and medicine. The colleges included, respectively, judges and physicians practicing in the city, as well as professors. At an early date, the student universities were subdivided into nations, also self-governing associations. (Similar arrangements also prevailed at Bologna and other *studia* of medieval origin in Italy.) In developments of a type common to the Italian *studia*, the autonomy of the academic corporations gradually yielded first to the power of the government of the city (in the case of Padua, the signoria of the house of Carrara) and then to the demands of the Renaissance state.

In 1405, Padua came under the political control of Venice; by the second half of the fifteenth century the administrative changes that would transform the medieval *studium* of Padua into the state university of the Venetian republic were already under way. Under Venetian patronage, the late fifteenth- and early sixteenth-century *studium* seems to have flourished, with numerous students and some distinguished professors; but a sharp disruption occurred in 1509, when Padua was temporarily lost to Venice in the War of the League of Cambrai. After the restoration of peace in 1517, Venetian administrative control over the university was strengthened and institutionalized by the establishment of the Venetian magistracy of the Riformatori dello Studio (officially in 1528, confirming earlier informal arrangements), responsible to the Senate. Thereafter, although the student universities and nations continued to have administrative functions and, on occasion, to make their wishes strongly felt, discipline, finance, and all but the most minor professorial appointments were essentially controlled by the Riformatori, and ultimately by the Venetian Senate, although frequently with input from the teaching faculty at Padua, and intermittently from other sectors of the university community.

At the local level the College of Philosophers and Physicians, as the doctoral college of arts and medicine was by this time grandly named, continued to be an influential body. Within the *studium*, this was chiefly because the college was the examining body for the Paduan degrees in arts, philosophy, and medicine. (College membership was limited to Paduan citizens or Venetians living in Padua; many professors were thus automatically excluded, although the first ordinary professors of medical *theoria* and *practica* were members ex officio.) In civic affairs, the college was influential because of close ties with the Paduan municipal council and because it supervised medical practice in the city.

From the restoration of Venetian power in 1517 until about 1545, the various bodies and individuals in a position to do so—the Riformatori, whether acting spontaneously or in response to wishes expressed by the faculty, the Paduan College of Philosophers and Physicians, and individual professors—engaged in a variety of initiatives designed to revive, improve, or extend the quantity, quality, and content of medical teaching. Among these endeavors belongs the endorsement of Alpago's version of the *Canon* by the College of Philosophers and Physicians.[56]

Turning from the standpoint of administrative to that of intellectual history, the decision of the college to endorse an improved version of the *Canon* may be viewed both as a result of developments extending back to the fifteenth century and as a forerunner of the deservedly more famous innovations in medical teaching of the 1530s and 1540s. Of the latter, a recent scholar has written: "It was within a relatively short period from the mid 1530s to the mid 1540s that several of the most fundamental changes occurred, including the transformation of anatomical teaching from a short annual event into a permanent major subject, the institution of a botanic garden under university auspices for the express purpose of teaching medical botany, and the systematic use of the hospital to teach nosology and therapy."[57] All of these developments involved the expansion or institutionalization of aspects of medical teaching based primarily on an immediate encounter with the objects of the physician's professional expertise: the human body, disease, and

---

[56] The document containing the endorsement of Alpago's work is printed in Francesca Lucchetta, *Il medico e filosofo bellunese Andrea Alpago († 1522) traduttore di Avicenna* (Padua, 1964), p. 90. For a summary of the early history of the Paduan *studium*, Siraisi, *Arts and Sciences*, pp. 15–31; for the fifteenth and early sixteenth centuries, *Storia della cultura Veneta*, vol. 3, pt. 2 (Vicenza, 1980), 608–47, and Ronald E. Ohl, "The University of Padua 1405–1509: An International Community of Students and Professors" (Ph.D. diss., University of Pennsylvania, 1980); on the College of Philosophers and Physicians of Padua, Palmer, *Studio of Venice*, pp. 17–18, and idem, "Physicians and the State in Post-Medieval Italy," in *The Town and State Physician in Europe from the Middle Ages to the Enlightenment* (Wolfenbüttel, 1981), for a useful discussion of the role of city colleges of physicians and their relations with governments in the sixteenth century.

[57] Bylebyl, "School of Padua," p. 342.

medications. Yet such an encounter did not preclude, but rather required, the simultaneous study of books on the subject; the extent to which an intimate involvement with the study of ancient texts, as well as of nature, was characteristic of Renaissance anatomy, botany, and concepts of disease and treatment is too well known to call for further emphasis here.

Hence, the developments of the 1530s and 1540s are in one way or another linked not only with the earlier history of the actual practice of dissection, teaching at the bedside, and compounding medications at Padua and in other north Italian schools, but also with the whole tradition of the teaching of *practica, anatomia,* or *chirurgia,* whether by physical demonstration, lectures on texts, or a combination of the two. Moreover, the growth of practical, anatomical, and surgical interests among the Paduan medical faculty from the middle years of the fifteenth century is now well documented.[58] It thus seems probable that a major motivation of the College of Philosophers and Physicians in recognizing the work of Alpago was to contribute to the teaching of *practica.* The appointment of Alpago himself as first extraordinary professor of *practica* suggests that the college perceived his contribution as primarily in that area;[59] in particular, it appears likely that the members believed his glossary of Arabic technical terms would help to unravel the confusions in botanical and pharmacological nomenclature for which the *Canon* had so often been criticized over the last thirty years.

The endorsement of Alpago's efforts is also a manifestation of faith that linguistic studies had a contribution to make to university teaching in scientific and technical subjects. As has recently been demonstrated, the general humanist enthusiasm for the improvement of Latin translation and the study of Greek texts in the original found specific application within university teaching of technical subjects at Padua in the 1490s. In that decade, not only were humanist Latin translations of Aristotelian works introduced to university audiences, but in some instances Aristotelian philosophy began to be taught from the Greek

---

[58] Tiziana Pesenti Marangon, "Michele Savonarola a Padova: l'ambiente, le opere, la cultura medica," *Quaderni per la storia dell'Università di Padova* 9–10 (1976–77), 45–102, and " 'Professores chirurgie' "; Tiziana Pesenti, "Generi e pubblico della letteratura medica padovana nel Tre- e Quattrocento," in *Università e società nei secoli XII–XVI, Atti del nono Convegno Internazionale di studio tenuto a Pistoia nei giorni 20–25 settembre 1979* (Bologna, 1983), 523–45; Ongaro, "La medicina nello Studio di Padova," pp. 80–99; L. R. Lind, *Studies in Pre-Vesalian Anatomy: Biography, Translations, Documents* (Philadelphia, 1975).

[59] Lucchetta, *Alpago,* document 13, p. 91.

text.[60] It is clear that medicine as well as philosophy was affected by these developments; indeed, Francesco Cavalli, reputedly the first to teach Aristotle from the Greek text, was also a physician and a professor of practical medicine.[61] The number of physicians involved in Greek textual studies probably always remained small, but the numerous humanist Latin translations of Greek medical works found their readership in university circles. Furthermore, although most medical, as most philosophical, teaching doubtless continued to be based on texts in Latin, once the teaching of Greek philosophical texts had been introduced, professors of medicine could count on getting at least a few students with some practice in studying scientific material in Greek, since philosophy was still normally required before proceeding to medicine. And some mid-sixteenth-century medical commentators certainly seemed to take it for granted that their presumably student readers would all be able to handle at least brief phrases or quotations in Greek.[62] No such chain of developments was to occur in the case of Arabic—indeed, the emphasis on Greek in some settings may have inhibited interest in Arabic—but the context and parallel help to explain the value set on Alpago's linguistic endeavors.

Finally, it seems likely that the approval extended to Alpago's work may also be placed in the context of an attempt to improve the teaching of medical *theoria*, for which *Canon* 1.1 served as a major text. As we have seen, medical *theoria* drew for its subject matter upon parts of Aristotelian natural philosophy that were considered relevant to medicine and upon the principles of Galenic physiology. While the structure of the university curriculum, and the opinion of physicians, classified philosophy as a necessary preparatory study for medicine (that is, in reality for medical *theoria*), the distinguished history of the Paduan philosophical faculty from the fourteenth to the early sixteenth century is certainly not suggestive of an ancillary role.[63] On the contrary, particu-

---

[60] Charles B. Schmitt, "Aristotelian Textual Studies at Padua: The Case of Francesco Cavalli," in *Scienza e filosofia*, ed. Poppi, pp. 287–313. Edward P. Mahoney, "Philosophy and Science in Nicoletto Vernia and Agostino Nifo," in *Scienza e filosofia*, pp. 135–202, points out that Nicoletto Vernia had already developed an interest in the Greek commentators on Aristotle, whom he apparently knew via the Latin translations of Ermolao Barbaro (ibid., p. 156) in the course of the 1480s.

[61] Schmitt, "Aristotelian Textual Studies," p. 294; on Cavalli, see Tiziana Pesenti, *Professori e promotori di medicina nello Studio di Padova dal 1405 al 1509* (Padua and Trieste, 1984), pp. 70–72.

[62] Greek phrases occur with a fair degree of frequency in the commentaries on *Canon* 1.1 of, for example, G. B. Da Monte and Giovanni Costeo—but they are usually very brief, and often involve no more than individual technical terms.

[63] On the relationship of philosophy and medicine in the Italian universities of this pe-

larly from the mid-fifteenth century, the teaching of medical *theoria* seems to have compared rather poorly in vigor and distinction either with philosophy or with *practica* and associated branches of medicine. Whereas, for example, in the early fifteenth century Giacomo da Forlì, one of the most distinguished and prolific authors to teach at Padua, held a chair in medical *theoria*, in subsequent generations the best-known and most productive professors held chairs either in medical *practica* (Michele Savonarola, Giovanni Arcolano, Alessandro Bene-detti) or in philosophy (Nicoletto Vernia, Agostino Nifo, Pietro Pomponazzi). Gabriele Zerbi did indeed occupy the first ordinary chair in medical theory, but his principal written work was on anatomy.[64] Moreover, in 1506 the position allocated to *theoria* in the curriculum was reduced when, as a result of an economic crisis brought on by war, the Venetian Senate suppressed one of the professorships in the subject. However, the revival of the university in 1517 included the restoration of the suppressed chair and the addition of two more teaching positions in medical *theoria*, actions that presumably indicated an official inten-tion to reinvigorate the teaching of that branch of medicine as well as to foster anatomy and *practica*, in which chairs were also added.[65] A similar purpose may be read in the appointment to the first ordinary chair in theory in 1524 of Matteo Corti, and still more that in 1543 of the noted Galenist and clinician Giambatista Da Monte.[66]

Within about a twenty-year period these men and their colleague Oddo Oddi each produced a substantial commentary on *Canon* 1.1. Da Monte's was the first part of an ambitious project to expand and reform the way the first book of the *Canon* was used in medical teaching. Dur-ing his tenure as first professor of *theoria* he followed up the customary lectures on *Canon* 1.1 by reintroducing lectures on *Canon* 1.2, and in-dicated his belief that *Canon* 1.3 (regimen) should be taught.[67] And he

---

riod, see Charles B. Schmitt, "Aristotle among the Physicians," in Wear et al., *Medical Renaissance*, pp. 1–15, 271–79.

[64] Ongaro, "La medicina nello studio di Padova," pp. 77, 80, 86, 87, 89, and Pesenti, *Professori e promotori*, pp. 35, 49, 187, 214, for the chairs held by the physicians men-tioned.

[65] Bertolaso, "Ricerche d'archivio," (1959–60), p. 18. The chair suppressed in 1506 was in *theoria extraordinaria*. According to Bertolaso, the chairs in theory revived in 1517 were one *ordinaria* and the other *extraordinaria*. The minor chair in *practica* devoted to lec-tures on *Canon* 3 was also suppressed in 1506 and restored in 1517.

[66] For the dates of appointment, Bertolaso, "Ricerche d'archivio," (1959–60), p. 23. Further biographical information about Da Monte and some of the other commentators on the *Canon* mentioned in this chapter in the context of the history of the Paduan or Bolognese curriculum can be found in Chapter 6.

[67] Da Monte, comm. *Canon* 1.2 (Venice, 1557), p. 8.

also lectured on *Canon* 1.4 (principles of therapy), which by his own account was seldom or never used as at Padua in his day (and elsewhere was taught by professors of *practica*). Discussion of some of the contents of the commentaries that resulted from these lectures is reserved for later chapters, but here their implications as far as the Paduan curriculum is concerned may be briefly considered. From one standpoint, Da Monte's activity with regard to the *Canon* involved no more than adherence to a neglected Paduan university statute of 1465, which mandated the teaching of the whole of *Canon* 1. Even when originally instituted, this statute may have been no more than the expression of a wish (perhaps a desire to perpetuate the unusual accomplishment of Matteolo Mattioli, who had lectured on all four parts of *Canon* 1 at Padua in 1464), since, as already noted, the commentary tradition suggests that it was never customary to lecture on the whole first book. Up until the middle years of the fifteenth century, however, *Canon* 1.1 and 1.2 were often lectured on together.[68]

But Da Monte's output of *Canon* commentary is also linked to his views on the proper structure and organization of medical education as these emerge from the commentaries themselves. Da Monte was profoundly critical of the notion that *theoria* was a study to be undertaken apart from and without direct reference to medical *practica*, as well as of the idea that nothing of any significance was to be learned from *theoria* and that what mattered was exclusively the study of *practica*. Accordingly, he disapproved more or less equally of the treatment of *Canon* 1.1 by most Latin scholastic commentators,[69] of those teachers of *theoria* among his contemporaries who confined their lectures on *Canon* 1 to the first fen,[70] and of students who tried to bypass *theoria* entirely.[71] In Da Monte's view, what was needed was a unified introductory overview of "universal medicine." This would from the beginning teach students method and principles as they related to *practica*—not only

---

[68] For Mattioli's lectures in 1464, see Pesenti, *Professori e promotori*, p. 134.

[69] For example, "alii semper soleant implicari quaestionibus inutilibus, ita ut scholares avertant," Da Monte, comm. *Canon* 1.1 (Venice, 1554), fol. 1r.

[70] *Canon* 1.2 "quatuor habet conditiones advertandas a nobis. Prima attinet maxime ad partem theoricam. Secundaque ea quae quaeruntur in hac secunda fen sunt valde necessaria futuris medicis, ut sine his nullus esse possit medicus. Tertiaque ordine doctrine necessaria continuetur primae fen. Quarta et ultima, quod cognitio earum quae traduntur in prima fen, sine cognitione eorum quae traduntur in hac secunda, omnino frustratoria et mutilata sunt." Da Monte, comm. *Canon* 1.2 (Venice, 1557), pp. 1–2.

[71] "Scio enim plures huc accedere sive ob paupertatem, sive ob imperitiam, sive malevolentiam, ut velint esse medici qui tamen nesciunt quam scientiam et dogma velint sequi; et cum accedunt ad dogmaticos medicos quaerunt receptas ab illis, vel contempta ratione et theorica accedunt ad empiricos." Ibid., p. 3.

principles of natural philosophy and the elements, temperaments, humors, members, virtues, and spirits, but also the rest of medicine: the dispositions of the body and their causes and signs, the conservation of health, and the alteration of bodily dispositions. In his opinion, therefore, Book 1 as a whole could supply the need for such a textbook of Galenic medicine, but not *Canon* 1.1 alone.[72]

Da Monte thought the separation between *theoria* and *practica* found in *Canon* 1.1 utterly wrong. Such a separation was, to his mind, an "Arab" innovation that had no precedent among Greek authorities and no counterpart in the real world of medical activity.[73] He likened the assertion that theory is separate from practice because someone who has studied the theory of temperaments does not necessarily know how to treat the sick to the statement that because a child who knows the elements of [Latin] grammar cannot necessarily speak grammatically, the elements are not part of grammar. The child learns the principles in order to be able to apply them later, and so does the medical student.[74]

---

[72] "Nam ubi medicus didicit totum artificium medendi in prima, secunda, tertia, et quarta fen, nihil aliud ipsi deest, quam ut dirigat studia sua ad opus in rebus particularibus quod divinus noster Avicenna fecit; nam ubi artificium in prima, secunda, tertia et quarta fen docuit, aggreditur tertium librum, ubi docet methodum illum universalem applicare particularibus." Ibid., pp. 8–9.

[73] Da Monte, comm. *Canon* 1.1 (Venice, 1554), fols. 8ᵛ–12ʳ. At fol. 10ᵛ: "Re vera quod haec sententia, quod medicina sit partim theorica, partim practica, est vulgata apud Arabes, et tuentur eam hac ratione qua movetur Avicenna, sed nullum Graecorum inveni qui ita diviserit medicinam in partem theoricam et practicam." This was not a new observation. Compare: "Iam autem intellexerunt quidam ex antiquis magistris de Salerno quod Galenus per hoc dictum suum innueret divisionem medicine in theoricam et practicam quam nequaquam invenimus haberi in aliquo librorum suorum qui usque hodie ad latinam linguam exiverint." Turisanus, *Plusquam commentum* 1.10 (Venice, 1512), fol. 9ʳ. Turisanus (Torrigiano), however, approved of the division and of Avicenna's role in disseminating it. According to Ludwig Englert, *Untersuchungen zu Galens Schrift Thrasybulos, Studien zur Geschichte der Medizin*, ed. Karl Sudhoff and Henry E. Sigerist, vol. 18 (Leipzig, 1929), p. 23, the origins of the division are probably Hellenistic.

[74] "Sed praeter authoritates Graecorum est ipsa ratio, et nescio quomodo tanti viri sint decepti, et praesertim Avicenna, qui dicitur etiam vir ingeniosissimus a suis adversariis . . . quaero a te [Avicenna] nunquid medicus quando ista principia considerat an absolute an respective considerat secundum rationem formalem subiecti? . . . nulla pars medicinae est theorica eo modo quo ipse intelligit, nam illud argumentum Avicennae quando dicit siquis novit elementa corporis et temperaturas, nescit tamen propterea operari et medicari, ideo non facit hoc ad operationem, vanissimum est; istud est similiter ac si quis dicat puer sciens elementa grammaticae nescit propterea loqui grammaticae, ideo elementa non sunt pars grammaticae, videtis quam hoc sit vanum, licet enim nesciat propterea puer loqui grammaticae, vanum tamen est dicere quod scire principia et temperaturas et ea quae multum remota sunt est pars theorica, pars autem quae est magis propinqua operationi est practica. . . . Dico igitur quod sententia Graecorum est magis

Da Monte's program for making use of *Canon* 1 thus involved employing the work to give beginning students a firm grasp of the scope of the various parts of medicine, of appropriate methodology, and of scientific and therapeutic principles, which they would subsequently see in operation and learn to apply for themselves as they moved through the more advanced part of their studies, and considered actual cases. In the interest of adapting *Canon* 1 to these goals, Da Monte was willing to modify it fairly drastically, as is shown by his advocacy of elimination of repetition from section to section,[75] by his rejection of Avicenna's opinions on various topics, and by his use of the framework of *Canon* 1.2 chiefly as the vehicle for attacks on scholastic medical authors and the expression of his own opinions rather than for the exposition of Avicenna (see Chapter 6).

Da Monte's endeavor to use *Canon* 1 as a unified introductory medical textbook may be related to the revival of the ancient fivefold division of medicine into physiology, pathology, semiotics, hygiene, and therapy. This scheme (which does, in fact, outline the content of *Canon* 1) was available through various texts translated into Latin during the Middle Ages, but apparently seldom used by fourteenth- and fifteenth-century scholastic physicians, who preferred the division into *theoria* and *practica*.[76] The replacement of the division into *theoria* and *practica* by the fivefold scheme and of teaching by commentary by direct exposition of the subject led ultimately to the production of textbooks of the variety known as "the institutes of medicine," of which Boerhaave's is the best known. Perhaps Da Monte's set of commentaries may be regarded as representing a very early stage in this process.[77]

---

docta, et magis secundum essentiam medicinae." Da Monte, comm. *Canon* 1.1 (Venice, 1554), fol. 11^r-v.

75 Ibid., fol. 14^r.

76 The fivefold scheme is found in the pseudo-Galenic *Introductio, seu medicus* (Kühn, 14:689–95). This work was translated into Latin by Niccolò da Reggio in the early fourteenth century and included in three editions of Galen's *Opera* in Latin published between 1490 and 1528. A new translation by Guinter of Andernach was included in all twelve collected editions of Galen's works published between 1541–42 and the end of the century. See Durling, "Census," p. 293, no. 134, and entries cited there. The fivefold division is also found in the commentary on *De sectis* translated into Latin in the early Middle Ages and again in the twelfth century by Burgundio of Pisa; see *Iohannis Alexandrini Commentaria in librum De sectis Galeni*, ed. C. D. Pritchet (Leiden, 1982), pp. vi–viii, 11–12. On the origins of the division, see Englert, *Untersuchungen*, p. 22.

77 Herman Boerhaave, *Institutiones medicae* (Leiden, 1707), is divided into sections on physiology, pathology, symptomology, hygiene, and therapy. According to G. A. Lindeboom, Boerhaave explained the phrase "institutiones medicae" to mean "the general aspects of theoretical medicine as well as the general precepts of practical medicine. On the basis of physiology the Institutes give general points of view on pathology, symp-

It is indeed possible that Da Monte's handling of *Canon* 1.1 was, at least in part, inspired by his reaction to a new and potentially rival general textbook, namely the *Physiologia* of Jean Fernel, first published in 1542. In general subject matter and arrangement, the *Physiologia* approximately parallels *Canon* 1.1, although with significant alterations: Fernel put anatomy first, and introduced a separate section on innate heat. Although Fernel's teaching can be described as generally Galenic, his idiosyncratic views on certain medical subjects long made him a symbol of neotericism in medicine.[78] Johannes Crato of Krafftheim, a pupil of Da Monte, has left an account of the rapid reception of Fernel's work at Padua, of Da Monte's interest in it, and of the eager pronouncement by Bassiano Landi that Fernel had superseded Avicenna. Yet Fernel's unorthodoxy was sufficient to make his work unacceptable to some Galenists. Da Monte may have wished to show that lectures on *Canon* 1 could be made to serve the purpose of providing teaching that was as unified and up-to-date as that of the *Physiologia*, and more authentically Galenic. Da Monte's ideas about the need to provide comprehensive and unified introductory medical teaching were carried a stage further after his death—and disseminated in northern Europe—by Crato. In 1587 there appeared at Frankfurt a work said to be by Da Monte and entitled *Universa medicina*. In this, Martin Weindrich, acting on Crato's suggestion, wove together excerpts from Da

---

tomology and therapy, which are to apply later to individual cases. So the term theoretical medicine, sometimes used for the Institutes, is less exact. Apparently the Institutes consisted of a course that formed an introduction to clinical medicine." *Herman Boerhaave: The Man and His Work* (London, [1968]), p. 58. A similar fivefold division, and title, had, however, been adopted much earlier by Daniel Sennert, in his *Institutionum Medicinae libri V* (Wittenberg, [1632]). Lester S. King, *The Road to Medical Enlightenment, 1650–1695* (London and New York, 1970), pp. 16, 181–83, provides other seventeenth-century examples of the concept and similar titles. Guinter (and Vesalius revising him) had, of course, used the title *Institutiones* in the 1530s, but for a work on anatomy, not general medicine.

There is little doubt that Da Monte thought of his commentaries on *Canon* 1 as a set. He lectured on *Canon* 1.2 immediately after *Canon* 1.1, referring on p. 1 of the former to his lectures "anno elapso." He had already expounded *Canon* 1.2, when he wrote on *Canon* 1.4: "Sed his latius egimus exponentes secundam partem primi libri Avicennae, ubi etiam de contagio abunde disseruimus," Da Monte, comm. *Canon* 1.4 (Venice, 1556), fol. 51ʳ. Vivian Nutton, "Montanus, Vesalius and the Haemorrhoidal Veins," *Clio medica* 18 (1983), 36, dates Da Monte's lectures on *Canon* 1.2 to 1545–46, from which it follows that the lectures on *Canon* 1.1 belong to 1544–45, and those on *Canon* 1.4, probably, to 1546–47. However, the author notes that Crato of Krafftheim believed the lectures on *Canon* 1.2 to have been given in 1548–49.

[78] The *Physiologia* was published in 1542 under the title *De naturali parte medicinae*; it was subsequently incorporated under the title *Physiologia* into Fernel's *Universa medicina* (Paris, 1554).

Monte's works, including his commentaries on the *Canon*, into a continuous narrative. The result is indeed something very like a general textbook of medicine.[79] At Padua, however, Da Monte's approach to the problem of unifying medical teaching left no lasting impression on the curriculum. Later commentators explicitly stated, as Da Monte had not, that *Canon* I as a whole encompassed the five parts of medicine, but *Canon* I.I alone continued to be the subject of lectures on Avicenna in the course on *theoria*. *Canon* I.2 again fell into disuse after Da Monte's death, although, as we shall soon see, it was briefly reintroduced early in the next century. His plea for more use of *Canon* I.4 at Padua appears to have met with little or no response.[80] And by the time the traditional statutory division between *theoria* and *practica* was finally abandoned at Padua in the 1760s, the age in which *Canon* I could be perceived as a viable textbook had long since passed.

Teaching the Canon at Padua, ca. 1550–1620

The international reputation of the University of Padua as a medical school stood high in the second half of the sixteenth and the beginning of the seventeenth century. Padua's renown rested largely upon the an-

---

[79] "Memini cum ante viginti octo annos *Physiologica* Fernelii prodissent et Argenterius sua quoque proferret, Montanum vehementer Fernelii atque adeo omnium conatum in dilucidandis scriptis veterum probasse, et nimio Argenterii reprehendendi morbo, quem ille prodit, graviter offensum esse. Bassianum vero Laudum [sic], virum ingeniosum et philosophicis studiis atque elegantioribus literis in primis politum, quem post meum ex Italia discessum atra dies abstulit, cum forte ad me venisset, et apud me Fernelii libri reperisset, totum cupide domi suae attente perlegisse, mihique illius iudicium exquirenti, hoc respondisse: 'Gallus iste ingenii et doctrinae luce atque ordine nobis Avicennam vel totum obscurabit, vel ut multos illius errores videamus, faciet.' Vere Bassianum iudicasse nec minus Fernelium quam Avicennam de arte medica bene mereri voluisse, monumenta ingenii, voluntatis speculum sunt. Quanto autem illustrius evidentiis omnia in Fernelio quam Avicenna appareant, qui non perspicit, ille sua quadam persuasione caecus est." Prefatory letter by Crato of Krafftheim in *Jo. Fernelii Ambiani Universa medicina* (Frankfurt, 1593), fol. a3ᵛ. See also *Medicina universa Johannis Baptistae Montani*, ed. M. Weindrich (Frankfurt, 1587). Crato (1519–85) studied in Italy and subsequently returned to Germany to become an imperial household physician. See R.J.W. Evans, *Rudolf II and His World* (Oxford, 1973), pp. 98–99.

[80] For example, Costeo, comm. *Canon* I.I (Bologna, 1589), p. 2, refers to *Canon* I as encompassing the five parts of medicine. It may be noted that the medieval statute requiring *ordinarii theorici* at Padua to lecture on "totum primum Canonis" was twice reissued in the sixteenth and early seventeenth centuries, although apparently ineffectually. See *Statuta alma universitatis D. artistarum et medicorum patavini gymnasii* (Venice, 1589), fol. 38ʳ, and *Statuta almae universitatis D. D. philosophorum et medicorum cognomento artistarum patavini gymnasii* (Padua, 1607), p. 80.

atomical studies carried on since the time of Vesalius by Realdo Colombo, Gabriele Falloppia, Girolamo Fabrizio d'Acquapendente, and Giulio Casseri. However, Venice and Padua were also important centers for the exchange of botanical and pharmacological information, activity of this kind being fostered both by the academic work of Prospero Alpini and Giacomo Antonio Cortusio and by the position of Venice as a mart of trade in medicinal substances as in so many other goods. Students also welcomed the opportunity to study with such practitioners of contemporary renown as Girolamo Mercuriale and Girolamo Capodivacca, and the ease with which they could gain practical experience of their own. At the same time, in the age of Zabarella and Cremonini the university was still a fairly important center of Aristotelian natural philosophy, a subject of renewed interest to some medical men, among them William Harvey (at Padua 1599–1602). And of course the Venetian and Paduan contacts made by Galileo during his sojourn at Padua (1592–1610) show the presence in those cities of a few intellectuals open to radically innovative scientific approaches.[81]

In medicine Galenism was still the reigning orthodoxy, despite the dissemination of views critical of various aspects of Galen's teaching. Challenges to Galen came from Vesalian anatomists, Paracelsians, modern Aristotelians, followers of Fernel and Argenterio, and various other medical innovators. Nonetheless, the chief effect of the medical humanism of the early sixteenth century had been to reinforce Galen's authority, and that authority still predominated at the century's end.[82]

[81] For an overview of anatomy at Padua in this period, see Ongaro, "La medicina nello Studio di Padova," pp. 89–112. For pharmacy and pharmacology at Padua and Venice, see Richard Palmer, "Pharmacy in the Republic of Venice in the Sixteenth Century," in Wear et al., *Medical Renaissance*, pp. 100–117, 303–12. For student opinion on the value of *practica* at Padua, Bylebyl, "School of Padua," pp. 351–52. On Zabarella, Cremonini, and the relationship between Aristotelian philosophy and the development of science at Padua, see Schmitt, *Aristotle and the Renaissance*, pp. 10–12 and bibliography cited there. Harvey's Aristotelianism is a major theme in Walter Pagel, *William Harvey's Biological Ideas* (Basel, 1958). On Galileo's circle at Padua and Venice, Antonio Favaro, *Galileo Galilei e lo Studio di Padova* (Florence, 1883) contains much detailed information. There is, of course, a bibliography of specialized studies on each of the figures mentioned, as well as a large older literature on Paduan anatomy and Aristotelianism, none of which I make any attempt to list here.

[82] For a general overview of the complex situation and interactions of Galenism and its critics in the period ca. 1540–1630, see Temkin, *Galenism*, pp. 134–73; and for discussion of selected themes, Andrew Wear, "Galen in the Renaissance," in *Galen: Problems and Prospects*, ed. Vivian Nutton (London, 1981), pp. 229–62. The continued dominance of Galenism in the medicine of the later sixteenth century is well brought out in Palmer, *Control of Plague*, pp. 254–66. The beginnings of dissemination of Paracelsan ideas in Italy in the late sixteenth century is traced in Palmer, "Pharmacy," pp. 110–17, and Marco

By that time, it is clear, the statutory public lectures on *theoria* and *practica*, especially those of *theoria*, had come to be widely regarded as providing only a beginner's introduction to even the book-learned parts of medicine, and as requiring much supplementation both by the study of other books and by other forms of instruction (including private lessons) and practical experience. But to the extent that the books assigned for the public lectures on *theoria* and *practica* were Hippocratic and Galenic in their teaching, they were not yet outmoded, and there was unlikely to be much essential conflict between their content, and that of lectures on them, and what was taught in other settings in the *studio*. As the dispute over the Arabs receded into the past, along with the height of the vogue for rhetorical and philological humanism in medicine that had engendered it, it seems to have become increasingly easy to accept the retention of *Canon* 1.1 and other parts of Avicenna's opus.

By about the 1550s, the victory of Galen over the Arabs was in one sense fairly complete: probably few physicians would thereafter have defended Avicenna as an independent authority against Galen. But a good deal of the evidence that had served to dethrone Avicenna as a prince of physicians in his own right could also be interpreted as offering reinforcement for the belief that the *Canon*, apart from its pharmacological sections, contained reasonably accurate summaries of Galenic teaching suitably simplified for student use. Thus, one result of the *querelle des arabes* had been to establish, with a degree of certainty and detail never before realized, the precise extent of Avicenna's dependence upon Galen, while the parallels between the two authors were laid out for all to see in some of the new Latin editions of the *Canon* (see Chapter 5). Furthermore, the attention devoted to the *Canon* by Da Monte, whose commentaries became well known,[83] provided a model of the way in which a Galenist and *modernus* of stature might lecture upon Avicenna without doing violence to his principles, and in itself constituted an endorsement of the continued usefulness of parts of the *Canon* as introductory textbooks. All these developments,

Ferrari, "Alcune vie di diffusione in Italia di idee e di testi di Paracelso," in *Scienze, credenze occulte, livelli di cultura*, Istituto Nazionale di Studi sul Rinascimento (Florence, 1982), pp. 21–29. The hostility of Cremonini to Galen and Galenism is brought out in Charles B. Schmitt, *Cesare Cremonini: Un Aristotelico al tempo di Galilei*, reprinted in his *Aristotelian Tradition*, pp. 3–21 (original pagination), and Bylebyl, "School of Padua," pp. 363–65.

[83] At any rate to later editors of and commentators upon the *Canon*; see, e.g., Cardano, comm. *Canon* 1.1, 1563, in his *Opera* (1663), 9:459, and Capodivacca, *Opera* (Frankfurt, 1603), p. 408.

along with the recognition that the differences separating Galen from some of the *moderni* were of a more radical nature than those between Galen and Avicenna, made it easier to defend the position that Avicenna and Galen were essentially aligned in a common tradition. Occasionally, moreover, the increasing familiarity of the notion that the ancients might in some respects have been superseded seems to have served to bolster claims that the Arabs had added original contributions of their own to the heritage they had received from the Greeks.[84]

This intellectual climate, as well as the vagaries of university politics, help to explain not only the survival of a place for Avicenna in the Paduan curriculum, but also its actual enlargement in the last decade of the sixteenth and first decade of the seventeenth century. Throughout the second half of the century, leading professors at Padua continued to lecture on the *Canon* and to preserve their lectures for publication. *Canon* 4.1 was the subject of surviving lectures given by Trincavella as first ordinary professor of *practica* in 1553, by Alessandro Massaria in the same position between 1587 and 1598, and by Capodivacca as ordinary professor of *practica* in second place in 1579.[85] During his long tenure as first ordinary professor of *theoria* (1563–92), Bernardino Paterno must have lectured on *Canon* 1.1 a number of times; his lectures are unusual in that they survive in three manuscripts as well as in a printed version (see Appendix 2).

Yet despite its presentation by these professors, the *Canon*, and *Canon* 1 in particular, probably played a fairly small part in the total educational experience of most students. As the representatives of the German Nation of arts and medical students remarked in 1596/97, students were drawn to Padua from afar not by lectures on books but by opportunities for practical training.[86] Furthermore, the public lectures on books in the statutory curriculum, which were regularly given (in 1583–84 the two principal professors of *theoria*, Paterno and Albertino

---

[84] Arguments of this kind were used by Giovanni Costeo in one of the prefaces to the Venice, 1564, edition of the *Canon*, and by Andrea Graziolo in the preface to his translation of *Canon* 1.1 (Venice, 1580). See Chapter 5, below.

[85] Trincavella, *Opera*, 3 vols. in 2 (Venice, 1599), 3:1; Massaria, *De febribus* (comm. Canon 4.1), in his *Practica medica* (Trèves, 1607), pp. 314ff.; Capodivacca, comm. *Canon* 4.1, Siena, Biblioteca Comunale, MS C IX 18, a. 1579. The version of Capodivacca's lectures on *Canon* 4.1 printed as *De febribus* in the *Practica* section of his *Opera* (Frankfurt, 1603), has a different preface (pp. 814–19) from that of the Siena manuscript. For Massaria's biography see *Biogr. Lex.* 4:161.

[86] *Atti della Nazione Germanica Artista nello Studio di Padova*, ed. Antonio Favaro, 2 vols. (Venice, 1911–12), Monumenti storici pubblicati dalla R. Deputazione Veneta di Storia Patria, vols. 19 and 20. Serie prima: Documenti, vols. 14 and 15, 2:77–78; the passage is discussed in Bylebyl, "School of Padua," pp. 351–52.

Bottoni, delivered eighty-six ordinary lectures each, and the two principal professors of *practica*, Girolamo Mercuriale and Capodivacca, eighty-four each), were by no means the only teaching by lecture available. There were also some public lectures on special books or topics: for example, in 1577, Paterno lectured on case histories from the Hippocratic *Epidemics*, and Capodivacca on his own "universal method" of curing diseases.[87] In addition, members of the medical faculty (and apparently other physicians and surgeons who did not hold official chairs) frequently conducted private lessons in which they appear to have concentrated on *practica*, taught topical specialties rather than by commentary, and used treatises by Galen or modern works as textbooks if any were needed. By the 1590s, some faculty members were cutting short the length of their public lectures in order to have more time for private precepting, private lessons were being scheduled at times that conflicted with public lectures, and students were neglecting the official public curriculum in favor of the informal study of *practica* and efforts to gain practical experience of their own. An attempt to restore the balance met with student resistance; the ensuing compromise allowed those who had completed the study of philosophy and *theoria* to attend private lessons and visit the sick, a result that must have contributed to the further relegation of *theoria* to the role of an introductory survey.[88]

On the occasions when student opinion on the curriculum made itself felt, it was usually on the side of the expansion of practical training or experience in one way or another. Thus, the members of the German Nation protested the attempt to get students to spend more time listening to public lectures and expended energy and funds in arranging or pressing for the performance of anatomies.[89] However, one cer-

[87] Venice, Biblioteca Correr, MS Dona dalle Rose 212, fols. 41, 42[r-v], report of Antonio Rosato, *bidello degli artisti*, for 1583–84, with list of lectures delivered. The lectures given in 1577 are noted in *Atti*, ed. Favaro, 1:108–9. These, however, were special arrangements made for a plague year. In normal years, professors who were designated *ordinarii* gave some "extraordinary" lectures in addition to their regular series; for example, in 1583–84 Paterno gave twenty-two extraordinary lectures and Mercuriale twelve.

[88] *Atti*, ed. Favaro, 1:77–80; *De gymnasio patavino Antonii Riccoboni commentariorum libri sex* (Padua, 1598), fol. 100[r-v]. Bylebyl, "School of Padua," pp. 351–52 (and for the earlier history of hospital precepting at Padua in the sixteenth century, pp. 348–50). Giulio Casseri, pupil and assistant of Fabrizio d'Acquapendente, conducted private anatomies for which he was paid by the students of the German Nation before he held any public teaching position at Padua; see Gweneth Whitteridge, *William Harvey and the Circulation of the Blood* (London and New York, 1971), pp. 28–29.

[89] See for example, *Atti*, ed. Favaro, 1:165, 210–11.

tainly cannot infer any general repudiation on the part of students of a bookish or scholastic approach to medicine, of teaching by commentary, or of the Arabs and their older interpreters.

Student patterns of book ownership can be reconstructed to some extent from the lists of books accumulated by the German Nation between 1586 and 1636 as the result of a regulation requiring members to donate to the Nation books that they would otherwise have sold upon graduation;[90] in addition, the Nation purchased some books on its own account, doubtless with the needs of its members in mind. By definition, the donated books were books that were no longer needed by newly fledged physicians; nonetheless, the spread of material is wide enough to lay to rest the supposition that particularly unwanted categories were being dumped on the Nation in disproportionate amounts. As one might expect, most of the medical books given to or bought by the Nation in this fifty-year period were either modern medical treatises (Fernel and Sennert being especially favored authors) or translations or editions of Greek medical classics. Yet the modern works included large numbers of commentaries, most on Greek medical works, but some on Avicenna and Rasis. In addition, there was significant representation of editions of the text of works of Arabic origin and of thirteenth- to fifteenth-century Latin scholastic medicine. As well as at least six copies of the complete *Canon* (three of which appear to have been large, and doubtless expensive, folio editions) and four of *Canon* 1.1, the Nation owned copies of the commentaries on *Canon* 1.1 by Da Monte (three copies), Oddo Oddi (three copies), Paterno, and Santorio; of Da Monte on *Canon* 1.2; and as part of larger collections of their works, of Trincavella (two copies) and Capodivacca (nine copies) on *Canon* 4.1. Medieval and early Renaissance authors represented included Arnald of Villanova, Bernard of Gordon, Torrigiano, Tommaso del Garbo, Giacomo da Forlì, and Michele Savonarola (there were at least six copies of Savonarola's *Practica*). In 1605, a single graduate presented the Nation with copies of the *Chirurgia* of Gui de Chauliac, one of Dino del Garbo's commentaries on the *Canon*, and Ugo Benzi's commentaries on the *Ars* and *Canon* 1.1, a gift suggesting that this student, at least, was more conservative than his preceptors.[91] In

---

[90] Ibid., p. 219 (1586). Thereafter donations of books were recorded annually; the books mentioned in this paragraph were culled from the lengthy lists that recur for each year in *Atti*, ed. Favaro, vol. 2 (for the years 1591–1615), and *Acta Nationis Germanicae Artistarum (1616–1636)*, ed. Lucia Rossetti (Padua, 1967). For an account of the Nation's library as a whole, see Lucia Rossetti, "Le biblioteche delle 'Nationes' nello Studio di Padova," *Quaderni per la storia dell'Università di Padova* 2 (1969), 53–67.

[91] *Atti*, ed. Favaro, 2:234.

1633 the largest amount expended for any single book purchase by the Nation itself went for the acquisition of "veteres Avicennae interpretes" in four volumes; and in 1635 the Nation bought a copy of the commentaries on the Hippocratic *Aphorisms* and *Prognostics* by Taddeo Alderotti.[92]

Further evidence that the Paduan attachment to teaching from Avicenna, already noted as idiosyncratic as early as the 1550s,[93] was not necessarily thereafter regarded with disfavor, even by a scholar whose ideas about medicine had first been formed north of the Alps, comes from a letter of Peter Monau written in 1576. Monau, a member of the circle of Crato of Krafftheim and like him keenly interested in every aspect of the contemporary medical scene, studied at Padua for a number of years in the 1570s and 1580s.[94] Writing to Crato, Monau remarked on the predilection in the Italian schools for teaching from the Arabs instead of "sweating over the books of the Greeks," as he himself had been wont to do. He added that he thought it showed poor judgment to reject the Arabs out of hand, since, despite their numerous errors, they had also contributed many things that the Greeks had omitted; and he reported that someone had told him that this was especially the case in the nomenclature of purgative and exotic drugs.[95] The comment occurs in a letter that is principally devoted to a detailed account of a dissection in which Fabrizio promised to provide ocular demonstration of the pores in the septum of the heart mentioned by Galen. Monau's comment about Avicenna's pharmacology therefore belongs in a context of which the most current anatomical findings and controversy were also part.

[92] *Acta*, ed. Rossetti, pp. 344, 370. The collection of older commentators on Avicenna may have been the edition of the *Canon* with commentaries published in Venice, 1523, although this was complete in five volumes, not four.

[93] "De more autem huius gymnasii Avicennam sequemur: ita enim olim per omnia gymnasia institutum erat." Trincavella, comm. *Canon* 4.1 (Padua, 1553), in his *Opera* (Venice, 1599), 3:1.

[94] On Monau, see Evans, *Rudolf II*, p. 203.

[95] *Johannis Cratonis . . . Consiliorum et epistolarum medicinalium liber sextus* (Frankfurt, 1671) (includes bk. 5), bk. 5, 345: "Arabum doctrinam ex veteri instituto in scholis Italicis proponi facile assentior. Mihi in Graecorum libris aliquandiu desudandum proposui. In his si quid assecutus fuero, forte ad alteros illos divertere non fuerit supervacaneum, quorum quidem universa dogmata, ut Fuchsius saepissime inculcat, uno quasi impetu rejicere minime consultum arbitror. Ut enim maxime in quibusdam aberrent, et minus feliciter in alienam linguam translati sint, quia tamen multa utilia, a Graecis praetermissa, ipsi in medium adferant, nemo negare potest. Et audivi judicium cuiusdam, qui affirmabat propter purgantium nomenclaturam, et exotericorum quorundam pharmacorum descriptionem, quorum nunc frequens admodum usus plurimi a nobis Arabes merito faciendos esse." I am grateful to Vivian Nutton for drawing my attention to this passage.

Hence, proposed or actual changes in the amount of time devoted by professors at Padua to public lectures on portions of the *Canon*, of which there were several between 1579 and 1602, were not, in the main, introduced because of controversies over the wisdom of teaching from Avicenna. Instead, the principal issues had to do with the need for coverage of particular kinds of medical subject matter, the proper balance between *theoria* and *practica* and between public and private instruction, scheduling problems, university finances, conflicts between the interests of the various groups affected—professors and the Paduan College of Philosophers and Physicians, the student university and the nations, the Riformatori dello Studio and the Venetian Senate—and competition for jobs between individuals. Nonetheless, these episodes are revealing of the current situation of the *Canon*.

After 1560, when the student universities lost the last vestige of their ancient right to elect professors, the power to appoint to all professorial positions, from the most junior to the most senior, as well as to erect or abolish chairs, lay in the hands of the Venetian government. This power was not exercised arbitrarily, however. From time to time, the Riformatori dello Studio, acting on behalf of the Venetian Senate, tried to trim the budget and to recruit distinguished teachers from other universities for senior positions (from which Paduans were excluded); but on many issues the Riformatori seem on the whole to have been quite responsive to representations from various interest groups within the *studio* and to have attempted to balance their respective needs.

A glimpse of how the process worked can be gained from the succession to the first ordinary professorship in *practica* in 1587. By that time, this chair was probably the most desirable position in the entire *studio*. In principle, the first ordinary chair in *theoria* ranked higher, but by around 1580 the salaries of the two professors—significantly larger than those of any of their other colleagues in arts and medicine—were equal.[96] Moreover, there can be little doubt that student demand for training that would prove directly useful in the exercise of the medical profession strengthened the position, reputation, and probably the income from private teaching of the professor of *practica* vis-à-vis his colleague in *theoria*. Hence, when Girolamo Mercuriale left the chair in *practica*, Bernardino Paterno, then holder of the first ordinary chair in *theoria*, sought to transfer to the vacant position. The Paduan officials known as moderators of the *studio* were apparently willing to gratify an

---

[96] Antonio Favaro, "Informazione storica sullo Studio di Padova circa l'anno 1580," *Nuovo archivio veneto*, n.s. 30 (1915), pt. 1, pp. 255, 258. On the relationship of the Venetian Senate and the *studio*, see Bylebyl, "School of Padua," pp. 343–45.

influential senior faculty member without much regard to the academic consequences, and recommended Paterno's appointment, with the proviso that Massaria should succeed Paterno in the position in *theoria*. When this recommendation reached the Venetian Senate, however, objections were raised on the grounds that almost all Paterno's teaching experience had been in *theoria*, whereas Massaria was experienced in both branches of medicine. As a result, and apparently with Paterno's agreement, Massaria got the position in *practica*, and Paterno retained the chair in *theoria* with an increase in salary. (In 1598, however, Massaria was earning more than Paterno's successor.)[97] This mutually satisfactory arrangement left Capodivacca, who also held an ordinary chair in *practica* and had hoped to succeed to the senior position, profoundly disgruntled. Since at least 1560, Capodivacca had been closely involved with the German Nation, whose friendship he carefully cultivated. Now, he orchestrated a student protest on his own behalf by refusing to lecture unless he got the first ordinary position in *practica* or unless the position of *supraordinarius* in *practica* was created for him. The Nation dutifully sent an emissary to Venice, but to no avail.[98] Perhaps the Venetians remembered the disastrous episode of 1576 when Capodivacca was one of a team of professors who denied the existence of one of the worst plague outbreaks of the century.[99] Subsequently, the special relationship with the Nation was inherited by Capodivacca's nephew Annibale Bimbiolo, whom the Nation staunchly, but fruitlessly, supported in the equally keen competition for succession to Capodivacca's own chair following the latter's death in 1589.[100]

In the 1560s and 1570s, those curricular changes at Padua that affected the teaching of the *Canon* all resulted in a decrease in the number of public lectures on that book. Thus a decree of 1579, designed as an economy measure, reduced the number of extraordinary chairs in medical *theoria* and *practica* from three to two each. The same decree formally abolished two positions especially assigned for the teaching of *Canon* 3 (parts of the body and their diseases). These two minor chairs in *practica*, carrying an insignificant salary for lecturers on holidays, were the last medical teaching positions to which the students retained

[97] Riccobono, *De gymnasio patavino*, fols. 69ᵛ–70ᵛ, 147ʳ⁻ᵛ. The story that Paterno himself endorsed Massaria, comes from Bernardino Gaio's preface to his edition of Paterno, comm. *Canon* 1.1 (Venice, 1596), fol. 3ᵛ; the edition is dedicated to Massaria.

[98] *Atti*, ed. Favaro, 1:33–34, 40–41, 44, 242–43. As a Paduan citizen, Capodivacca was ineligible for the first position (although he had taught *in concorrenza* with Mercuriale); doubtless he hoped an exception would be made in his case.

[99] See Palmer, *Control of Plague*, pp. 242–54.

[100] *Atti*, ed. Favaro, 1:272, 276, 290.

the right of election, and had seldom been occupied since that right was removed in 1560.[101]

The trend toward reduction in the number of chairs was, however, reversed in 1591. In that year, a dogal decree reintroduced one lectureship on *Canon* 3, with the explanation that experience had shown that the chair "of 3 Avicenna is very useful and necessary for the practice of medicine, which is the end and perfection of that science," and that the small sum of money saved by the abolition of the chair was not worth the damage done to the curriculum.[102] The appointment of a second lecturer on *Canon* 3 followed in 1598;[103] and in the following year the salary of Antonio Negro, holder of the first chair, was raised to 80 fiorini, quadruple the amount he had been allotted in 1591 (the increase still left him near the bottom of the scale).[104] From 1602, when, as we shall see, Negro was promoted to another position, there was only one lectureship on *Canon* 3. Given the content of that book, it was inevitable that lectures on it would cover some of the same subject matter as those parts of the regular three-year cycle in *practica* that dealt with diseases from the head down to the heart, and the heart down to the feet. However, Andrighetto Andrighetti, who lectured on *Canon* 3 throughout the first decade of the seventeenth century, did not attempt to expound the whole book in any one year. Instead, he taught on selected special topics, presumably using sections of *Canon* 3 as his text— skin diseases in 1603–1604, diseases of the eye in 1604–1605.[105] Andrighetti's decision to limit his subject matter doubtless enabled him to treat the chosen topics in more detail than there was time for in the other public lectures on *practica*. Perhaps as a result, his lectures were in sufficient demand to appear a threat to his colleagues; such at any rate seems to be the inference from the official warning given him in 1608 against lecturing in the morning hours and encroaching on the material assigned to other professors.[106]

[101] Bertolaso, "Ricerche d'Archivio" (1959–60), pp. 32–33; Riccobono, *Gymnasio patavino*, fol. 78ᵛ; AAUP 507, "Decreto del Senato 1579, per levar molte cattedre superflue" (eighteenth-century copy). The number of extraordinary chairs seems subsequently to have gone back from time to time to three each in *theoria* and *practica*.

[102] AAUP 669, fol. 237ʳ, copy of dogal decree of May 6, 1591: "vedendosi per esperienza che fra tutte le altre [that is, chairs that had earlier been abolished] quella del 3° d'Avicenna e molto utile et necessaria per la practica di medicina, che e fine et perfettione di quella scienza."

[103] Ibid., fol. 233ᵛ, 14 October 1594.

[104] Ibid., 28 October 1599.

[105] Bertolaso, "Ricerche d'archivio" (1959–60), p. 33. Andrighetti, or Aldreghetti, d. 1631; see Papadopoli, *Historia Gymnasii Patavini*, 1:357.

[106] ASV, Riformatori dello Studio di Padova, *busta* 419, Rectors to Riformatori, 9 November 1608.

A larger change in the place of Avicenna in the curriculum than the restoration of the minor lectureships on *Canon* 3 was proposed in 1600. In that year, Orazio Augenio, Paterno's successor as first ordinary professor of *theoria*, petitioned the Riformatori for the reestablishment of public lectures on *Canon* 1.2.[107] Augenio pointed out that such lectures were required by the university statutes and had been given by the "ancients" Giacomo da Forlì and Ugo Benzi and, most recently, by Da Monte, as could be seen from the latter's commentary. The neglect of *Canon* 1.2 was, in Augenio's view, much more serious than that of *Canon* 1.3 and 1.4, which were also prescribed by statute: *Canon* 1.3 (regimen) could be omitted with little harm, and the *theorici* covered essentially the same subject matter as *Canon* 1.4 (principles of therapy) when they lectured on Book 3 of the *Ars*. But the failure, since Da Monte's time, to lecture on *Canon* 1.2 had done great damage, since this part of the work dealt with subjects—diseases, symptoms, and their causes, and diagnosis by pulse and urine—of such importance that no one should call himself a medical doctor who had not studied them.[108]

Augenio apparently took it for granted that revived lectures on *Canon* 1.2 would take their historic and statutory place as part of the curriculum in *theoria*; indeed, his motivation in proposing the change was probably at least in part to restore *theoria* to some of its former importance. But the subject matter of *Canon* 1.2 was of interest not only to teachers of *theoria*. Moreover, to propose the introduction of what was in effect a major new course into the core of the curriculum was necessarily to raise questions of scheduling and curricular balance. Accordingly, the first response of the Riformatori to Augenio's petition was to instruct the rectors of the university to poll the entire medical faculty for their opinions on the issue and also to respond themselves.[109]

[107] The history of Augenio's request, of the establishment of the chair, and of its subsequent fate is recounted in Bartolo Bertolaso, "La cattedra 'De pulsibus et urinis' (1601–1748) nello Studio Padovano," *Castalia: Rivista di storia di medicina* 16 (1960), 109–17, based chiefly on documents in AAUP 651, 667, 669. In addition, a collection of letters conveying to the Riformatori faculty opinions about the proposed chair survives in ASV, Riformatori dello Studio di Padova, *busta* 419. I am deeply grateful to Richard Palmer for drawing my attention to the latter collection, on which the following discussion is based.

[108] ASV Riformatori 419, letter from Orazio Augenio, no date. On Augenio, *DBI* (Rome, 1962), 4:577–78.

[109] In an undated covering letter the rectors informed the Riformatori that replies from all the doctors teaching in the studio had been obtained, with the exception of Niccolò Trivisano, who was away, and Giovanni Pietro Pellegrino, who was ill. Most of the letters are undated; however, one from the rectors giving their own opinion on the issue is dated 3 April 1600. According to the *rotulus* for 1599–1600, edited in Antonio Favaro,

The replies collected reveal something of the complexity of the re-lationship between the official curriculum of public lectures and the in-formal and unregulated aspects of Paduan medical teaching. Professors and rectors were unanimous in endorsing the importance of the pro-posed subject matter: not surprisingly, none of them could conceive of a medical education that did not involve the study of pathology and se-miotics. But they were also in general agreement that these subjects were in fact already being taught, normally in private lessons, but oc-casionally in public lectures offered at will by members of the faculty on holidays when regular lectures were not scheduled. Of the profes-sors of *practica* who responded, three (including both the *ordinarii*)—Er-cole Sassonia, Eustachio Rudio, and Giovanni Tommaso Minadoi[110]—took pains to emphasize that they gave such instruction to their private pupils. The question to which the respondents addressed themselves, therefore, was not whether the students should be introduced to hith-erto neglected material, but whether it would be desirable to substitute public lectures on an officially prescribed text for more informal kinds of instruction. On this issue, they were divided. Of the thirteen faculty members who responded, eight favored and five opposed the institu-tion of a new chair, although this simple classification does not do jus-

---

Galileo Galilei a Padova: Ricerche e scoperte, insegnamento scolari, Contributi alla Storia dell'Università di Padova (Padua, 1968), 5:109–11, the medical faculty then consisted of: theory, ordinary, in first place: Orazio Augenio; theory, ordinary, in second place: Emi-lio Campilongo; practica, ordinary, *in paritate*: Ercole Sassonia and Eustachio Rudio; anatomy and surgery: Girolamo Fabrizio d'Acquapendente; theory, extraordinary, in first place: Annibale Bimbiolo; theory, extraordinary, in second place: Niccolò Trivi-sano; *practica*, extraordinary, in first place: Tommaso Minadoi; *practica*, extraordinary, in second place: Alessandro Vigonza; *practica*, extraordinary, in third place: Pietro Pelle-grino; lecture on Book 3 of Avicenna, in first place: Antonio Negro; lecture on Book 3 of Avicenna, *in concorrentia*: Andrighetto Andrighetti; lecture on simples: Prospero Al-pini; demonstration in the botanic garden: Giacomo Antonio Cortusio. ASV Riforma-tori 419 contains signed responses from all of the above except Trivisano, Pellegrino, Fa-brizio, and Cortusio; however, there are two unsigned letters that presumably can be ascribed to the two last named. There is also a letter from Tarquinio Carpenedo, whose name appears as third extraordinary professor of theory in a copy of the original printed *rotulus* for 1603–1604 in Biblioteca Correr, MS Dona dalle Rose 212, 122.

[110] On the life and writings of Sassonia (1551–1607), see *Biogr. Lex.* 5:182; Rudio (d. 1611), ibid., 111; Minadoi (d. 1615), ibid., 4:245. Minadoi had some interest in Near Eastern culture; he came from Rhodes and served the Venetian consulate in the Levant, and is best remembered as the author of a *Historia della guerra fra Turchi et Persiani . . . cominciando dall'anno MDLXXVII* (Rome, 1687; there are other early editions). The front matter of this volume includes a two-page vocabulary of Turkish, Arabic, and Persian words. According to Charles Patin, *De Avicenna oratio habita in Archi-Lycaeo Patavino di X Nov. 1676* (Padua, 1678), p. 28, Minadoi was the author of an oration on Avicenna, but I have been unable to find a copy.

tice to their academic ingenuity in devising a range of variant schemes.[111] Yet their replies show that they all took it for granted that public and private teaching would continue to exist side by side and that both offered complementary advantages.

One objection to the establishment of a new ordinary chair or to the insertion of additional material to be covered within existing regular public lectures, whether in *theoria* or *practica*, was that either action was likely to involve the expansion of the cycle of lectures from three years to four, thus imposing upon the students a delay in achieving professional qualification and an additional financial burden. Another, as just noted, was that material on diseases and symptoms was already adequately covered in private lessons or holiday teaching. Those who found private teaching insufficient did not cast aspersions on its quality. Instead, they stressed the advantage of regular scheduling offered by public lectures, and pointed out that private teaching did not afford sufficient time to cover the material completely and did not reach all students. Thus, Sassonia remarked that knowledge of the subjects in question was as essential a tool for the physician as logic for the philosopher, so that they should be taught every year; Tarquinio Carpenedo, from the lowly position of third extraordinary professor of *theoria*, emphasized the importance of reaching beginners, which could only be done by instituting public lectures. Other respondents noted, however, that some instruction on these topics was already being given in the existing public lectures. Prospero Alpini, professor of simples, remarked that the subject of urines was treated by *theorici* in lecturing on the *Aphorisms* and by *practici* in lecturing on fevers (that is, *Canon* 4.1). Alpini added, justifiably, that written works based on the public lectures at Padua of distinguished members of the medical faculty—Da Monte, Trincavella, Mercuriale—showed that they had not neglected diseases, their causes and symptoms, and pulse and urine.[112] Eustachio Rudio similarly held that all good *practici* had always taught these sub-

---

[111] Those opposed were Campilongo, Rudio, Minadoi, Vigonza, and Alpini.

[112] "Etenim theorici, quum aphorismos Hippocratis interpretantur saepius de urinis et aliis excrementis agere coguntur. . . . Practici cum de febribus agunt coguntur itidem ad ipsarum notitiam illustrandam disserere de pulsibus ac de excrementis. . . . Non minus quoque, qui particulares morbos tractant, ad ipsorum accuratam dignotionem coguntur docere morborum symptomatumque omnium cum differentias, tum causas. Montani Veronensis olim in hoc gymnasio professoris extant lectiones impressae olim studiosis medicinae publicatae, de pulsibus et urinis, et aliis excrementis, de symptomatibus, de morbis, et de causis. Trincavellius in lectionibus de febribus de pulsibus atque urinis accuratissime egit. Mercurialis de iisdem accuratissimos tractatus habuit. Alii itidem plures idem fecerunt." ASV Riformatori 419, Prospero Alpini. Alpini was the only respondent to write in Latin. On Alpini, a leading Renaissance botanist, see *DBI* 2:529–31.

jects, presumably in both their public and private capacities.[113] Alessandro Vigonza, second extraordinary professor of *practica*, pointed out that not only the writings of the faculty but also Padua's record of production of distinguished physicians were evidence that the present system of public, as well as private, instruction assured adequate attention to this branch of training.[114]

One possible implication of Augenio's proposal was that material that was being taught, privately and to some extent publicly, by professors of *practica* (and which certainly pertained to *practica*) would henceforth either be assigned to *theoria* or to a newly created special lectureship. The academic and economic objections of *practici* to such a possibility (as well as the small esteem in which some of them held their colleagues in *theoria*) were rather frankly expressed by Vigonza with remarks to the effect that if what was wanted was a few general lectures about the importance of studying diseases and so on, then these could be entrusted to the *theorici* as the statute provided and could be easily fitted in without expanding the course of study beyond three years; but the establishment of a new chair for substantial and detailed lectures on these topics would oblige the *practici* to face additional competition without any corresponding advantage to the students.

The rectors, too, showed their determination to keep the material out of the hands of the *theorici*. In forwarding the results of the poll, they declared that the faculty opinions showed that a new lectureship was necessary, which was also their own view; even if the *theorici* did touch on the subjects in question, their teaching was not likely to be very useful in an area that really concerned the treatment of diseases.[115] The rectors added that the new chair should be set up with lectures to be given on the numerous holidays, since at those times the absence of competing lectures by other professors of medicine would free all the

[113] "La dottrina di Galeno dei morbi et symptomi . . . esplicata ad ogni accuratezza dai buoni pratici, li quali parimente nella esposizione delle febri trattano dei polsi et delle orine, sicome si ha sempre osservato dai pratici passati, et hora." ASV Riformatori 419, Eustachio Rudio.

[114] "La esperienza, vera maestra delle cose, ci ha pur mostrato, che nel corso di tanti anni quantunque non e stato in questo studio dottore alcuno destinato a cosi particolar lettura, sono non dimeno quindi usciti medici di nome e di fama celebri in Italia et altrove." ASV Riformatori 419, Alessandro Vigonza.

[115] The Riformatori "vederano la necessita della lettione proposta, cosi conoscevano che si conviene dar questo carico a principal soggetto, et che intende bene le curationi di morbi et che habbia oltre la theorica con la esperienza del medicar dato honorato saggio di se stesso, perche seben li theorici nelle loro lettioni ne dicono alcuna cosa, non la trattano pero ex professo, da che ne nasce il poco frutto che si fa." ASV Riformatori 419, rectors.

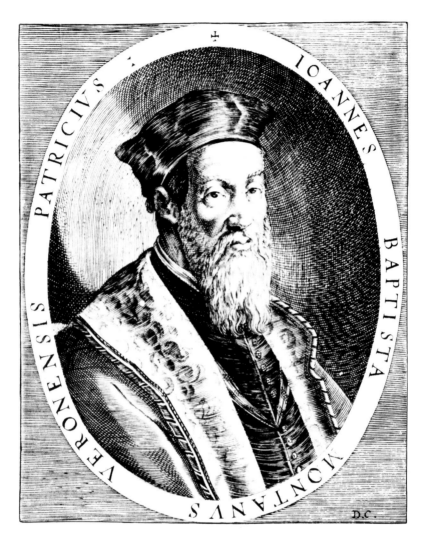

GIAMBATISTA DA MONTE
(Portrait file, New York Academy of Medicine)

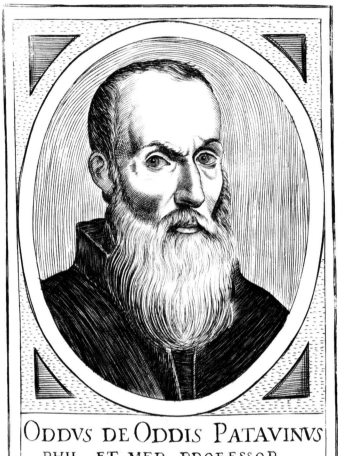

ODDVS DE ODDIS PATAVINVS
PHIL ET MED PROFESSOR

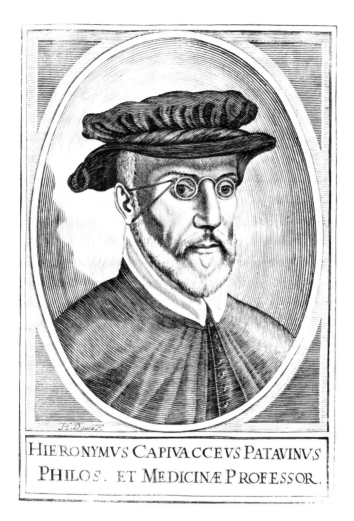

HIERONYMVS CAPIVACCEVS PATAVINVS
PHILOS. ET MEDICINÆ PROFESSOR.

ODDO ODDI (*at left*) and GIROLAMO CAPODIVACCA
as portrayed in J. F. Tomasini, *Illustrium virorum elogia iconibus
exornata* (Padua, 1630) (Special Collections, Columbia University)

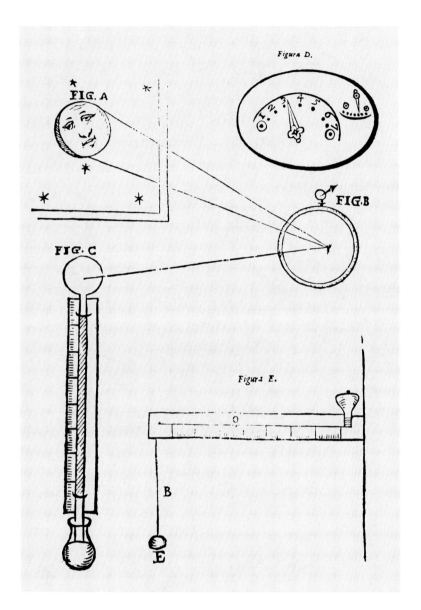

A physical demonstration for Santorio's students. The notion that the earth was affected by celestial heat emanating from all of the heavenly bodies provided a physical basis for much astrological teaching. Without rejecting the concept, Santorio tried to find a way to assess it by measurement. He devised this equipment for a demonstration of the insignificance of any supposed lunar heat when compared with that of the sun (see text and n. 195, p. 289). Illustration from Santorio, comm. *Canon* 1.1 (Venice, 1646), cols. 109–10. (New York Academy of Medicine)

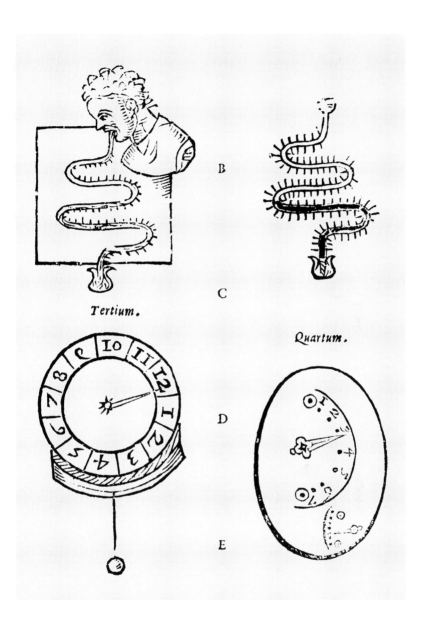

B

C

Tertium.

Quartum.

D

E

Santorio's thermoscopes and pulsilogia, used to estimate
variations in body heat. Illustration from Santorio, comm. *Canon* 1.1
(Venice, 1646), cols. 307–308.
(New York Academy of Medicine)

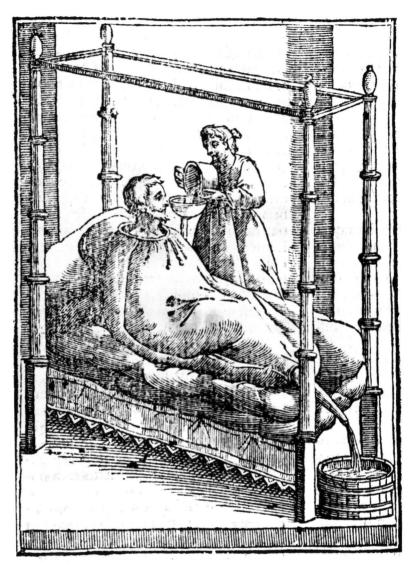

Hydrotherapy by Santorio. Illustration from Santorio,
comm. *Canon* 1.1 (Venice, 1646), col. 567.
(New York Academy of Medicine)

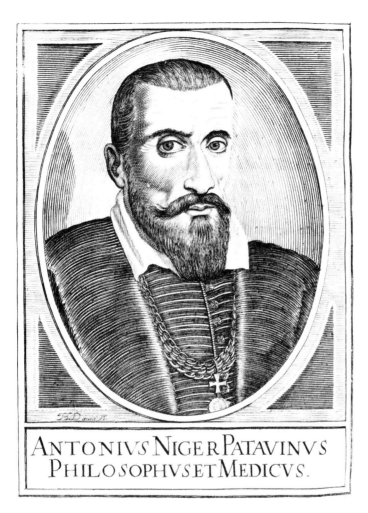

ANTONIVS NIGER PATAVINVS
PHILO SOPHVS ET MEDICVS.

ANTONIO NEGRO, successful candidate
for a new medical chair that called for lectures on the *Canon*
(see Chapter 4), as portrayed in Tomasini's *Elogia*
(Special Collections, Columbia University)

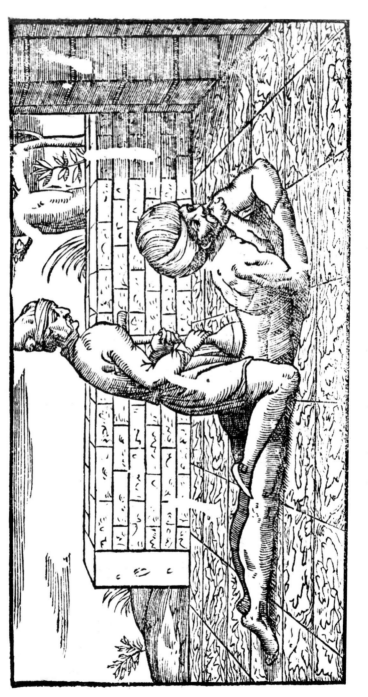

Arab medicine in the eyes of a sixteenth-century illustrator:
one of a set of illustrations used in several successive editions of the *Canon*
(this one from the Venice 1595 edition)
(New York Academy of Medicine)

medical students to attend. Presumably because this letter did not produce the hoped for response, after some months the rectors wrote
again, in stronger terms, pointing out that the reason so many lecturers
were maintained at the public expense was to teach the scholars how to
treat the sick, and complaining that lack of necessary lectures as well as
of professors of name and reputation were damaging the *studio* and
causing students to go elsewhere.[116] Again, they repeated a plea that the
lecturer to be appointed should be someone with a knowledge of practice as well as theory, and went on to recommend Antonio Negro for
the position, describing him as a man of about forty, skilled in *theoria*
and especially outstanding in practice, and well liked by the students.
It will be remembered that Negro was the holder of the senior of the
two recently revived lectureships on *Canon* 3; although the students
had not recovered their earlier right to elect the holders of these chairs,
this recommendation suggests that the student university continued to
consider itself in a special way the patron of these lectureships. Thus,
in the hands of the rectors, the attempt of the elderly Augenio (who
reminisced about having attended Da Monte's lectures on *Canon* 1.2)
to restore an aspect of the traditional curriculum in *theoria* turned into
a campaign to obtain a new chair that would break down the division
between *theoria* and *practica*, and to staff it with a popular young teacher
whose main experience was in *practica*.

Amid all these other considerations there was also the issue of
whether or not the *Canon* constituted an appropriate textbook. It may
be presumed that Rudio's and Alpini's opposition to the proposed new
chair was at least partially inspired by lack of enthusiasm for the *Canon*,
since both of them stressed the importance of studying Galen's books
on diseases, symptoms, and causes. Rudio, indeed, specifically asserted
that Galen's works on these subjects were so clear that they did not require any explanation by lecturers who drew on philosophy. He added
that works of Galen were much more useful and necessary for all parts
of medicine than the *Canon: De temperamentis, De naturalibus facultatibus,* and *De usu partium* for physiology; *De locis affectis* and *De crisibus*
for semiotics; and *Methodus medendi* for therapy. In Rudio's view, the
original compilers of the official curriculum in *theoria* and *practica* had

---

[116] "Perche non peraltro con tanto dispendio publico . . . mantengono tanti lettori, se
non per insegnar alli scolari la cura delle infirmita . . . certe non sappiamo perche lezione
tanta necessaria sia fin' hora stata cosi trascurata, come che all'incontro tante altre ve ne
sono, che gia fu delito, che si levassero come infruttuose, ne e alcun dubbio, che il mancamento delle lettioni necessarie et il mancamento de dottori di nome et riputazione in
questo studio e causa della poca quantita de scolari," ASV Riformatori 419, the rectors,
March 29, 1601.

117

selected *Canon* 1.1 and the other textbooks in order to explain to students two particularly compressed and obscure compendia, and had assumed that anyone who seriously intended to become a good physician would in time read all the works of Galen on his own.[117] Minadoi noted that the proposed lecturers would have to expound everything Galen had written on the subjects, as well as *Canon* 1.2.[118]

Explicit support for the *Canon* was avowed only by Augenio himself and Annibale Bimbiolo, although Vigonza noted his acceptance of it as a text for use by *theorici*. Augenio's conviction that *Canon* 1.2 was a useful textbook treating essential subject matter was not part of any general campaign to enlarge the study of Avicenna; as we have seen, he found no fault with the practice of passing over other sections of Book 1. However, Bimbiolo, by now first extraordinary professor of *theoria*, submitted an elaborate scheme for interweaving the study of works of Galen and Hippocrates pertaining to diseases, symptoms, pulse and urines with that of portions of the *Canon*, all within the space of three years; the teaching of *Canon* 1 was to be expanded in the first year, that of *Canon* 4 in the third, and *Canon* 5 (compound medicines) was to be introduced in the second. Thus, Bimbiolo concluded triumphantly, all the medicine, both theoretical and practical, of all the authors and all five books of the *Canon* would be expounded in the *studio* every year.[119]

---

[117] "Questi libri di Galeno, nei quali egli tratta queste materie tutte sono tanto chiari et aperti che no han bisogna di espositione appresso quelli chi cossegono la philosophia . . . se si volesse explicare tutti li libri di Galeno appartenenti ad un buon medico ve ne sono di molto piu utili, et necessarii alla medicina, come sono nella parte physiologica li tre libri *De temperamentis*, li tre *De facultatibus naturalibus*, et quasi divinissimi diciasette libri *De usu partium*. Nella parte symiotica praestantissimi i sei libri *De locis affectis* et li tre *De crisibus*, et nella parte curatrice quei mirabilissima et necessariissima quatordici libri *De methodo medendi*. Et tutti questi sono piu necessarii et piu difficili delli proposti per la nuova letura. Non dimeno si nostri maggiori in cio prudentissimi et occultatissimi, per non dar longa noia et incommodita alli poveri scolari, s'hanno contentati di far esplicar pubblicamente alli theorici solo li *Aphorismi*, come oscurissimi, et *l'Ars parva* di Galeno, et la prima fen del primo libro d'Avicenna, come dei libri compendiosi brevissimi et oscuri, et alli pratici li morbi particolari et le febri, penssando ch' chi desidera di farsi perfetto medico possa da per se veder col tempo tutti li scritti di Galeno," ASV Riformatori 419, Eustachio Rudio.

[118] ". . . con assidua diligenza tutto quello che da Galeno in diverse sue opere, et da Avicenna nel primo libro nella fen 2," ASV Riformatori 419, Gio. Tommaso Minadoi.

[119] "Il primo anno li libri di Galeno, *De differentiis* et *causis morborum*, et *symptomatum*, non partendosi ponte da quello che scrive Avicena [*sic*] nella prima fen del primo libro, nella quarta dottrina.

"Il secondo anno il quinto libro di Avicenna, nel qual tratta de medicamentis compositis, et arte compendorum medicamentorum; et appresso qualche altro trattato, de arte consultandi, o simile.

"Il terzo anno De urinis et pulsibus, De venenis, et De decoratione, non partendosi

In a separate letter, Bimbiolo put in a plea for the job, if a new ordinary professorship of pulse and urines was set up; he hoped to hold it in conjunction with his present position in *theoria* and stressed his experience in both branches of medicine (adding the inevitable allusion to his relationship to the late Capodivacca).[120] For the remainder of the respondents, including the rectors, the issue of the *Canon* as a textbook was not sufficiently controversial to be worth mentioning. Doubtless they took it for granted that the *Canon* would have a place, but also that it would need to be extensively supplemented by direct study of works of Galen, by personal instruction from experienced practitioners, and by more or less supervised contact with patients.

The Riformatori eventually resolved the issue by recommending the institution of a new chair, which was formally set up in 1601. The subject matter to be covered was diseases and their causes and symptoms, and diagnosis by pulse and urine, all of which was to be treated within a single academic year. *Canon* 1.2 was officially prescribed as the text, but teaching was not to be confined to lectures: the holder of the chair was also obliged to provide demonstrations on diagnosis by urine and pulse at the hospital of San Francesco. The rectors were gratified and Annibale Bimbiolo presumably disappointed by the appointment of Antonio Negro to the new position at the respectable salary of 300 fiorini per year. (By way of comparison, in 1598 the second ordinary professor of *theoria* got 400 fiorini, and the first extraordinary professor of *practica* 200.)[121]

The chair established for Negro, which combined lectures on *Canon* 1.2 with clinical instruction and demonstration in a hospital, lasted only until his death in 1626. Thereafter the lectures on causes and symptoms of diseases were quietly reabsorbed into the regular curriculum, and the hospital instruction on pulse and urine continued separately.[122] The episode of the institution of this chair, like that of the restoration of the lectures on *Canon* 3, testifies primarily to the importance attached to expanding the public curriculum in *practica*. It is instructive

---

ponte da quanto scrive Hippocrate et Galeno in piu libri, et Avicenna nel quarto suo libro.

"Et cosi ogni anno nel studio verrebbono esplicati tutti li cinque libri di Avicenna, et tutta la medicina, se theorica come prattica, de tutti gli auttori; et massime se fosse datto tal carico a dottor essercitato, che havesse letto et theorica et prattica." ASV Riformatori 419, Annibale Bimbiolo.

[120] ASV Riformatori 419, Annibali Bimbiolo, inc. "Havend'io Annibale Bimbiolo humilissimo servo. . . ."

[121] Bertolaso, "La cattedra 'De pulsibus,' " p. 113. For the 1598 salaries, Riccobono, *De gymnasio patavino*, fols. 146ᵛ–47ᵛ.

[122] Bertolaso, "La cattedra 'De pulsibus,' " pp. 113–14.

to note that neither the continued use of Avicenna nor teaching by commentary on traditionally assigned books seemed incongruous with this goal, although both were evidently considered in need of supplementing. Meanwhile, the task of *theoria* had apparently been reduced to the provision of introductory generalizations. Some attempt to redress the balance upset by the introduction of the additional chairs in *practica* using Avicenna was made in 1602, with the institution of a new chair of *theoria* offering lectures, on festival days only, on the standard rotation of *Canon* 1.1, *Aphorisms*, and *Ars*. However, the insignificance of this gesture is revealed by the lecturer's salary—a meager 25 fiorini per year.[123] Thereafter, no further efforts were to be made by university authorities at Padua to revitalize or extend either the teaching of *theoria* or lectures on the *Canon*. Between 1611 and 1625, Santorio Santorio made a noteworthy effort to combine some use of demonstrative experiments and instrumentation with scholastic commentary in his lectures on the *Canon* (the content of which will be discussed in subsequent chapters), but this endeavor involved no formal curricular change.

Teaching the Canon at Bologna and Padua after the 1620s

The tapering off of the publication of commentaries after the 1620s may be thought to mark the end of any real influence of the *Canon* on European medical thought. Various factors combined to bring about this result. Of these, the most important, of course, was the gradual replacement of Aristotelian natural philosophy and Galenic physiology. Although more remains to be learned about the whole process of the reception of new scientific ideas in these areas in Italian medical and academic circles, it is, for example, clear that by 1650 there had occurred, to quote two recent scholars, "extremely deep permeation of the idea of circulation among Italian intellectuals."[124] And the careers and contributions to zoology and physiology of M. A. Severini, Borelli, and Malpighi are further evidence, if any be needed, of the presence of scientific vitality and international contacts within Italian university faculties of medicine in the mid- and later seventeenth century.[125]

[123] Bertolaso, "Ricerche d'archivio" (1959–60), p. 28.

[124] Charles B. Schmitt and Charles Webster, "Harvey and M. A. Severino: A Neglected Medical Relationship," *Bulletin of the History of Medicine* 45 (1971), 49.

[125] Ibid., pp. 49–75, on Severino. A mass of information about the intellectual milieu of Malpighi and Borelli is contained in Howard B. Adelmann, *Marcello Malpighi and the*

But resistance to all forms of intellectual change also remained strong within the faculties of medicine for much of the seventeenth century, as Malpighi's troubles with his colleagues at Bologna show.[126] Moreover, traditionalism was reinforced by the increasing provincialization and contraction that overtook the north Italian universities in the same period. Despite the existence of some advanced scientific circles in the university medical milieu, the general picture at Bologna and Padua, as elsewhere, was of diminution in student enrollment and loss of the ability to attract students from abroad. (The rise of Leiden as an international center of medical education played a part in the latter.) The training of local medical practitioners, always an important function of the Italian faculties of medicine, was now predominant. The tendency, always present, for graduates of local origin to monopolize the public lectureships and treat them as sinecures seems to have become harder to keep in check.[127] Statutory lectures often appear to have been perfunctory—one professor at Bologna in the 1640s proposed to expound the first three *doctrinae* of *Canon* 1.1 in one day[128]—and were sometimes omitted entirely. Such conditions provided modernists as well as the slothful with ample opportunity to avoid spending time giving or hearing lectures on the traditional books. Some teachers continued conscientiously to provide fuller treatments of the *Canon*, but if the lists of lecture topics submitted by members of the Bologna faculty in the 1640s and the lectures delivered by Girolamo Santa Sofia at Padua in 1651 are anything to go by, the content provided was likely to be

---

Evolution of Embryology (Ithaca, 1966), vol. 1, pt. 1, "The Life and Works of Marcello Malpighi."

[126] Ibid., 1:128–34, referring mostly to events of the 1650s.

[127] Complaints about lack of students and irresponsibility on the part of lecturers can be traced back as far as the fifteenth century in the north Italian universities (see, for example, Ohl, "The University of Padua," pp. 47–49). But there seems little doubt that decline in numbers of students after 1600 was also accompanied by a loss of international appeal; see, e.g., for details regarding Bologna, Adelmann, *Malpighi*, 1:52–66.

[128] ASB, Assunteria dello Studio, Serie di annue lezioni, Busta 1, fol. 447[r–v]: "Continuatio explicationum supra 4m fen libri primi Avicennae de quibus in publicis scholis hora 3a matutina sermonem habebit Franciscus Caelius per totam diem 28 Martii" (thirty-nine heads follow); fol. 448, lectures on *Canon* 1.1–3 to be given for whole of 19 December 1646, by Franciscus Caelius; fol. 450, *explicationes* of *Canon* 1.4 to be given by Franciscus Caelius for the whole of 20 December 1642 (twenty-six headings); fol. 454, Franciscus Caelius on *Canon* 1.4 for the whole of 23 June 1643 (thirty-four headings). Professors were obliged to submit schedules of their forthcoming lectures to the Assunteria, the regulatory magistracy established to oversee the universities, in an effort to oblige them to fulfill their statutory obligations; Giorgio Cencetti, *Gli archivi dello Studio Bolognese* (Bologna, 1938), p. 93.

121

wholly routine, almost all effort to introduce innovative material having been abandoned.[129]

However, there were also teachers who met their obligation to lecture on Canon 1.1 by simply substituting modern physiological and other scientific content. Such, at any rate, was the procedure of Lorenzo Bacchetto, who occupied the humble place of third extraordinary professor of theoretical medicine at Padua in 1687.[130] He circulated a printed prospectus of his lectures in which he announced his intention to perform various experiments; to draw on the works of Gilbert, Bacon, Boyle, Gassendi, Harvey, Van Helmont, Mayow, and other modern authors; and to discuss such topics as the number of the elements, air pressure and the barometer, Mayow's ideas on respiration, and the circulation of the blood. It is evident from this list of topics, and from the fact that Bacchetto devoted almost half his prospectus to the subject matter of the doctrina on the elements, that he intended to use Canon 1.1 as the framework for a survey of recent work in general physical science as well as physiology. No doubt his course would have been a stimulating intellectual experience, although perhaps not very helpful to a student whose goal was to pass an examination, however cursory, on Canon 1.1.[131] Essentially similar, although somewhat less radical, was the solution adopted by a more distinguished figure in the

[129] Ibid., fols. 447 (Franciscus Caelius on Canon 1.4, n.d.), 448 (same on Canon 1.1, 1646–47), 450 (same on Canon 1.4, 1642), 454 (same on Canon 1.4, 1643), 493, 498 (Pompeius Bolognettus on Canon 4.1, n.d.), 496^r–97^v (same on Canon 1.4, n.d.), 506 (Ercole Betti on Canon 1.1, n.d.), 515–16^v, 518 (Franciscus Sacentus on Canon 1.4, n.d.), 595 (Franciscus Severinus on Canon 1.1, n.d.), unnumbered small sheet (same on Canon 1.1.4, chap. 2, 1643), another unnumbered small sheet (same on Canon 1.1–1.4, n.d.), 596 (same on Canon 1.1.6.1, 1649?), 600 (same on Canon 1.1.5.1, 1643), 624 (same on Canon 1.1, 1648?). Each of these schedules consists of lists of lecture topics, none of which indicates any intention to depart from routine treatment or introduce contemporary material. Of course, it is possible that any professor infected with modernism might not have wished to let the Assunteria know his plans. Santasofia's commentary is contained in WL MS 4353. Conceivably, his provision of separate sections on innate heat and spirits (which are not accorded separate chapters in the text of Canon 1.1) should be perceived as a reflection of sixteenth-century interests.

[130] Facciolati, Fasti, 2:371.

[131] ASV Riformatori 452 (printed rotuli and synopses of courses), Explicationem in primam fen primi libri Canonis Avicennae incipiet Laurentius Bacchettus Patavinus publicus medicinae theoricae professor (n.d.). These course outlines, unlike those from Bologna, seem to have been intended for distribution to students. Most are for courses on law. The only other one here on Avicenna (Io. Pompilio Scoto, olim Duglassi, on Canon 1.1, 1693) is in the main much more conservative, although it does indicate an intention to compare atomist with Aristotelian theories. Bacchetto's endeavor may be compared to the lectures on Aristotle's Meteorologica given in 1714–15, described in Dooley, "Science Teaching."

history of medicine, G. B. Morgagni, when called upon to lecture on *Canon* 1.1 at Padua early in his career. Morgagni laid more emphasis on physiology and less on general science than Bacchetto had apparently done, provided his pupils with a cursory account of traditional as well as lengthy descriptions of modern ideas, and spoke of Avicenna with respect as a personage of historical importance. (On the content of Morgagni's lectures, see Chapter 6.)

By the early eighteenth century, educational reformers were calling for the abandonment or drastic overhaul of the traditional university curriculum in medicine, as in other subjects. What, demanded Scipione Maffei rhetorically in 1713, would an educated foreigner think if he looked over a list of the courses at Padua and found chairs dedicated to lecturing on Avicenna?[132] Only in the second half of the century, however, were the goals of the reformers finally achieved in the Italian universities.[133] At Padua, lectures on *Canon* 1.1 and on the other books in *theoria* finally gave way to courses designated physiology and pathology in 1767.[134] Lectures on *Canon* 1.1 and 1.4 were at last abandoned at Bologna in 1716 (only to be replaced by lectures on Galen's *Methodus medendi*).[135]

But there is a sequel. Among the various reports on university conditions produced in the eighteenth century was one submitted to the Assunteria di Studio of Bologna between 1735 and 1737. In it, Matteo

[132] Maffei's recommendations for the reform of the *studio* of Padua are edited in Biagio Brugi, "Un parere di Scipione Maffei intorno allo Studio di Padova sui principi del Settecento," *Atti del R. Istituto Veneto di Scienze, Lettere ed Arti* 69 (1909–10), pt. 2, 575–91. For Maffei's opinion of the current curriculum in medicine, see p. 578. His proposals for its reform involved reducing the number of chairs in theory and *practica*, extending the length of the anatomy course, restoring a separate chair in surgery, and adding chairs in chemistry and "neoteric medicine" (pp. 580–81, 591). Alexander Knips Macoppe, *Pro empirico secta adversus theoriam medicam: praelectio habita in Archilyceo Patavino* (Padua, 1717) is an attack by a professor in the university on medical theory as a discipline, as well as on Galenists and Paracelsians, and a plea for a new kind of medical *theoria* based on (p. 84) experimental knowledge and "accuratissimae historiae humani corporis."

[133] Bartolo Bertolaso, "Ricerche d'archivio su alcuni aspetti dell'insegnamento medico presso la Università di Padova nel Sette- ed Ottocento," *Acta medicae historiae patavina* 5 (1958–59), 1–30; Baldo Peroni, "La riforma," pp. 115–74, and Alessandro Visconti, "L'opera del Governo Austriaco nella riforma universitaria durante il ventennio 1752–1773," *Contribute alla storia dell'Università di Pavia* (Pavia, 1925), pp. 175–237; Francesco Torra et al., *Storia della Università di Napoli* (Naples, 1924), pp. 304 (regarding the establishment of a chair of the Institutes of Medicine by 1703) and 433–72; Visconti, *Storia*, p. 109; Simeoni, *Storia*, 2:110–11.

[134] Bertolaso, "Ricerche d'archivio" (1958–59), p. 8. The chair of *practica* was abolished at Padua in 1806, but a modern (1695) textbook on fevers was being used in 1771 (ibid., pp. 8–9).

[135] Dallari, *Rotuli*, 3:1, 260–61.

Bazzani and Giacomo Bartolomeo Beccari deplored the absence of a chair of "animal economy, a title essential and extremely important for a proper grasp of physiological medicine." Under this modern-sounding title, they proposed the restoration of the teaching of *Canon* 1.1.[136] In justice to Beccari it should be noted that he had active scientific interests and a concern for the reform of science teaching. One can only conclude that he took for granted that the traditional titles of the chairs had really become simply a designation of subject matter, and a memorial to a text of historical importance. The plea was successful, and *Canon* 1.1 continued to find a nominal place in the official curriculum at Bologna until 1800.[137]

As Bacchetto and Morgagni demonstrated, a determinedly modernist lecturer could adapt the traditional curriculum—or rather its husk— to his own needs. By long tradition, teaching by commentary was nothing if not adaptable to individual interests and changing circumstances, and this adaptability may have helped to ensure its survival. Furthermore any decision to adopt a new textbook would obviously have opened up the possibility of conflict and might also have raised fears about the possible introduction of heterodox scientific or religious ideas. Nonetheless, it is difficult to see the last century of continued reliance on *Canon* 1.1 at Padua and Bologna as the sole officially endorsed university textbook in physiology otherwise than as a mark of intellectual stagnation and administrative timidity. By contrast, Renaissance teaching based on the *Canon* was still part of the mainstream of contemporary medicine. A closer look at the editions and commentaries that were the products of Renaissance and early seventeenth-century use of Avicenna's work is now called for.

[136] ASB, Assunteria dello Studio, Diversorum, Letture, 1st folder, 1735–37 on cover; the report of Bazzani and Beccari occupies four unbound folios: "[Medicina teorica] riman priva del titolo che racchiude l'animal economia: titolo essenziale ed importantissimo per ben apprendere la medica fisiologia, senza di cui lui e impossibile il diventare un buon teorico, e percio titolo da aggiungersi alla teorica medicina; o per dir vero da restituirsi alla medesimo, giacchè anticamente leggersi sulle cattedre . . . , e noi ci rammentiamo benissimo di averlo insegnato pubblicamente, allorchè costumarsi di leggere la prima Fen, ossia parte del primo libro di Avicenna, comprensiva della prementionata animali Economia, che poscia fuor di dovere ne fu levata, ed . . . omessa. . . . E che la medicina theorica debbe introdursi con la prima Fen del primo libro d'Avicenna." (fols. 1ᵛ–2ʳ).

[137] For the careers of Bazzani (1674–1749) and Beccari (1682–1766), see *Biogr. Lex.* 1:342, 349. For the restored lectures, Dallari, *Rotuli* 3:2, annually from 1737 until 1800. However, by 1790 the lectures were not actually being given; see Adelmann, *Malpighi*, 1:101. At Pisa in the 1730s the public lectures often only lasted for fifteen minutes (AAUP Università, 3:1, 49ʳ).

PART III

The *Canon* and Its Renaissance Editors, Translators, and Commentators

5

Renaissance Editions

Writing in 1674, Georg Jerome Welsch of Augsburg was able to look back on a century and a half of efforts to provide western Europe with a Latin version of the *Canon* more satisfactory than Gerard of Cremona's translation. The history Welsch recounted was one of projects planned but never started, or started but never completed, or completed but never published; of fresh translations of small portions of the work; of massive editions of the whole adorned with every resource of sixteenth-century scholarship save direct retranslation of the entire text from Arabic. Hence, the call for a new or emended Latin version of the *Canon*, already, as Welsch noted, heard in medical humanist circles in the early sixteenth century, was still being expressed by the learned Orientalists of Welsch's own day. By the 1670s, however, medical interest in the *Canon* was no longer sufficient to encourage such an undertaking. From the standpoint of late seventeenth-century scholarship in Oriental languages, this history must have seemed one of failure, or at any rate of very partial and circumscribed success; nor can one say that Welsch's own edition and translation of two brief chapters of the *Canon* materially altered the situation.[1] Yet the sixteenth- and seventeenth-century Latin editions of the *Canon*, including editions of a kind Welsch found beneath his notice, such as reprints of sections of the bare Gerard of Cremona translation for student use, served generations of medical teachers and students. In themselves, these editions have much to tell us about

---

[1] *Canon* 4.3.2.21–22, ed. and tr. Welsch (Augsburg, 1674), preface, sig. b1ʳ–cʳ. On Welsch, and this edition, see C. F. von Schnurrer, *Bibliotheca Arabica* (Halle, 1811), pp. 452–54, no. 395. *Canon* 2, ed. and tr. Kirsten (Breslau, 1609), pp. 7–8, and *Canon* 1, 2, and 4.1, tr. Plemp (Louvain, 1658), fols. 2ᵛ–3ʳ, also survey textual work on the *Canon* to the time of writing. Among the seventeenth-century Arabists who are said by Plemp and Welsch to have contemplated editing or translating the *Canon* are Erpenius (Thomas van Erpe, 1584–1624) and Athanasius Kircher. The extent to which Avicenna, or the *Canon*, was of serious interest among early Orientalists merits further investigation, although the topic goes beyond the scope of the present work and the competence of the present author. It is clear that the usefulness of Arabic for medicine was long a standard theme in arguments for the expansion of Arabic studies, and that some of those few who pressed for the introduction of the teaching of Arabic in northern European universities did so in large part because of presumed benefits for medicine; for examples, see Alastair Hamilton, *William Bedwell the Arabist, 1563–1632* (Leiden, 1985), pp. 7–8.

127

Renaissance medical learning and Avicenna's place therein. And Renaissance commentary and teaching based on the *Canon* is scarcely explicable without some account of their history.

Between 1500 and 1674, some sixty editions of the complete or partial text of the *Canon* were published (see Appendix 1). Apart from one edition of the entire work in Arabic, and two others of sections of the Arabic text with Latin translation, all of these publications were in Latin; in the great majority of cases their context was the continued use of the *Canon* in university medical training, especially in Italy. (The count of Latin editions would be considerably higher if every edition of a commentary that also included some passages from the text were included.)[2] The emphasis of both Avicenna's detractors and his defenders upon the faults of his twelfth-century translator fostered the belief that a more satisfactory presentation of the text of the *Canon* would enable the real usefulness of Avicenna in medicine to be properly appreciated once more. A medical milieu in which the *Canon* was still too useful and too firmly entrenched to be abandoned but in which its presentation had come to seem old-fashioned, if not worse, provided a ready market for editions of the work that could claim in some way or another to be improved or purified. Translators, scholarly editors, and publishers hastened to supply this market. Thus, whereas the editions of the *Canon* issued in the early years of the sixteenth century served simply to perpetuate approaches to the work developed in the schools of western Europe between the thirteenth and the mid-fifteenth century, the later printing history of the *Canon* in the West is marked by a series of attempts to improve the accuracy or comprehensibility of the text.

After about the 1520s, although excerpts from the Gerard of Cremona translation without revision or editorial additions continued to be published for students, a number of scholars devoted themselves to the preparation of editions that, in one way or another, reflect an endeavor to apply humanist learning to the *Canon* itself. The efforts of

---

[2] See the introduction to Appendices 1 and 2, below. The editions in Arabic referred to are that of the whole work (Rome, 1593) (von Schnurrer, pp. 449–51, no. 393); *Canon* 2, ed. and tr. Kirsten (Breslau, 1609) (von Schnurrer, pp. 451–52, no. 394); and *Canon* 4.3.2.21–22, ed. and tr. Welsch (Augsburg, 1674). To the number of editions printing portions of the text of the *Canon* in Arabic could be added Werner Rolfinck, *Liber de purgantibus vegetabilibus* (Jena, 1667). The author of this work made use of the Rome, 1593, edition of the *Canon*, and called on Johann Ernest Gerhard for assistance in correcting the passages in Arabic reproduced. However, the book is a general work on vegetable purgatives, and draws upon other authors who wrote on this subject in Arabic, as well as Avicenna. There are also fourteen incunabular editions of the *Canon* in Latin and one in Hebrew (GW nos. 3113–27).

these scholars often struck contemporaries as flawed and partial (the difficulty of producing a new version of the *Canon* apparently seldom inspired the reflection that the achievement of Gerard of Cremona, however imperfect, deserved some respect). This dissatisfaction in turn encouraged yet other schemes, not all of which were realized, for further work on the *Canon*. Hence, far from perpetuating an unchanging and monolithic tradition, the European printing history of the *Canon* includes a wide range of different material and displays an equally wide range of apparent editorial objectives, attitudes toward Avicenna as a medical author, and in some cases methodologies of revision. Especially worthy of note are those publications that attempt to provide an improved Latin text or to accompany it with up-to-date apparatus of various kinds, an enterprise in which, collectively, a good deal of time and effort on the part of scholarly editors, revisers, and in a few instances translators, and of money on the part of publishers was evidently invested. Yet even routine reprintings of short excerpts from the *Canon* commonly prescribed as textbooks merit attention to the extent that such reprintings provide a clue to the call for copies of the work in the schools.

Among the editions, a handful were the product of a group of sixteenth-century Italian scholars, most of them associated with the University of Padua or with Venice, to present the *Canon* in a form consonant with the tastes and scholarship of their environment. Of all the Latin editions of the work, this group of publications yields the most information about the ways in which the *Canon* was studied and expounded in sixteenth-century universities. Accordingly, I shall first broadly survey the output of *Canon* editions in an attempt to classify them by type and chronology, and then return to a discussion of the characteristics of the innovative editions produced in Italy or with the participation of Italian professors of medicine. What follows is, however, very far from being a complete account of the career of the *Canon* as a Renaissance Latin medical book since, although valuable studies by Francesca Lucchetta, Marie-Thérèse d'Alverny, and Luis Garcia Ballester have illuminated some attempts to revise the Latin text of the *Canon*, much remains to be learned about the textual history of the Latin versions of the work.[3]

---

[3] Lucchetta, *Alpago*; d'Alverny, "Avicenne et les médecins de Venise"; d'Alverny, "Les traductions d'Avicenne (Moyen Age et Renaissance)," in *Avicenna nella storia della cultura medioevale*, Problemi attuali di scienza e di cultura dell'Accademia Nazionale dei Lincei, Quaderno no. 40 (Rome, 1955), pp. 71–87, at pp. 84–87; and d'Alverny, "Andrea Alpago, interprète et commentateur d'Avicenne," in *Atti del XII Congresso internazionale di filosofia* (Florence, 1960), 9:1–6; L. Garcia Ballester, "The Circulation and Use of Med-

In content, the Latin editions of the *Canon* published after 1500 fall into six categories: the complete text in the translation produced in the circle of Gerard of Cremona before 1187, without commentary and with no recent "modernization" of text or apparatus; one or more of the five books into which the *Canon* is divided, accompanied by Latin commentary written between the thirteenth and fifteenth centuries; the complete *Canon* or a major portion of it with textual revisions and apparatus contributed by late fifteenth- or sixteenth-century medical scholars; one or more of the short sections of the work used as university textbooks, either alone or in compilations of brief texts such as the *articella*; compendia or collections of maxims based on the *Canon*; and, finally, retranslations of portions of the work.

Broadly speaking, these publications may be divided into three chronological groups, each marked by a different distribution of the various kinds of content just indicated. However, the identification of these groups should not be allowed to obscure the extent of overlap between them, or the presence of elements of continuity through all three. With one exception, the first group of twenty-two editions published between 1500 and 1525 essentially perpetuates approaches to and presentations of the *Canon* that had developed, most notably perhaps in the schools of northern Italy, but also in Montpellier, Paris, and other Western university centers between the thirteenth and fifteenth centuries. Among the twenty-nine Latin editions published between 1526 and 1608, attempts to revise the text or presentation predominate. Most of the latter productions can, once again, be associated with the learning of the north Italian universities; moreover, this group, which includes the editions that are the main subject of the present discussion, coincides chronologically with an active phase in the production and publication of commentaries on the *Canon* in the Italian schools (to be discussed in the next chapter). Finally, a small group of nine editions was published between 1609 and 1674. They included efforts by northern European Arabists to provide a better Latin text of the *Canon*, efforts that were in some respects more far reaching than earlier endeavors of that kind; but by the time these works appeared, neither the medical content of the *Canon* nor a pedagogical and investigative methodology based on the exposition of ancient scientific authorities aroused much further interest. The survival of parts of the Latin *Canon* in various university curricula until well into the eighteenth century

---

ical Manuscripts in Arabic in Sixteenth-Century Spain," *Journal for the History of Arabic Science* 3 (1979), 183–99, at p. 189, and Garcia Ballester, *Los Moriscos y la medicina*, pp. 24–31.

was insufficient to stimulate demand for fresh Latin editions after the mid-seventeenth century.

In the period 1500–1525, the appearance of two editions of the complete Gerard of Cremona text without commentary, both in the first decade of the century,[4] was overshadowed by a considerably larger number of publications of the text accompanied by the expositions of its principal thirteenth- to fifteenth-century commentators. Perhaps because he accomplished the unusual feat of writing commentaries on all five books, Gentile da Foligno's expositions seem to have been especially favored by the *Canon*'s early sixteenth-century editors. As already noted, even Gentile probably did not in fact quite accomplish the monumental task of commenting on the entire *Canon* since his exposition of Book 3 is apparently incomplete. However, his prolixity, and that of other authors whose commentaries were used to supplement his, was sufficient to preclude the presentation of the complete *Canon* with commentary in a single volume. Thus, to choose only one of several examples, Books 3 and 4 with the commentaries of Gentile and the French physician Jacques Despars, supplemented for parts of Book 4 with those of Dinus Florentinus (probably Dino del Garbo), and Giovanni Matteo Ferrari da Grado, published at Venice about 1505, occupy three large folio volumes.[5] The culmination of this approach to the *Canon* came in 1523, with the appearance from the Junta press of Venice of a set of five massive tomes, which announced itself as presenting the entire *Canon* along with the expositions of all its principal interpreters. The roundup of commentators included all those so far mentioned, as well as Taddeo Alderotti. There seem to be no editions of the complete *Canon* or of the whole of any of its five books subsequent to the Junta volumes of 1523 that are adorned with commentaries written before 1500; separate editions of such commentaries (some of which, as noted, include portions of text), which were issued rather frequently between the introduction of printing and the mid-1520s, appeared much less often thereafter.[6]

---

[4] *Canon* (Venice, 1505) and *Canon* (Venice, 1507; facsimile, Hildesheim, 1964). The majority of the Latin incunabular editions also contain the entire Gerard of Cremona translation without commentary.

[5] The impression that Gentile's commentaries were printed as an accompaniment to the text of the *Canon* more frequently than those of other fourteenth- or fifteenth-century authors in the period ca. 1500–1525 is based on volumes included in Appendix 1 on the principles indicated in the introduction thereto; Gentile's works would not necessarily predominate if all early sixteenth-century printings of commentaries on the *Canon* written before 1500 were taken into account.

[6] However, a few early commentaries continued to be printed from time to time. For examples, see Chapter 6, n. 22.

If the goal of those responsible for the editions just described appears to have been to flank the *Canon* with the fullest possible scholastic commentary, others in the early years of the century followed another practice that also had earlier antecedents: to make Avicenna's medical thought accessible by means of drastic abbreviations or rearrangements of the Latin text. Thus, the preface to a small volume of *Flores Avicennae* published at Lyon in 1508 refers to the importance in medicine of aphoristic works that can readily be committed to memory, and to the example of the Hippocratic writings.[7] The task of abbreviation was undertaken with such enthusiasm that Avicenna's chapter on the elements (*Canon* 1.1.2) was compressed from about 550 words in the full Gerard of Cremona version into 53 in the *Flores*. This compendium was twice reissued, in 1514 and again in 1528, in an expanded version that included similar treatment of other works by Avicenna. A like emphasis upon the goal of easy memorization is found in the dedicatory letter that Pietro Antonio Rustico prefaced to his *Memoriale medicorum canonice practicantium*, published in 1517 and intended to help students at the University of Pavia, where Rustico was a professor. Rustico's first two sets of *canones* are based on *Canon* 1.4 and 4.1, which he broke down into axioms grouped in numerous brief sections. A similar emphasis upon conciseness is present in the title of a "very brief" so-called "alphabetized" *Canon* published in 1520, although the contents of the work are actually a kind of index.[8]

In the early years of the century, too, excerpts from the *Canon* commonly used as university textbooks were printed several times as part of the *articella*, the celebrated collection of brief medical textbooks first formed, probably in southern Italy, early in the twelfth century and subsequently expanded by the inclusion of additional works.[9] For ex-

[7] *Flores Avicenne* (Lyon, 1508). The preface is by Michael de Capella, *artium et medicine magister*.

[8] *Textus principis Avicenne per ordinem alphabeti in sentencia reportatus*. This is the third of five separately foliated booklets in a work entitled *Habes humane lector Gabrielis de Tarrega Burgdalensis civitatis medici regentis et ordinarii opera brevissima theoricam et prathicam* [sic] *medicinalis sciencie . . . amplexancia* (Bordeaux, 1520 and 1524). Yet other works outlined for students the teaching of Avicenna along with other major medical authors. I mention only one of these, as an example, here: Alfonso Bertocci's *Methodus generalis et compendiaria ex Hippocratis, Galeni, et Avicennae placitis deprompta ac in ordinem redacta . . . Alfonsi Bertotii opera hinc inde collecta* (Venice, 1556). To the general category of compilations, collections of excerpts, and abbreviations making extensive use of the Canon apparently also belong the *Metaphora medicine* (1522) and *Modus faciendi cum ordine medicandi* (ca. 1527) of the Spanish Franciscan Bernardino de Laredo, which I have not seen and cite from López Piñero, *Ciencia y técnica*, p. 340.

[9] The *Canon* excerpts were not part of the *articella* as it existed in the twelfth or thirteenth century, and are not found in incunabular editions of the *articella* (Klebs 116.1–6).

ample, *Canon* 1.1–2, 1:4, and 4.1 are found in an *articella* published at Pavia in 1506 with a dedicatory letter by Pietro Antonio Rustico, and reissued at Venice the following year. Another version of the *articella*, printed at Lyon in 1515 and subsequently reissued several times, included the same portions of the *Canon* and, in addition, 4.3–5 (surgery).[10] Although *Canon* 1.1 was printed in these collections as, since the early fourteenth century, it had usually been taught, with the omission of the section on anatomy, the texts printed in the *articella* are excerpts from, not abbreviations or rearrangements of, the text of the Gerard of Cremona translation.

Thus, the salient features of the various types of *Canon* edition that appeared most frequently in the first twenty years of the sixteenth century—scholastic commentaries, aphoristic presentations, and the incorporation of sections of the *Canon* into the *articella*—all testify to the continuing vitality in those years of long-established forms of medical education.

The first person to undertake a new translation of the *Canon* into Latin was apparently Girolamo Ramusio (1450–86). Trained as a physician at Padua, Ramusio was also a poet with connections in literary and philosophical circles. From 1484 until his death he served as *medico condotto* to the Venetian community at Damascus. There, in the brief space of eighteen months, he produced a translation of *Canon* 1 directly from the Arabic; this was never published, although Antonio Graziolo had access to the work in manuscript while preparing his own version of *Canon* 1 (Venice, 1580).[11] Hence, the credit for the first printed edition of the *Canon* to show awareness of humanist scholarship or criticism must go to Symphorien Champier, whose activities as a critic of the Arabs have already been discussed, and to Pietro Antonio Rustico. An edition of the complete Gerard of Cremona text published at Lyon in 1522 claimed in its title to be corrected "from errors and every barbarism in all parts" by Rustico, and was preceded by a set of "notes, errata, and castigations" by Champier.

Of much greater long-term influence than the Champier-Rustico edition was the version of the entire *Canon* emended and provided with a glossary of Arabic terms by Andrea Alpago, prepared for publication by his nephew Paolo Alpago, and first published at Venice in 1527.[12]

---

[10] *Articella* (Lyon, 1515); reissued Lyon, 1519, 1525, 1534.

[11] On Ramusio, see Francesca Lucchetta, "Girolamo Ramusio," *Quaderni per la storia dell'Università di Padova* 15 (1982), 1–60. Ramusio's translation survives as Paris, Bibliothèque Nationale, MS arabe 2897, which I have not seen. I am grateful to Charles B. Schmitt for supplying a description.

[12] *Canon,* ed. Alpago (Venice, 1527), also included Alpago's versions of two short

The history of Alpago's long residence in the Middle East as a physician in the service of the Venetian Republic, and of the formal endorsement of his version of the *Canon* by the Paduan College of Philosophers
and Physicians has been recounted by Francesca Lucchetta and was discussed in the last chapter.[13] Alpago's work was the basis of most subsequent major Latin editions, and inspired several others produced in
negative response to his efforts. Moreover, almost all later commentators on the *Canon* made use of the *versio bellunensis*, that is, of Alpago,
whose family came from Belluno. Paolo Alpago's own awareness of
the probability of large demand for the new version is doubtless reflected in his care to secure privileges from the pope, the king of France,
and the Venetian Republic, granting him exclusive rights over the
printing for a period of ten years.[14] This first edition of Alpago's work
was published by the Junta press of Venice, which, the reader will recall, had only four years earlier issued the most majestic of the editions
of the unrevised text with all its major thirteenth- and fifteenth-century
commentators. In 1544 Paolo published a second edition, also with
Junta, which included some further textual revisions, additions to Andrea's glossary of Arabic terms, a life of Avicenna translated by Nicolò
Massa (d. 1569),[15] and a set of illustrations showing a physician manip-
ulating dislocations.

But dissatisfaction with the results of Alpago's efforts manifested itself almost immediately. In 1530 there appeared a new translation of
Canon 1.4 by Jacob Mantino, a Jewish physician active in Venice.[16] In
a letter of dedication to Doge Andrea Gritti, Mantino explained that
owing to the difficulty of finding equivalents for Arabic idioms in
Latin, the Gerard translation was marred by many major errors. Al-

---

medical works by Avicenna, namely *De medicinis cordialibus* (that is, *De viribus cordis*) and
the *Cantica*, both of which had been printed, in earlier versions, in some of the previous
editions of the *Canon* (see Klebs, p. 69).

[13] Lucchetta, *Alpago*, pp. 35–56.

[14] The privileges are printed at the beginning of the 1527 edition.

[15] On Nicolò Massa's career and writings, see Richard Palmer, "Nicolò Massa, His
Family and His Fortune," *Medical History* 25 (1981), 385–410. Regarding biographies of
Avicenna included in editions of the *Canon*, see below, in this chapter.

[16] For the career of Mantino (d. 1549), at one time a papal physician who also translated
works of Averroes and became involved in the controversy over Henry VIII's divorce,
see D. Kaufman, "Jacob Mantino. Un page d'histoire de la Renaissance." *Revue des études
juives* 28 (1893), 30–60, 207–38. On Mantino's part in the Renaissance effort to produce
new editions or translations of works of Averroes (which in some ways quite closely parallels the treatment accorded Avicenna), see Charles B. Schmitt, "Renaissance Averroism Studied through the Venetian Editions of Aristotle-Averroes (with Particular Reference to the Giunta Edition of 1550–2)," reprinted in his *Aristotelian Tradition*, p. 129
(original pagination).

pago, whom Mantino characterized as a distinguished physician equally learned in Latin and Arabic, had removed some of these, but many remained to cloud the true meaning of the work. Mantino claimed to have freed *Canon* 1.4 from these errors by translating it afresh not from the original Arabic, but from Hebrew (the *Canon* existed in Hebrew not only in numerous manuscripts, but also in print; an edition was published at Naples in 1491).[17] Mantino announced his intention to go on to translate the other parts of the *Canon* most frequently studied "in the public schools," namely 1.1 and 4.1, although he appears only to have completed the former. His version of *Canon* 1.1 and 1.4 enjoyed considerable success. The latter was printed at least four more times and was disseminated across Europe (Ettlingen, 1531; Paris, 1532 and 1555; The Hague, 1533).[18] Although Mantino's translation of *Canon* 1.1 seems to have been printed only twice, both times in the Veneto (Venice, ca. 1540; Padua, 1547), it was influential, judging by the rather numerous references to it by subsequent editors and commentators. Thus, for example, the sections of the commentary on *Canon* 1.1 by Oddo Oddi (Venice, 1575) are headed by the passages commented on in both the "translatio [*sic*] bellunensis" and the "translatio Mantini," and Oddo frequently weighed the merits of the two versions.

Recourse was had to the medieval Hebrew translations as a means of improving the Latin text of the *Canon* quite frequently throughout the sixteenth century. In Italy, this strategy was facilitated by the presence of a Jewish medical community reinforced by recent exiles from the Iberian peninsula.[19] Amatus Lusitanus, one of the most distinguished Jewish physicians of the period, who spent a number of years in Italy and knew the Italian medical scene well, believed that Andrea Alpago himself (as well as the mid-sixteenth-century editor Benedetto Rinio) had on occasion restored passages from the Hebrew. He was contemptuous of their efforts, while praising those of Mantino, whom he described as "most skilled in many languages." Lamenting Mantino's untimely death, Amatus expressed the hope that others would carry on his work on the *Canon*, although Amatus believed it was more likely

[17] GW 3113. See also Moritz Steinschneider, *Die hebräischen Übersetzungen des Mittelalters und die Juden als Dolmetscher* (Berlin, 1893; facsimile, Graz, 1956), pp. 683–85.

[18] Mantino also translated a chapter on headache from *Canon* 3, printed in Cornelius Baersdorp, *Methodus universae artis medicae* (n.p., 1538).

[19] See P. C. Ioly Zorattini, "Gli Ebrei a Venezia, Padova e Verona," *Storia della cultura veneta*, vol. 3, pt. 1 (Vicenza, 1980), 560–67; also Emilia Veronese Ceseracciu, "Ebrei laureati a Padova nel Cinquecento," *Quaderni per la storia dell'Università di Padova* 13 (1980), 151–68.

that the necessary linguistic skills would be found in Germany than in Italy; however, among scholarly physicians in Italy he thought Bartolomeo Eustachi best equipped to undertake the task.[20]

Willingness to rely on the Hebrew translation to emend the Latin translation of the *Canon* was by no means confined to Jewish or *converso* circles. Outside them, however, the help of a Jewish physician was usually needed to interpret the Hebrew text. The most celebrated instance of this kind is probably Vesalius' reliance on the assistance of Lazaro Ebreo de Frigeis for the Arabic names of bones "ex Hebraeo Avicennae interprete."[21] Somewhat similarly, in 1531 Dionysius Coronaeus wrote to Symphorien Champier from Rome describing his study of a "very old" manuscript of the *Canon* in Hebrew, with the aid of a Jewish physician on the difficult passages. Coronaeus described the translation contained in his manuscript in glowing terms, claiming it to be superior to the recently published Alpago version.[22] Subse-

[20] Faxint dii ut nobis aliquem arabice et latine loquentem mittant medicum, qui Avicennam latiniorem ac incorruptiorem faciat; confecerat nam opus hoc Jacobus Mantinus Hebraeus, vir multarum linguarum peritissimus, ac medicus doctissimus, qui iam nonnullas partes Avicennae doctissime interpretatus fuerat, veluti primam fen primi libri, et quartam primi, et primam fen quarti, ac nonnulla alia, nisi malus quidam genius eum a tam felici successu retraxisset. . . . At ut verum fateamur, hoc hodie Germanis, utpote viris doctissimis et linguarum peritissimis, debetur; si cui tamen Italorum opus hoc committi deberet, id merito committi posset hodie Bartholomeo Eustathio, illustrissimi Urbinatis Ducis medico ingeniosissimo, ac doctissimo, et multarum linguarum peritissimo." *Curationum medicinalium Amati Lusitani medici physici praestantissimi tomus primus* (Venice, 1566), scholium to *Cent.* 1.1, pp. 37–38. And: "... unde satis conscius sum quod Belunensis, et Rinus ipse, ac iis alii similes viri, suas in Avicenna restitutiones ab Hebraico contexto, vel saltem ad eius enarratoribus, emendicarunt, non vero a puro fonte Arabico eas contraxerunt, quem si recte callerent Avicennam de novo interpretarentur, et tam ingentem errorem non praetermitterent, ut alios propter infinitos sileam; non deerit tamen aliquis qui brevi Avicennam ex integro nobis latinissimum et sincerum ac purum pro veritate Arabica reddat; sed mea sententia pro hac conficiundo opere non unius viri, sed duorum et trium labor emergat, decet." Ibid., 2:94–95, *Cent.* 7.54. The first *centuria* of Amatus was composed in 1551. On Eustachi, who is best remembered today as an anatomist, see *DSB*, 4:486–88.

[21] "His [Latin and Greek names] succedent Hebraea, sed et aliqua ex parte adhuc arabica ex Hebraeo Avicennae interprete propemodum omnia, insignis medici mihique familiaris amici Lazari Hebraei de Frigeis (cum quo in Avicenna versari soleo) opera desumpta." Andreas Vesalius, *De humani corporis fabrica* (Basel, 1543), p. 166. On attempts to identify Lazarus de Frigeis, see Shelomo Franco, "Ricerche su Lazaro ebreo de Frigeis medico insigne e amico intimo di André Vésal," *La rassegna mensile di Israel* 15 (1949), 495–515. Most recently, it has been suggested that Lazarus is to be identified with Giovanni Battista Freschi Olivi, a convert from Judaism who received a medical degree from Padua in 1551; before his conversion he bore the name of Lazarus and practiced medicine. See *Quaderni per la storia dell'Università di Padova* 14 (1981), 159–60.

[22] Coronaeus' letter is printed as part of the front matter of *Canon* 3.1.4, tr. Cinqarbres (Paris, 1572), pp. 9–13.

quently, Coronaeus brought the manuscript to Paris, where, a generation later, it served as the basis for translations of three short excerpts by Jean Cinqarbres, regius professor of Hebrew at Paris, which were published there in 1570, 1572, and 1586.[23] The first of these was dedicated to the dean of the College of Physicians at Paris and described as a specimen of a larger future work. But the Cinqarbres translations seem never to have achieved either the circulation or the influence of those of Mantino, no doubt chiefly because the portions selected for translation were not those most frequently studied in the schools.

Georg Jerome Welsch hazarded the guess that the translation of the *Canon* that Julius Caesar Scaliger, around 1551, told Lorenz Gryll that he had made into "pure and terse Latin" from "Punic" ("ex Poenorum lingua") may have been from Hebrew. The story that the elder Scaliger had purified, or perhaps retranslated, the text of the *Canon* evidently spread on the basis of this report. Two scholars who worked on the text of the *Canon* in the seventeenth century, Welsch and V. F. Plemp, were both rightly skeptical of the claim, since it was denied outright by Joseph Scaliger. The latter, however, did assert that his father had known some Arabic, enough to make useful annotations in his own copy of the work, and added that Julius used to commend the reading of Avicenna as essential for the physician.[24] In 1580, as we shall see, Andrea Graziolo drew on the help of a Jewish physician familiar with the *Canon* in Hebrew when preparing his own Latin version of *Canon*

[23] In a dedicatory epistle prefaced to *Canon* 3.2, tr. Cinqarbres (Paris, 1570), fols. 2ʳ–3ᵛ, Cinqarbres explained how he purchased the manuscript thirty-six years after Coronaeus brought it from Rome to Paris.

[24] *Canon* 4.3.2.21–22, ed. and tr. Welsch (Augsburg, 1674), preface c 1ʳ; *Canon* 1, 2, 4.1, tr. Plemp (Louvain, 1658), prologue, fol. 3ʳ. In the course of a kind of medical grand tour of Europe financed by Jacob Fugger, Gryll, a pupil of Leonhart Fuchs and subsequently a professor at Ingoldstadt, visited the elder Scaliger at Agen. The information that "Is [Scaliger] Avicennae libros praecipuos ex Poenorum lingua in purum et tersum latinum sermonem convertit" presumably came from Scaliger himself. *Oratio de peregrinatione studii medicinalis . . . autore Laurentio Gryllo* (n.p., 1566), bound with *Laurentii Grylli . . . De sapore dulci et amaro* (Prague, 1566), fol. 7ʳ (and for Gryll's career, fol. 2ʳ⁻ᵛ). According to Joseph Scaliger, "Non repurgavit Avicennam pater Julius Scaliger, quanquam nonnulla forte haud spernenda in suo Avicennae libro annotaverat veluti scholia, quippe qui Arabicae linguae satis peritus esset, ut et vulgarium linguarum, plures loqui sciens quovis alio coaetaneo ac contemporaneo. Nescio num istum Avicennam cum scholiis nobis suffuratus fuerit plagiarius ille Constantinus qui nunc Montalbani medicinam facit. Hoc scio, non excudi Venetiis, ut ille dicebat tamen. Julius Scaliger Avicennae lectionem medicis omnibus tanquam pernecessariam commendabat nec quenquam in magnum medicum evadere posse existimabat, qui tam doctum opus non legisset." *Scaligerana, Thuana, Perroniana, Pithoeana, et Colomesiana* (Amsterdam, 1740), 2:25–26. Nutton, "John Caius and the Eton Galen," shows how important a hand-annotated copy of a printed edition could be for sixteenth-century medical scholarship.

1.1; and at the beginning of the seventeenth century, Fabio Paolino again turned to a Jewish collaborator to verify a passage. As Welsch noted, Paolino's co-worker Moses Alatino began to translate the *Canon* from Hebrew into Latin; however, this translation appears never to have been published.[25]

The wide dissemination of Mantino's translations and the frequent expressions of respect for the Hebrew version may perhaps serve as an indication of the very limited role of Arabic studies in the approach to the *Canon* in sixteenth-century medical circles outside Spain. Certainly, among Italian learned physicians Ramusio and Alpago were highly unusual in their substantial command of Arabic gained by residence in Arabic-speaking countries. Sixteenth-century Italian physicians were, perhaps, not much more likely to know Hebrew than they were to know Arabic, but in this regard they had the advantage of the presence of scholarly Jewish medical men who owned and used Hebrew medical manuscripts.

Until about mid-century a somewhat different situation prevailed in Spain, owing to the survival of elements of Arabic scientific culture. The medical curriculum prescribed in Spanish universities made use of the same Arabo-Latin works taught elsewhere in Europe; in Spain as elsewhere these works were fiercely attacked by humanist enthusiasts for Greek medicine. However, Arabic still survived as a spoken language; medical manuscripts in Arabic were preserved and circulated; some Judeo-*conversos* knew Arabic well; and a few Christian learned physicians could read some Arabic, even though, as Nicolas Clenard scornfully remarked, they did not know any Arabic grammar. In Spain, therefore, the development of a humanistic approach to the *Canon*, stressing its value as a guide to Galen and the need to remedy the faults of the old translation, took place in the context of relatively easy access to Arabic manuscripts and to fluent or native Arabic speakers.[26]

---

[25] " . . . quare Avicennas hoc titulo ornavit in *Canone*, cum secundum versionem Alatini Hebraei medici, hominis eruditissimi, apud quem manuscriptus extat codex Avicennae ex Arabica in Hebraeum linguam conversus a Rabi Moyse Aegyptio, quem mihi ille ostendit, ita sit titulus." *Praelectiones Marciae, sive Commentaria in Thucydidis Historiam, seu narrationem, de peste Athenensium ex ore Fabii Paulini Utinensis* (Venice, 1603), p. 181; *Canon* 4.3.2.21–22, ed. and tr. Welsch (Augsburg, 1674) b 4ᵛ. Moses Alatino's (1529–1605) testimony to his own translation of Book 1 of the *Canon* from Hebrew into Latin is noted in *Galen's Commentary on the Hippocratic Treatise Airs, Waters, Places in the Hebrew Translation of Solomon Ha-Me'ati*, ed. and tr. Abraham Wasserstein, *Proceedings of the Israel Academy of Sciences and Humanities*, vol. 6, pt. 3 (Jerusalem, 1982), p. 191. Alatino also translated this Galenic commentary from Hebrew into Latin.

[26] Garcia Ballester, *Los Moriscos*, pp. 19–51, provides an account of the limited inter-

Hence, in preparing his own version of *Canon* 1.1 (Valencia, 1547/
48), Miguel Jerónimo Ledesma, a professor of medicine at Valencia
who had been educated at the humanist center of Alcalá, was able to
draw not only upon Alpago's version (of which he was critical), but
also upon a "very old" (and perhaps Arabic?) manuscript in his own
possession, as well as upon the assistance of an associate "equally
skilled in the Arabic language and in medicine."[27] By these means Ledesma succeeded in producing what seems to be the only independent
new translation of a substantial section of the *Canon* directly from Arabic to appear in the sixteenth century. He accompanied his work with
a brief commentary, the main purpose of which appears to be to endorse Avicenna by demonstrating his dependence on Galen. Ledesma,
an ardent Platonist, was however occasionally critical of Avicenna because of his Aristotelianism.[28] Death prevented Ledesma from proceeding any further with his work on the *Canon*.[29] Judging by the in-
frequency with which it is cited in later editions and commentaries, his
version of *Canon* 1.1 did not achieve much circulation outside Spain.[30]
After about 1560, moreover, the increasing hostility of political and religious authorities to any manifestations of Arabic culture put an end to
any further developments along the same lines.[31]

Whether or not Mantino, Ledesma, and Cinqarbres succeeded in improving on Alpago's emendations of Gerard of Cremona, Alpago's
version, unlike any of theirs, encompassed the entire *Canon*. It was the
basis of yet another Junta edition published in 1555, with editorial ad-

---

action between Latin academic and Morisco culture in sixteenth-century Spanish medical
circles. Clenard's remark is quoted on p. 22.

[27] *Canon* 1.1, tr. Ledesma (Valencia, 1547–48), fols. 2ᵛ–3ʳ: "Cui labori praesto fuit ve-
tustissimus noster codex Avicennicus manu scriptus, longe a vulgato dissidens. Item Andreas Bellunensis novus interpres, atqui is aliquando Gentilis, aut Nicoli, aut alterius
cuiuspiam sententiam verius sequitur quam veritatem. Quibus praeter peculiaria nostra
investigandis linguarum proprietatibus studia, adde consultum fuisse socium Arabicae
linguae non minus quam rei medicae peritum." On Ledesma and his version, see Garcia
Ballester, *Los Moriscos*, pp. 24–28.

[28] "Hoc dixerim quia Avicenna philosophorum maximum appellat Aristotelem, Pla-
tonem autem unum ex primis philosophis, cuius sententiam apertiorem quidem esse sentit Aristotelica, at non aeque veram atque illam, nos vero longe veratiorem Platonis et
Galeni sermonem censemus." *Canon* 1.1, tr. Ledesma (Valencia, 1547–48), fol. 81ᵛ.

[29] Ibid., fols. 117ᵛ–[18ʳ].

[30] For example, I have not noticed any allusion to it in the prefaces of Kirsten (1609),
Plemp (1658), or Welsch (1674), all of which, as several times mentioned, contain much
information about earlier editions.

[31] Garcia Ballester, *Los Moriscos*, pp. 17, 55–57, 310–40. For the general cultural situation in Spain after the 1520s, see J. H. Elliott, *Imperial Spain* (New York, 1966), pp. 211–
14, 222–24.

ditions by Benedetto Rinio of Venice.[32] The most important new features of the Alpago-Rinio version were the insertion of Alpago's emendations into the body of the text and the provision of innumerable cross-references keying the *Canon* to passages in Greek and other medical authors. Printed for the first time with the *Canon* in this edition were Alpago's translations of two other short medical works by Avicenna.[33] This first Alpago-Rinio version was reissued almost unchanged at Basel in 1556. In 1562, however, Junta published a revised edition with the claim that it incorporated fresh emendations drawn by Rinio from manuscripts given him by Alpago's heirs.[34]

It might seem that the Alpago-Rinio presentation was destined to become the "revised standard version" of the Latin *Canon*. But in 1564 a major rival appeared in the shape of a two-volume edition of the *Canon* and the four short medical works prepared by Giovanni Costeo and Giovanni Mongio and published, also at Venice, by Valgrisio. It is, indeed, hard to avoid the impression that this edition was deliberately designed to compete with the revised Alpago-Rinio edition put out by Junta in 1562. Giovanni Costeo was a professor in the faculty of medicine at Bologna from 1581 until his death in 1603.[35] His best-known work was a set of "physiological disquisitions" (Bologna, 1589), which is in fact a commentary on *Canon* 1.1. Mongio appears to

[32] Rinio was a collateral descendant of an earlier Benedetto Rinio, author of an illuminated manuscript book of simples now in the Biblioteca Marciana (Lat. VI.59 [2548]), which was at one time in the younger Rinio's possession. See Ettore de Toni, "Il libro dei semplici di Benedetto Rinio," *Memorie della Pontificia Accademia Romana dei Nuovi Lincei*, 2nd ser., 5 (1919), 171–279, 7 (1924), 275–398, 8 (1925), 124–264, at 5 (1919), 173. The Rinio with whom we are here concerned apparently died before 1566, when his son Fabrizio prepared his father's brief *Tractatus de morbo gallico* for publication; see *De morbo gallico omnia quae extant*, 2 vols. in 1 (Venice, 1566), 2:14. That Rinio was a practicing physician is indicated both by this treatise, which is in fact a *consilium* for a priest, and also by his ownership of a collection of treatises on empirical medicine, namely *Benedicti Victorii Faventini . . . Opera* (Venice, 1550). The copy of the latter work at the New York Academy of Medicine contains Rinio's ownership signature and recipes in his hand on front and back flyleaves.

[33] *De removendis nocumentis, quae accidunt in regimine sanitatis* and *De syrupo acetoso*. Alpago's translation of these two works was first published along with his translation of two Arabic commentaries on parts of the *Canon* (Venice, 1547).

[34] "Novissime autem idem Rinius in hac editione toto volumine summa iterum diligentia perlecto, adhibitis etiam exemplaribus manu Alpagi scriptis (quorum copiam nuper nobis fecerunt eius haeredes) innumeris pene aliis tum castigationibus, tum locorum citationibus . . . illustravit." Title page, *Canon*, ed. Rinio (Venice, 1562).

[35] According to *Biogr. Lex.* 2:89–90; however, his name can be found in the Bologna *rotuli* only for the years 1581–98, when he held an extraordinary or supraordinary lectureship first in practical, and later in theoretical, medicine; see Dallari, *Rotuli*, vol. 2, under the years indicated.

have practiced medicine in Venice and Padua.[36] Costeo and Mongio printed the text in the Gerard of Cremona translation and supplied variant readings from both Alpago and, where available, Mantino; they also appended substantial annotations to most sections of the text. In addition, they provided each of the first four books of the *Canon* with its own preface in the shape of a letter from either or both of them to a different medical personality. Two of the individuals thus honored were professors of medical theory at Padua, and another held a similar position at Pavia; the fourth was the Paduan botanist Giacomo Antonio Cortusio. Book 1 was dedicated to Bernardino Paterno, the first professor of medical theory at Padua from 1563 until his death in 1592, and author of a commentary on *Canon* 1.1.[37] Paterno, at one time Costeo's teacher,[38] evidently had a more than nominal interest in the edition prepared by his former pupil; it was apparently on his advice that the editors decided to print the Gerard translation, relegating emendations to the margin, rather than incorporating them into the body of the text as Rinio had done.[39]

Nonetheless, in the eyes of Paterno and other contemporaries, the Costeo and Mongio edition still left room for improvement. In 1580, yet another version of Book 1 was produced by Andrea Graziolo, whose project acquired, as he informed his readers in his preface, the enthusiastic support not only of his own preceptor, Oddo Oddi,[40] but also of Paterno, Niccolò Sanmichele, and Fracastoro. It would thus appear that Graziolo's work was begun before Oddo's death in 1558, and was originally intended to improve upon the various Alpago and Al-

---

[36] C. G. Jöcher, *Allgemeines gelehrten Lexikon* (Leipzig, 1751), 3:615.

[37] On Paterno, in addition to Bertolaso, "Ricerche d'archivio" (1959–60), p. 23, see J. F. Tomasini, *Illustrium virorum elogia iconibus exornata* (Padua, 1630), pp. 151–53. The others are Niccolò Sanmichele and Francesco Modegnano, identified as professors of theory at Padua and Pavia respectively (although Sanmichele is not listed as a professor by Bertolaso). On Cortusio, from 1590 the third head of the Paduan botanic garden, see G. B. de Toni, "Spigolature Aldrovandiane XIX: Il botanico Giacomo Antonio Cortuso nelle sue relazione con Ulisse Aldrovandi e con altri naturalisti," in *Monografie storiche sullo Studio di Padova: Contributo del R. Istituto Veneto di Scienze, Lettere ed Arti alla celebrazione del VII Centenario della Università* (Venice, 1922), pp. 217–51.

[38] *Canon* (Venice, 1595), 1:101–2, referring to Paterno's time as a professor at Pisa, which, according to Fabroni, *Historiae academiae pisanae*, 2:468, occupied the years 1555–58.

[39] "Institutum autem in primis tuum sequuti, Paterne clarissime, antiquam versionem delegimus, puriorem certe et plerunque meliorem nisi paulo esset obscurior. Sed iam illustravimus varia lectione adhibita, quam in libri margine . . . apposuimus." *Canon* (Venice, 1564), dedication to Paterno preceding Book 1.

[40] *Canon* 1, tr. Graziolo (Venice, 1580). Graziolo referred to Oddi as his preceptor in his preface to the reader.

pago-Rinio editions—whence perhaps Graziolo's emphasis upon his use of wholly different sources, namely the *Canon* in Hebrew and in the translation left in manuscript by Ramusio.[41] But the project was evidently not completed until after the appearance of the first Costeo and Mongio edition in 1564, both because Graziolo asserted that he had only recently received the Ramusio manuscript—that is, presumably shortly before 1580—and because he identified the source of the manuscript as Sanmichele, a recipient of one of Costeo and Mongio's dedicatory letters. Presumably if the Ramusio manuscript had been in Sanmichele's possession when Costeo and Mongio were at work, he would have made it available to them. It thus seems reasonable to assume that Graziolo's efforts were perceived by his backers as an advance not only over those of Alpago and Rinio, but also over those of Costeo and Mongio. Furthermore, the personal, institutional, and regional links between the scholars involved in one way or another in the Costeo and Mongio and Graziolo editions[42] suggest that the sense of the importance of an improved understanding of the *Canon*, manifested in the endorsement given to Andrea Alpago's work by the Paduan College of Philosophers and Physicians in 1521 (in which Oddo Oddi took part),[43] was still very much alive in some Paduan professorial circles in the 1550s through the 1570s.

Graziolo's version of Book 1 was never reprinted. Of the two competing major editions of the complete work, that of Costeo and Mongio seems ultimately to have been the more successful. Rinio's revised edition was reprinted once by Junta in 1582. Thereafter, that press took over the edition of Costeo and Mongio, which subsequently appeared, revised and elaborated, in 1595 and again in 1608. The 1595 edition was characterized by revisions by Costeo, by the participation of Fabio Paolino of Udine, and by the publisher's reuse of supplementary material from earlier editions of the *Canon* from the same press. Attention is drawn to Costeo's revisions both on the title page and in the latter's single preface (now addressed to his colleagues in the College of Philosophers and Physicians of Bologna); their presence is signaled throughout Book 1 by references to his own "physiological disquisitions," published in 1589, and by the expansion of some of the annotations.

The multiple prefaces by Costeo and Mongio were dropped, pre-

---

[41] These and other statements in Graziolo's preface are discussed in d'Alverny, "Avicenne et les médecins de Venise," pp. 182–84.

[42] Similar ties bound some of those involved in the Alpago and Rinio editions. Lucchetta, *Alpago*, pp. 61–62, draws attention to the personal links betwen Paolo Alpago and Nicolò Massa; and we have seen that Rinio had the confidence of Alpago's heirs.

[43] Lucchetta, *Alpago*, p. 90.

sumably in the interests of modernization and in favor of the contributions of Fabio Paolino (1535–1604). The latter, who held a public lectureship in Greek at Venice, is perhaps best remembered as a Greek scholar, as the founder of the short-lived Accademia Uranica or degli Uranici at Venice, and as the author of a massive commentary on a single line of Virgil, which, according to D. P. Walker, presents "with remarkable completeness, not only the theory of Ficino's magic, but also the whole complex of theories of which it is a part."[44] However, Paolino also obtained a medical degree at Bologna and wrote medical works. Paolino's acknowledged contributions to the 1595 edition of the *Canon* consisted of an ode on the merits of Avicenna addressed to Lorenzo Massa,[45] an essay in Avicenna's defense addressed to "scholars of medicine" (*studiosis medicinae*), a complicated set of tables outlining the *Canon* and the medical *Isagoge* of Johannitius and intended to show that the plan of the two works was essentially the same, and a disquisition on the etymology and meanings of the word *canon* designed to justify its use in the title of Avicenna's work. From the earlier Junta editions came Nicolò Massa's life of Avicenna, a poem on the *Canon* by I. M. Rota first included in the edition of 1562 (a few lines in praise of Rinio that had accompanied this in the 1562 edition having been omitted), and the set of illustrations showing a turbaned physician reducing dislocations. The 1608 edition is a reprinting of that of 1595 with only minor changes.

So far as I have succeeded in determining, the two editions of the work of Costeo, Mongio, and Paolino were put together without reference to the most remarkable accomplishment in the Renaissance printing history of the *Canon*, namely the publication of that work in Arabic in Rome in 1593 by Giovan Battista Raimondi for the Stamperia Orientale Medicea. A remark of Paolino's in his prefatory letter to the 1595 edition to the effect that he foresaw that a good translation of the

[44] D. P. Walker, *Spiritual and Demonic Magic from Ficino to Campanella* (reprint; Notre Dame, 1975), p. 126. On Paolino and the Uranici in general, see ibid., pp. 126–42. Walker also throws light on a possible reason for the interest of Paolino in the *Canon* when he notes on p. 162, "Erastus' most violent attack on Ficino is as a follower of Avicenna." On Paolino's career, see G. G. Liruti, *Notizie delle vite ed opere scritte da' letterati del Friuli* (Venice, 1760), 3:352–72, and Pietro Someda da Marco, *Medici Forojuliensi dal sec. XIII al sec. XVIII* (Udine, 1963), pp. 70–71. The date of Paolino's death is established as 16 September 1604, by ASV, Provveditori alla Sanità, Reg. 832, *Necrologio*, anno 1604. I have not seen this document and owe the reference, as also the information that the dates of Paolino's lectureship in Venice are established by documentary evidence as 1588–1604, to Richard Palmer.

[45] Lorenzo Massa was a nephew of Nicolò and a successful Venetian official; see Palmer, "Nicolò Massa."

Canon would shortly be made by scholars who had learned Arabic may perhaps imply awareness of the Rome edition and of the aids to the study of Arabic also published by the Medici press. He may even have intended to embark on such a translation himself, since according to a late source he is said to have learned Arabic. However, his acknowledged contributions to the 1595 edition show no signs of knowledge of that language, and indeed include a comment that leaves little doubt that he did not know it at that time.[46] Furthermore, as already noted, a section of Paolino's commentary on Thucydides' description of the plague in Athens (Venice, 1603) shows that when he wrote that work he relied on consultation with a Jewish physician who owned a Hebrew translation to verify the text of the *Canon*.[47] As for Costeo, it is certainly conceivable that the printed Arabic text was not available when he was making his last revisions sometime between 1589 and 1595. This could scarcely have been the case when the 1608 edition was prepared (the Rome, 1593, edition was available to Peter Kirsten by 1609).[48] But by 1608 Costeo and Paolino (and probably also Mongio, who seems not to have taken part in the 1595 revision) were dead, and their work was simply reissued without significant alteration. Since the Venice, 1608, edition was the last major scholarly publication of the *Canon* to be produced in Italy, it is appropriate to defer consideration of the impact of Raimondi's Arabic publications upon the study of the *Canon* in European medical schools until the story of the Latin editions published in Italy is brought to a close.

After 1608, these editions all consisted of small volumes produced to supply the market among students created by the continued survival of parts of the *Canon* in the curriculum of the Italian universities, notably Padua. Thus, editions of *Canon* 1.1 appeared at Vicenza in 1611, along with Galen's *Ars*; at Padua "for the use of the University of Padua" in 1636; with the *Aphorisms* of Hippocrates and the *Ars* at Padua in 1648. Both *Canon* 1.1 and 4.1 were included along with the *Aphorisms* and the *Ars* in a little book called *Schola medica* published at Venice in 1647. *Canon* 4.1 was also published by itself at Padua in 1659. All of these presumably cheap little books presented the Gerard translation without

---

[46] "In quo melius fortasse, et gratius fecissent, si vicem tanti scriptoris, et optime de se meriti dolentes, Arabum percepta lingua, in qua aureum illius esse dicendi genus tradunt, latine eum loqui explosa barbarie fecissent, quod tamen auguror brevi fore." Paolino, prefatory epistle to "medicinae studiosis," *Canon*, ed. Costeo, Mongio, Paolino (Venice, 1595). The statement that Paolino learned Arabic comes from Liruti, but Paolino's own use of the word *tradunt* in this passage does not appear to imply personal knowledge.

[47] Paolino, *Praelectiones Marciae*, p. 181.

[48] *Canon* 2, ed. and tr. Kirsten (Breslau, 1609), p. 7.

scholarly apparatus. Usually, *Canon* 1.1 was printed without the anatomical chapters traditionally omitted in lecturing (although they are present in the edition published at Padua in 1648). As a result, the author of a preface included in two of these editions could without any apparent sense of incongruity refer to Avicenna's "opusculum."[49] The author of the preface to the edition of *Canon* 1.1 issued at Padua in 1636 referred approvingly to the "prudent institution of our ancestors" that had secured for Avicenna a place in the curriculum of the Italian schools.[50] The editors of the *Schola medica* displayed a somewhat more realistic appraisal of the actual nature of their readers' interest in Avicenna by including a list of "points for examination that are commonly propounded to degree candidates in the most famous schools" (*puncta quae laureandis proponi solent in celeberrimis collegiis*.)[51]

Looking back over the history of the publications of the *Canon* in sixteenth- and seventeenth-century Italy, one is struck by the prominent role played by the Junta press of Venice in the production of major new Latin editions of the *Canon*. Junta was responsible for the most lavish and comprehensive of the editions with older commentary (1523), for both the editions prepared by Paolo Alpago (1527, 1544), for the first edition of Mantino's translation of *Canon* 1.4, for three of the four editions of Rinio's work (1555, revised 1562, 1582), and for the revised and expanded Costeo, Mongio, and Paolino edition and its reprinting (1595, 1608). The Junta press was one of the largest Venetian printing and publishing houses, so that its predominance in the publication of the *Canon* may be merely a reflection of the firm's general position. Yet the successive editions of the *Canon* were issued across a period in which the general tendency in the Venetian book trade was toward contraction in the numbers of medical and related titles published and expansion of the religious list (the latter no doubt in response to the shifting demand, the official constraints, and the economic opportunities associated with the Counter Reformation). Given the rep-

---

[49] Preface to edition of Vicenza, 1611, reprinted before *Canon* 1.1 in *Schola medica* (Venice, 1647) (the sections of the *Canon* in *Schola medica* are separately paginated). Books such as these presumably served the need supplied in the preceding century by the *articella*, the abbreviations and compendia, and perhaps also the translations of Jacob Mantino, all of which circulated in small and doubtless inexpensive volumes. That there was also some market among students for the large folio editions with extensive modern apparatus is indicated by the gifts of such volumes to the library of the German Nation at Padua, discussed in the preceding chapter.

[50] "Prudenti majorum instituto usque ad nostram memoriam Avicennae dogmata Italiae Gymnasia retinuerunt." *Canon* 1.1 (Padua, 1636), p. 3.

[51] *Schola medica* (Venice, 1647), p. 143. The *puncta* from the two sections of the *Canon* occupy pp. 143–45.

utation of the Venice branch of the Junta press for a certain pragmatism in the selection of titles for publication, their output of editions of the *Canon* surely suggests the existence not merely of a market for copies but of a steady demand for continued revision and updating on the work's presentation from the 1520s to the end of the century.[52] While such demand was not necessarily confined to the Italian schools, the program of publication was presumably chiefly stimulated by local conditions.

In turning at last to the edition of the *Canon* in Arabic published by G. B. Raimondi in 1593, we encounter a deservedly famous episode in the development of Arabic studies in Europe, in which Raimondi's achievement in printing Arabic scientific books and that of Robert Granjon in incising an Arabic typeface superior to any produced earlier are notable landmarks.[53] Raimondi's accomplishment, however, appears to have had relatively slight impact on the medical scene. This was largely a consequence of the very different priorities of the Medici press and of Raimondi's incompetence in business; but it also reflected

[52] Paolo Camerini, *Annali dei Giunti.* I. *Venezia,* pt. 1 (Florence, 1962), p. 23, characterizes the publication policy of the Venetian branch as "fondata su libri di facile smercio." Much information about the Venetian book trade is contained in Martin Lowry, *The World of Aldus Manutius: Business and Scholarship in Renaissance Venice* (Oxford, 1979), and Paul F. Grendler, *The Roman Inquisition and the Venetian Press, 1540–1605* (Princeton, 1977). According to Grendler, the Giunti (Junta) press specialized in liturgical works, for which there was a large demand, and averaged a total of about ten editions a year, in all categories, throughout the sixteenth century; a normal press run was about 1,000 copies (pp. 4, 5, 10). The same author's survey of imprimaturs for new titles in Venice between 1551 and 1607, shows that in this period the average annual output of religious titles rose from 15.6 to 34.9 percent of the total number of editions, while the proportion of medical and related titles declined from 7.1 to 3.7 percent (ibid., p. 132).

[53] On Raimondi and the Stamperia Orientale Medicea, see J. R. Jones, "The Arabic and Persian Studies of Giovan Battista Raimondi, ca. 1536–1614" (M. Phil. diss., Warburg Institute, University of London, 1981); G. E. Saltini, "Della Stamperia Orientale Medicea e di Giovan Battista Raimondi," *Giornale storico degli archivi toscani* 4 (1860), 257–308; Berta Maria Biagiarelli, "La Biblioteca Medicea Laurenziana. Una nova sala per l'altrezzatura della Stamperia Orientale (sec. XVI)," *Accademie e biblioteche d'Italia,* anno 39, n.s., 22 (1971), 83–99; A. Bertolotti, "Le tipografie orientali e gli orientalisti a Roma nei secoli XVI e XVII," *Rivista europea* 9 (1878), 217–68. All of these articles make use of the substantial collections of Raimondi's papers that survive in the six *filze* of the Stamperia Orientale Medicea in the Archivio di Stato, Florence, and in a number of manuscripts in the Biblioteca Nazionale Centrale, Florence; the latter are fully described in Jones, "Raimondi," Appendix IV. On the development of Arabic studies in sixteenth- and seventeenth-century Europe in general, see Johann Fück, *Die arabischen Studien in Europa bis in den Anfang des 20. Jahrhunderts* (Leipzig, 1955); also Klein-Franke, *Die klassische Antike,* pp. 43–95, and Karl H. Dannenfeldt, "The Renaissance Humanists and the Knowledge of Arabic," *Studies in the Renaissance* 2 (1955), 96–117.

the nature of the demand for the *Canon* within the medical community. The Stamperia Orientale Medicea, established by Cardinal Ferdinando de' Medici in 1584 under papal auspices and for missionary ends, had as its primary purpose the printing of the gospels and other apologetic material in Arabic for distribution in the Middle East. However, Raimondi also printed Arabic grammars and scientific books in Arabic, namely Euclid's *Elements*, Edrisi's *Geography*, and the *Canon*. The scientific and the religious publications were primarily intended for distribution among schismatic Oriental Christians and Moslems in the Middle East, on the theory that the usefulness of works in the first category would ensure them a welcome that would somehow be extended to those in the second. The accession of Cardinal de' Medici as Grand Duke of Tuscany ended his active support of the enterprise. In 1596, Raimondi undertook to buy the press, but as he proved unable to meet the terms agreed on, in 1610 it reverted to Medici ownership, with Raimondi as curator for life. After his death in 1614, the press ceased to function, and the typefaces, manuscripts, and printed books belonging to it were returned for storage to its grand-ducal owner.[54] Throughout its brief history, the press was plagued by financial problems, since the output never seems to have brought the return envisaged in various agreements dividing the books to be sold between Raimondi and the Cardinal–Grand Duke. The latter divested himself of the press in 1596 in part because it represented a constant drain on his resources; Raimondi was unable to meet the terms of his purchase contract because he was not making sufficient profit to do so.[55]

There is no doubt that Raimondi's own concerns were to some extent scientific as well as religious. In his youth, he supposedly had mathematical and alchemical interests.[56] Furthermore, the importance of Arabic sources for science was one—but only one—of eleven reasons put forward by Raimondi that Arabic studies should be fostered at Rome (of the other ten reasons, eight had to do with religion and two with the dignity of the city of Rome). The sciences that Raimondi thought would gain most benefit from the encouragement of the study of Arabic were mathematics and medicine.[57] While there appears to be no evidence that Raimondi himself had any medical training, he was clearly appreciative of Arabic medicine. The *Canon* was the largest project undertaken by the press[58] and the most important scientific work of Arabic origin to be printed there. Medical books constituted

[54] Saltini, "Della Stamperia Orientale," pp. 257–98.   [55] Ibid., pp. 276–80.
[56] Ibid., pp. 264–65.   [57] Jones, "Raimondi," p. 190.
[58] Fück, *Die arabischen Studien*, p. 54.

one of the largest categories, with forty-one titles, of the impressive library of Arabic manuscripts collected for the press from sources in the Middle East. (For purposes of comparison it may be noted that books on Islam comprised forty-six items, books on mathematics over fifty, and books on philosophy nineteen.)[59] Raimondi tied his esteem for Arabic medicine especially to pharmacology, remarking that the Arabic language was "useful for the knowledge of the science of medicine, the Arabs having found doses and measures of drugs and medicaments, and there being in this profession eminent authors known among us, such as Avicenna, Rasis, Mesue, Alfarabi, and others, but very badly translated on account of the small knowledge until now of this language."[60] Furthermore, his interest in Arabic technical vocabulary in anatomy is evident in the lexical lists on this subject that he compiled, alone or in collaboration with others.[61]

Moreover, translation as well as printing was mentioned as part of the *Canon* project when it was set in motion by an order of Cardinal de' Medici in 1584.[62] The committee named to supervise the work included one medical member, namely Gian Battista Lucchese, identified as physician to Cardinal Savello. Dr. Lucchese's role must have been to give technical advice on medicine; J. R. Jones has drawn attention to

[59] Florence, BNC, MS II.III.13 (Magl. cl. 3, 130), "Raimundi (Jo. Baptistae) Catalogus codicum orientalium." The book lists occupy fols. 8ᵛ–49ᵛ; Arabic medical books, fols. 11ᵛ–13ʳ; books on Islam, fols. 23ᵛ–24ᵛ; mathematics, fols. 27ʳ–29ᵛ; philosophy fols. 8ᵛ–9ʳ.

[60] ASF, SOM, *filza* 3, document 21, plea for establishment of a chair of Arabic in Rome: the Arabic language "E utile per la cognitione della scientie, di medicina havendo gli Arabi ritrovati le dose e misure dei farmachi, e medicamenti." For a similar statement by Jakob Christmann, contemporary proponent of the study of Arabic in Germany, see Jones, "Raimondi," p. 22.

[61] Florence, BNC, MS II.III.15 (Magl. cl. 3, 119), "Raimundi (Jo. Baptistae) Excerpta vocabulorum Arabicorum anatomes etc. et fragmenta ex Avicenna cum latina versione eiusdem." The anatomical vocabulary occupies fols. 1ʳ–6ᵛ, 11ʳ–20ʳ. Jones believes that these and other lexical lists in Raimondi's hand were the result of teamwork ("Raimondi," p. 126).

[62] ASF, SOM, *filza* 3, document 20, fol. 1ʳ⁻ᵛ: "Comando che con l'occasione similmente del detto Patriarca si traducessero fidelmente et perfettamente l'opere d'Avicenna et si stampessero in Arabico et in Latino, al questo fu dato ordine et si institui una congregatione in casa del detto Patriarca et si comincio questa fatica a 17 d'Agosto del 84. Nella congregatione intervengono:
Il Patriarca soppradetto
Gio. Battista Lucchese, medico dell'Illustrissimo Signor Cardinale Savello;
Paolo Orsino di natione Turco ma fatto christiano;
Gio. Battista Raimondo."
Katherine Tachau was kind enough to recheck this passage for me. The document appears to be a rough draft.

the presence in one of Raimondi's personal notebooks of a Latin translation of a few short passages from the first two *doctrinae* of Canon 1.1,
along with the Arabic text, which clearly show that Raimondi planned
to do the actual translating himself.[63] The method adopted in these passages, as Jones has pointed out, was to use the translation of Gerard of
Cremona with Alpago's emendations as a base, and add a few further
emendations, so perhaps it would be more appropriate to speak of a revised rather than a new translation.[64] But Raimondi's effort (unlike
those of Rinio, Costeo, Mongio, and Graziolo) was based on direct
confrontation of the existing Latin version with an Arabic text that Raimondi fully understood. Hence his procedures were not much different from those used to produce some of the "new" Renaissance translations of Greek medical texts. However, any plans Raimondi may
have entertained for publishing a translation came to nothing.

There is, moreover, some evidence that Raimondi had contacts with
a few medical men, who drew upon his collection of Arabic manuscripts and his expertise. Thus, in June 1596, Francisco Capitano borrowed a copy of "Avicenna" in Latin from Raimondi, returning it the
next month.[65] In June 1602, Capitano borrowed *Canon* 3 in Arabic, and
in August, *Canon* 1 (he returned both volumes together in October). In
1611, Mario Sclepani, *medico*, wrote to Raimondi from Naples describing his own struggle to learn Arabic, which he had wanted to know
ever since he started to study philosophy and medicine, and asking Raimondi's advice about a point of translation. Sclepani expressed the
conviction that just as, in the fifteenth century, Medici patronage of
Greek scholarship had contributed much to the advance of philosophy,
medicine, and other sciences, so now their patronage of the spread of
knowledge of Arabic would lead to similar benefits, chief among
which he counted the advantage for medicine of the possibility of a
faithful Latin translation of the *Canon* and other Arabic works "which
we use in practice." Sclepani's remarks must have rung ironically in the
ears of Raimondi, who, over time, had found Medici patronage to be

[63] Florence, BNC, MS II.III.15 (Magl. cl. 3, 119), fols. 10ᵛ–7ʳ. Raimondi's translation
of the chapter on the elements (*Canon* 1.1.2) is edited, with the Arabic text, in Jones,
"Raimondi," Appendix VI.

[64] Jones, "Raimondi," p. 126. A further glimpse of Raimondi's method is provided by
BNC Florence, MS II.III.14 (Magl. cl. 3, 129), fols. 165ʳ–68ᵛ, in which fragments of the
Canon in Arabic alternate with Italian translation. The same manuscript contains a note
(fol. 126ᵛ) of an instance in which Avicenna openly differed from Galen.

[65] ASF, SOM, *filza* 2, document 24, list of books loaned by Raimondi, 1591–1605.
There are about twenty borrowers in all, many of them borrowing several books on different occasions. By no means are all the books Arabic. Capitano seems to be the only
borrower of the *Canon* on this list.

somewhat unreliable. Perhaps that accounts for the slightly acerbic tone of Raimondi's reply, in which he informed Sclepani unsympathetically that he had access to many aids to learning Arabic (presumably the grammars published by Raimondi himself) that had been unavailable when he, Raimondi, first began to study the language. Still, he commented on Sclepani's comments on the resemblances between Arabic and Hebrew patiently enough, and sent him a copy of the *Canon* in Arabic, a vocabulary, and a grammar. Sclepani's specific inquiry displayed an interest in the *Canon* as a source of Arabic pharmacology rather than as a compendium of Galenic theory; he wanted to know the Arabic term for and the meaning of a plant name latinized as *anarcine* in *Canon* 5, whether the same Arabic term occurred in *Canon* 2, and how the plant in question was described in the Arabic herbal in Raimondi's possession. To this inquiry, Raimondi's reply was full and detailed, and included a translation of the appropriate entry from his Arabic herbal.[66] This exchange of letters certainly suggests that Raimondi had at least some reputation among the contemporary Italian medical community as a source of information about Arabic medical terminology.

One might expect that Raimondi's printed Arabic *Canon* would have had far wider influence among physicians than he himself could ever have had as an individual. Such does not seem to have been the case, at any rate as far as the Italian universities were concerned. This conclusion rests not only on the absence of reference to his work in the late sixteenth- and seventeenth-century editions produced in Italy, but also on the lack of any display of knowledge of or interest in Arabic linguistics or philology in the commentaries of Italian provenance in this period. Thus, in the 1620s Santorio Santorio, a commentator noteworthy both for scholastic learning and for scientific innovation, solved problems of interpretation by comparing different Latin versions of the *Canon*.[67] Of course, one must remember that the pharmacological portions of the work, where new linguistic information was most likely to be thought useful, were not usually the subject of commentary because they were not assigned as textbooks.

In reality, it seems likely that the European distribution of Raimondi's edition was extremely limited. The Stamperia Orientale never worked out a wholly satisfactory means of distributing its products. The plan was that some of the books would be shipped in bulk to the Middle East. Direct distribution in the Middle East was always diffi-

---

[66] ASF, SOM, *filza* 5, fols. 327ʳ–28ᵛ, letter of Mario Sclepani, medico, to Raimondi, dated from Naples, 4 February 1611; fols. 329ʳ–32ʳ, two drafts, or copies, of Raimondi's reply, dated from Rome, 26 April 1611.

[67] Santorio, comm. *Canon* 1.1 (Venice, 1646), col. 72, for example.

cult, in part because permission from often hostile local authorities had to be secured and in part because misprints on the title pages of the *Canon* and the Euclid are said to have given a poor impression of the books.[68] Books were also to be sent for sale at the Frankfurt book fair, and in addition, some were sold or given to individuals by Raimondi in Rome.[69] As already mentioned, ownership of the books was at different times differently divided between the Ferdinando de' Medici and Raimondi, and Raimondi was supposed to recoup an income from the sale of his allotment.

In the case of the *Canon* the edition was, for the time, ambitiously large, so it is clear substantial demand was envisaged. Raimondi was originally instructed to print 1,000 copies at the cardinal's expense, but allowed to print more at his own expense if he wished[70] (presumably for sale for his own profit). Accordingly, he printed 1,750 or 1,760 copies.[71] Raimondi certainly shared Ferdinando de' Medici's missionary goals, but it seems possible that his desire to print copies over and above the cardinal's estimate was also inspired by the hope that the book might, in addition, find some market among European medical practitioners. In the event, about half the edition was never sold at all, in either East or West: in the eighteenth century 810 copies were still in the possession of the grand duke of Tuscany.[72] The fate of the rest of the copies—over 900 of them—cannot be determined, but apparently few were sold in Europe. Repeated visits to the press from a Flemish book merchant inquiring when the *Canon* would be ready for sale doubtless confirmed Raimondi's optimistic evaluation of the demand for the book. Alas, the Fleming lost patience and entered into a conspiracy with an employee of the press who stole about sixty-five copies, which ended up at the Frankfurt book fair on sale at a cut price. When Raimondi's authorized representative arrived at the fair with bales of copies of the *Canon* the following year, 1594—a season in which, admittedly, the fair was poorly attended owing to torrential rain and political troubles in eastern Europe—he found that the sale of those sixty-five copies had been sufficient to kill the demand for any

[68] Flück, *Die arabischen Studien*, p. 55; Saltini, "Della Stamperia Orientale," p. 27.

[69] Sclepani was not the only such case, but will serve as an example; see n. 66, above. For others, ASF, SOM, *filza* 2, document 25, fols. 6ᵛ, 7ʳ, 14ʳ, 32ʳ.

[70] ASF, SOM, *filza* 3, document 16, letter from Cardinal de' Medici to Raimondi, undated.

[71] Bertolotti, "Le tipografie orientali," p. 220.

[72] Saltini, "Della Stamperia Orientale," p. 293. In 1690, moreover, much of the material from the press, which presumably may have included yet more copies of the *Canon*, was destroyed by fire (ibid., p. 292). I have not attempted to investigate when the copies of the work found in major European libraries today were acquired.

more, especially at the full price. He was able to dispose of only one copy, which went to English merchants doing business with Levantine and North African merchants.[73] Whether Raimondi was able to sell copies of the *Canon* in any number thereafter is not known, but his continued financial straits seem to make it unlikely. The *Canon* was his most expensive item[74] and the sale of any significant number of copies would presumably have improved his fortunes.

The failure to market any substantial number of copies of the Arabic *Canon* in Europe contrasts strongly with the repeated issue and presumably successful sale of editions of the *Canon* in Latin by the hard-headed businessmen of the house of Junta. Raimondi's inability to sell his books to European physicians was no doubt in large part because such sales were for him a very secondary objective, if indeed they were ever deliberately planned at all, and because his scholarly idealism predominated over his business sense. But demand was in any case inevitably limited because few professors of medicine or medical practitioners knew Arabic. Of the many university-trained physicians and medical students who still valued the *Canon*, who believed that modern scholarship either had enhanced or was about to enhance its value, and who wanted to be assured that the editions at their disposal embodied the latest results of scholarship in Latin form, very few were likely to make a personal commitment to the arduous task of mastering Arabic. For the great majority, their own intellectual capabilities, limited access to Arabic books and teachers (even in the seventeenth century), and above all, their scientific and professional priorities must all have dictated a decision to rest content with Latin and perhaps some Greek. As Pietro Castelli put it, in a description of the qualifications of the ideal physician first published in 1637, a physician "cannot be deficient in Latin without great turpitude; he cannot be deficient in Greek without a certain turpitude. . . . But although I would greatly commend anyone who was skilled in Arabic . . . , I praise his knowledge, I do not require it."[75] Raimondi's correspondent, the Neapolitan physician

---

[73] Raimondi prosecuted both his disloyal employee and the Flemish merchant, and many of the documents of the case are preserved in the original or in contemporary copies in ASF, SOM, *filza* 1, pt. II. Bertolotti, "Le tipografie orientali," gives a detailed account of the episode. The evidence of Nicandro Filippini, Raimondi's authorized emissary to the Frankfurt fair, is contained in a deposition in ASF, SOM, *filza* 3, document 25; the interrogation of Gaspare the Fleming is recorded in ASF, SOM, *filza* 1, pt. II, fols. 234^r–241^r, documents 80–81.

[74] Fück, *Die arabischen Studien*, p. 53; Raimondi's price for the *Canon* was 18 scudi per copy.

[75] After stressing that literary elegance, in any language, should not be required of a physician, Castelli added: "sermone latino non possit carere . . . sine magna turpitudine,

Sclepani, was perfectly correct in suggesting that the chief use of the printed *Canon* in Arabic for European medicine would be to serve as a basis for translation—and for that few copies were needed. Thus, use of the printed Arabic *Canon* as a source was one of the features distinguishing some partial translations produced in northern Europe between 1609 and 1674.[76] These, however, came too late to have much actual impact on medical teaching and practice.

The four seventeenth-century editions or translations of parts of the *Canon* issued in northern Europe are the product of a scholarly milieu in many ways very different from that of the earlier (or the contemporary Italian) publications of the work. The late sixteenth and early seventeenth centuries were a time in which classical studies developed new techniques of editing and criteria of scholarly rigor, and the study of Oriental languages by Europeans was greatly advanced. In both these developments, Joseph Scaliger was a figure of great influence; by 1600, the University of Leiden, at which he taught, had become the chief center of Oriental studies in Europe.[77] Although the scholars responsible for the northern European translations and editions of parts of the *Canon* had medical qualifications and medical interests, the context of their work was primarily that of contemporary developments in classical and Oriental studies, rather than that of medical science. All four of these editions contained a new Latin translation of a section of the *Canon* made directly from the Arabic; two of them also edited the corresponding portions of the Arabic text. The supplementary mate-

Graeco non sine turpitudine solum. . . . Sed equidem illum quoque mirum in modum commendarem qui Arabici peritus esset sermonus . . . verum scientiam laudo, non requiro." *Petri Castelli . . . Optimus medicus, in quo conditiones perfectissimi medici exponuntur* (1637), in Hermann Conring, *In universam artem medicam . . . introductio* (Helmstadt, 1687), pp. 28–29. A somewhat similar assessment to Castelli's was reached by Jan van Beverwijck: "Doctrina autem in medico requiritur non vulgaris. Primum linguarum cognitio. Et de Latina quidem silere praestat, quam pauca dicere. Graeca absque maxime rerum ignoratione carere non potest. . . . Arabicae linguae ac Arabum medicorum, qui Graecis non pauca addidere, ex puris potius fontibus quam depravatis interpretum rivulis haurienda, scientiam medico admodum necessariam esse." *Joh. Beverovicii Medicinae encomium* (Rotterdam, 1644), p. 51.

[76] In the prefaces to their editions and translations Kirsten (1609), Plemp (1658), Rolfinck (1667), and Welsch (1674) all acknowledged the use of the edition of Rome, 1593.

[77] On Scaliger, see Anthony Grafton, *Joseph Scaliger: A Study in the History of Classical Scholarship. I. Textual Criticism and Exegesis* (Oxford, 1983). On Arabic studies in the Netherlands, Fück, *Die arabischen Studien*, pp. 64–79; and J. Brugman and F. Schröder, *Arabic Studies in the Netherlands*, Publications of the Netherlands Institute of Archaeology and Arabic Studies in Cairo (Leiden, 1979), 3:3–21, 48–49. On the related development of Hebrew studies at Leiden, see also Aaron L. Katchen, *Christian Hebraists and Dutch Rabbis* (Cambridge, Mass., 1984), pp. 1–100.

rial provided by the editors and translators is without precedent in the history of printed editions of the *Canon*: in three or four cases it included, in addition to useful summaries of the history of textual scholarship on the *Canon*, discussions of Arabic manuscripts used, as well as scholia dealing with problems of Arabic philology or manuscript readings. Of the scholars responsible, Peter Kirsten (1575–1640), who published an edition and translation of *Canon* 2 in 1609, had studied several other Oriental languages besides Arabic.[78] While he believed *Canon* 2 to be highly useful for medical practice, and had been told by Joseph Scaliger himself that "a true physician could better do without Latin than without Arabic or Greek,"[79] Kirsten valued the knowledge of Arabic at least as much for religious purposes as for science and medicine. His version of Book 2 of the *Canon* was one of a set of supplements to illustrate his Arabic grammar; others contained annotations on the four gospels and lives of the evangelists in Arabic.[80]

A project more exclusively medical in scope was undertaken by Vopiscus Fortunatus Plemp, a professor of medicine at Louvain who is chiefly remembered for his initial opposition to and subsequent acceptance of Harvey's teachings. For thirty years Plemp labored over the preparation of an edition and translation of the complete *Canon*, which he planned to publish with Arabic and Latin on facing pages, accompanied with copious scholia. However, the volume finally issued in 1658 contained only his Latin translation of Books 1 and 2 and Book 4, Part 1, along with relatively brief annotations of those sections. Plemp explained to his readers that he had resigned himself to the initial publication of only this portion of his work on account of the lack of locally available Arabic type, the small number of people in Christendom who knew Arabic (and the even smaller number who might be expected to know it in the future) and, above all, the representations of his publisher.[81]

---

[78] Kirsten, *Grammatices*, 1:3. On Kirsten (1577–1640), who became rector of the University of Breslau, see Jöcher, *Lexikon*, 2:2105–7.

[79] " 'Verus medicus potius linguam latinam carere posset, quam vel Arabicam, vel Graecam,' " Kirsten, *Grammatices*, 1:7. This may be contrasted with the more pragmatic views of the physician Pietro Castelli (see n. 75, above).

[80] *Petri Kirsteni . . . Notae in Evangelium S. Matthaei ex collatione textuum arabicorum, aegyptiacorum, hebraeorum, syriacorum, graecorum, latinorum* (Breslau [1611]), and *Petri Kirsteni . . . Vitae Evangelistarum quatuor: nunc primum ex antiquissimo codice manuscripto arabico Caesario erutae* (Breslau, [1608]). Use of Arabic in connection with biblical studies was often advocated in the seventeenth century; the brief lives of the evangelists presumably came from an Oriental Christian source.

[81] *Canon* 1, 2, 4.1, tr. Plemp (Louvain, 1658), fol. 2[v]. On Plemp (1601–71), who was a

No further volumes of Plemp's edition and translation ever appeared, but in the following year, 1659, Pierre Vattier, physician to the duke of Orleans and the author of treatises and translations, some of them in French, on various aspects of Middle Eastern or Moslem culture, published at Paris a Latin translation of some excerpts from *Canon* 3.1 having to do with mental disease.[82] In his preface, Vattier made a point of stressing that his translation from Arabic was completely his own, and that he had not followed the practice, so common even among great men in the past, of simply making interpolations in an older translation.[83] Finally, at Augsburg in 1674, Welsch, a practicing physician who had studied at Padua, published his edition and translation of two chapters of *Canon* 4.3 on parasites.[84] In Welsch's translation, the two chapters occupy four pages; they are accompanied by more than 450 pages of commentary and addenda, many of which seem designed to appeal to Arabists, philologists, mythologers, and historians at least as much as to physicians.

Each of these four scholars, Kirsten, Plemp, Vattier, and Welsch, presented his work as a "specimen" or portion of a larger project, but none of them appears to have produced any more work on the *Canon.* Whether their editions aroused much interest in northern European medical schools or among scholars of Oriental languages, I am not in a position to say, although the former seems improbable. Certainly, their efforts had little impact upon the practice of lecturing on the *Canon* in the medical faculties of the Italian universities. Alone among this group, Plemp chose to translate parts of the *Canon* still prescribed as textbooks, and as G. B. Morgagni had occasion to remark, Plemp's translation did not displace that of Gerard of Cremona in the Italian schools.[85] Conceivably the appearance of Plemp's work may have been

---

professor at Louvain from 1633 until his death, see G. A. Lindeboom, *Dutch Medical Biography* (Amsterdam, 1984), cols. 1544–46.

[82] On Vattier, see Moritz Steinschneider, *Die europäischen Übersetzungen aus dem Arabischen bis Mitte des 17. Jahrhunderts,* Sitzungsberichten der Kais. Akademie der Wissenschaften in Wien, Philosophisch-Historische Klasse, 149 (Vienna, 1904), p. 79, no. 117.

[83] "Novam hanc versionem a me non ex vetere interpolatam, sed vere ac plane novam factam esse. Hoc ideo dico, quod ex eiusmodi interpolatione magni viri non parvam nec sane immeritam laudem consecuti sint, Iacobus Sylvius ex Mesue librorum trium, Vesalius ex nono Rhasis ad Almansorem; vanitatis tamen in hoc cujusdam non absolvendi, qui ex Arabico horum autorum sermone Latinum suum expressisse videri quasi voluerint, qui neque aspexerant unquam, neque si aspexissent, ullam eius literam legere potuissent, homines alias quidem doctissimi, sed in Arabum idiomate prorsus hospites, magis ingenue facturi." *Canon* 3.1 (excerpts), tr. Vattier (Paris, 1659), dedicatory letter.

[84] Welsch (1624–77) was the author of a number of other medical works, all of which appear from their titles to be on practical aspects of medicine; see *Biogr. Lex.,* 6:236–37.

[85] "Quem librum Vopiscus Fortunatus Plempius, ante hos quinque et quinquaginta

155

a factor in discouraging further reprintings by Italian presses of any of the major editions of the *Canon* produced in the second half of the sixteenth century, but given other seventeenth-century developments it scarcely seems necessary to invoke this explanation.

Thus, the output of *Canon* editions after 1608 reflects, on the one hand, an outgrowth of a development of Arabic studies that doubtless came too late to have much impact on medical learning and, on the other, the durability of sections of the oldest Latin translation of the work as introductory medical textbooks and, in a sense, as medical classics. Quite different in character from either of these types is the series of publications of the complete *Canon*, or a major part of it, that began in 1522 with the first edition to show awareness of humanist criticism of Avicenna and ended with the appearance of the last major edition to be published in Italy in 1608. Most of the scholars involved in the production of this group of editions were primarily concerned with the *Canon* as a means of transmission of Galenic medical teaching and Greco-Arabic pharmacology, rather than with the study of Arabic. But they were equally far from commending the *Canon* solely as a book to be assigned to students because the tradition was bequeathed by "the prudent institution of our ancestors."

Instead, diverse though the editions they produced were, the Italian scholarly editors and revisers (and doubtless also their publishers) seem to have shared two common goals. The first was to present the *Canon* in a form that would be of practical use to the professors of medicine and graduate physicians who probably constituted the chief market for editions of the complete work or a major part of it. The second was to bring humanist medical learning to bear on the *Canon* itself, thus validating its continued study. The most obvious way to achieve both these goals was, of course, by the presentation of a Latin text that was improved in any or all of several senses: truer to the original, truer to Galen, clearer, or stylistically more elegant. But the validation of the *Canon* depended not only upon the revision of the text but also on the provision of supplementary material—indices, glossaries, references, introductory essays, or explanatory notes—which would both facilitate consultation of the work and aid the reader in its interpretation. The editions under discussion reveal a succession of editorial strategies all designed to accomplish the goals just outlined. While the textual revisions did not wholly satisfy contemporaries, some of the editors

---

annos, ex arabico, non indiserte latinum fecit; nostra, tamen, haec celeberrima academia vetustissimo, atque adeo primo omnium interprete utitur Gerardo Carmonense." Morgagni, comm. *Canon* 1.1, *Opera postuma* 4:16.

must be judged to have been rather successful in deploying their supplementary material to reinforce the position of the *Canon* in the medical learning of the second half of the sixteenth century.

Concerning the character of the revisions of the text, only a few general observations can be made. As noted earlier, much remains to be learned about the textual history of the *Canon* in Latin; the fundamental need is further investigation of the Gerard of Cremona version in the light of the original. Moreover, except for the work of Alpago, none of the other sixteenth-century revisions or partial translations, whether from Arabic or Hebrew, seems to have been studied in detail from a textual standpoint. But from what has already been noted, it is apparent that no sixteenth- or early seventeenth-century edition of the *Canon* published in Italy contains an entirely new translation made directly from Arabic alone. Alpago's published work on the *Canon* consists of emendations to the Gerard of Cremona version, accompanied by a glossary of technical terms and an explanatory note. Graziolo's version of Book I is different from that of Gerard, but not, as will become apparent, translated directly from Arabic. With the exception of the work of Ledesma in Spain, the other partial translations published in the sixteenth century—those of Mantino and, in France, Cinqarbres—were made from Hebrew.

Nonetheless, the claim that the text is revised, corrected, or improved is a prominent feature of almost all the editions of the complete *Canon* and of a good many of the partial editions published between 1522 and 1608. I have not succeeded in determining whether this claim refers to actual textual emendations in the earliest of these editions (Champier and Rustico, 1522); comparison of a few selected passages shows only the Gerard translation, and there appear to be no typographical indications of textual emendation. It is possible that Rustico's "castigations" are all incorporated into the front matter. The extent of Andrea Alpago's published revisions is made perfectly clear, both editorially and typographically, in the first two editions of his work, those prepared for the press by his nephew Paolo. The title of the 1527 edition refers to "correction" and "restitution," the privileges accompanying the work refer to "castigations and expositions," and the text itself is headed "translated by master Gerard of Cremona" (*translatus a magistro Gerardo Cremonensis*). In both editions, Alpago's emendations are clearly indicated in the margin and keyed to the text with various typographical devices. The scope of Alpago's alterations was, however, obscured, advertently or inadvertently, by the editorial procedures of Benedetto Rinio. An advertised feature of the latter's editions was, as noted, the removal of Alpago's emendations from the margin and their insertion into the body of the text. This freed Rinio's margins for copious citations of Greek and other medical authors, but it also made it impossible to determine the extent of Alpago's corrections without comparison with another edition. Costeo and Mongio, by reverting to the Gerard translation with alternative readings from Alpago (and, where applicable, Mantino) in the margins, once again provided their readers with the opportunity to distinguish both the source and the extent of suggested changes. There is some justification, therefore, for Johann Georg Schenk's view, stated in his *Biblia iatrica* (1609), that the Costeo and Mongio edition was the best available.[86]

Rinio, Costeo, and Mongio claimed to have added further emendations of their own. In some cases these appear to have taken the form of supplying translations of Arabic words hitherto only transliterated, especially as regards the simples in Book 2. How new these contributions were, how accurate, and what level of linguistic knowledge they represented must be left to others to determine. Costeo, at any rate, indicated that in emending in this fashion he usually followed the judgment of "more learned interpreters," who remain unidentified.[87] In the general theoretical treatise that opens *Canon* 1, Costeo and Mongio offered very few suggestions for improvement of their own, relying almost entirely on Alpago and Mantino. And in this part of the work the emendations by Alpago and Mantino seldom seem to have involved radical shifts in meaning. Rinio, Costeo, and Mongio all clearly assumed that their readers would have some interest in Arabic technical anatomical and botanical vocabulary—an interest that was, after all, shared to an extent even by Vesalius and Aldrovandi. Yet in many instances it is hard to see how Costeo and Mongio's edition of the list of simples in *Canon* 2, *Tractatus* 2, which presented Gerard's text flanked with a few of their own and many of Alpago's emendations in the mar-

---

[86] *Biblia iatrica, sive bibliotheca medica* . . . *auctore Joanne Georgio Schenkio* (Frankfurt, 1609), pp. 80–82.

[87] "Nunc autem demum a Benedicto Rinio Veneto . . . lucubrationibus illustrata. Qui et castigationes ab Alpago factas suis quasque locis aptissime inseruit: Et quamplurimas alias depravatas lectiones in margine ingeniosissime emendavit. . . . Plurimis etiam arabicis vocibus nunquam antea expositis, latinum nomen invenit: Indicemque latinum medicamentorum simplicium in secundum librum composuit." Title page, *Canon* (Venice, 1555); and: "Sed eam illustravimus varia lectione adhibita quam in libri margine tum ex Bellunensis correctione, et Mantini versione; tum ex variis vetustis codicibus; tum ex nostra et aliorum coniectura apposuimus. Difficiliores interdum Arabicas in contextu voces latinas reddidimus, ut facilior et expeditior legendi esset cursus; sequuti hac in re et doctiorum interpretum et Bellunensis iudicium; ita tamen ut antiqua vocabula in margine integra adhuc sint conservata, et asterisco indicata." Costeo, dedicatory letter to Paterno, preface to Book 1, *Canon* (Venice, 1564).

gin, could have been of much more practical use in identifying plants or their medicinal properties than the Gerard of Cremona translation alone. That Costeo and Mongio were aware of this problem is suggested by their deliberate repudiation of the task of studying the vocabulary of *Canon* 2 in the light of either Greek or contemporary botanical pharmacology.[88]

Moreover, in the case of Rinio, Costeo, and Mongio it seems clear that their emendations, however arrived at, should not necessarily be equated with substantial mastery of Arabic such as that obtained by the elder Alpago. This conclusion seems to be reinforced by the intermittent development and chiefly religious focus of Arabic studies in sixteenth-century Italy;[89] by even the younger Alpago's apparent inability in later life to translate a written narrative from Arabic, to which Francesca Lucchetta has drawn attention;[90] and by the admitted ignorance

---

[88] One brief example of the type of emendations supplied to the text of *Canon* 1.1 by Alpago and Mantino will have to suffice; it comes from the end of the first chapter on humors: "Sunt autem quidam hominum qui opinantur corporis virtutem sanguinis sequi multitudinem, et ipsius debilitatem sequi eius paucitatem. Sed non est ita.[h] [quod cum attenditur, est dispositio eius quantitatis, quae de eo corpus ingreditur.] Et sunt quidam, qui opinantur quod, quum humores aucti fuerint aut diminuti, † postquam corpora humanae secundum[i] [comparationem] fuerint, qua debent in quantitate unius ad alterum, sanitas erit conservata, sed non est ita; humores nanque praeter istud† [mensuram in quantitate conservatam] habere debent; non in compositione alterius humoris, immo in se, cum custodia mensurationis quam habent in comparatione unius ad alterum. Adhuc quidem remanserunt de rebus humorum quaestiones, quae non medicis, sed tantum pertinent philosophis. Ideoque eas praetermisi." Except for the words in square brackets, the foregoing is the Gerard of Cremona translation; Costeo and Mongio supplied the following marginal annotations:

    h. B[elunensis, i.e. Alpago] immo quid de eo attenditur vel consideratur est dispositio
        quam corpus ex eo fugit vel nutritur.
    † Mant. dum tamen servetur inter eos ea proportio, quae humanis corporibus debetur,
        in sua quantitate; sanitas, etc.
    i. B. proportionem
    † Mant. certam quantitatem ac mensuram.
    Canon, ed. Costeo and Mongio, 1.1.4.1 (Venice, 1595), 1:23.
For Costeo and Mongio's avoidance of full responsibility for editing *Canon* 2, see ibid., 1:259–60. Aldrovandi copied a list of Arabo-Latin names of simples from *Canon* 2 and some excerpts from Alpago's glossary into one of his notebooks, namely Bologna, Biblioteca Universitaria, MSS Aldrovandi 136, vol. XIII, fols. 6ʳ–57ʳ.

[89] See Fück, *Die arabischen Studien*, pp. 35–55; and Dannenfeldt, "Renaissance Humanists," passim.

[90] Lucchetta, *Alpago*, p. 39, basing the conclusion on the assertion in Massa's life of Avicenna that the Arabic manuscript had been supplied for the 1544 edition by Paolo (having previously belonged to Andrea) Alpago, but that no one could be found who was able to translate it; see *Vita*, tr. Massa (1544), fol. 24ʳ (the life is placed at the end of this edition of the *Canon* in a separately foliated section). See also in the same sense d'Al-

of that language of Nicolò Massa, whose Latin version of an Arabic life of Avicenna was based on an intermediary translation into Italian,[91] and of G. B. Da Monte, one of the most distinguished sixteenth-century Italian commentators on the Canon.[92] Presumably, if these men had considered command of Arabic to be essential for their work they could have acquired it, since most of them were resident in Padua or Venice, and Venetian trade contacts with Arabic-speaking countries were frequent. Joseph Scaliger, indeed, appeared to imply that his father had gained some familiarity with the language in just such an informal way, since he associated Julius' purported acquaintance with Arabic with his facility in learning vernaculars.[93] Of course, in other cases, some command of spoken Arabic might have been a far cry from the ability to read medieval philosophical and scientific texts. In any case, those who edited or commented on the Canon in the Veneto after Alpago seem not to have seen their task as imposing any personal responsibility for the further development of Arabic studies.

Graziolo not only made no secret of his own ignorance of Arabic, but also implied that he had no contact with anyone who did know it.[94] M. T. d'Alverny has drawn attention to his own explanation of how in these circumstances he managed to produce a translation clearly different from that of Gerard of Cremona.[95] Graziolo stated that he had carefully studied all previous interpreters of the Canon, especially the annotations of Alpago, and had drawn on the assistance of the Jewish physician Jacob Anselmo, who could read the Canon in Hebrew (as Graziolo presumably could not). It was only when his work was already well advanced that he secured access to Ramusio's manuscript containing Canon 1 in Arabic with Ramusio's Latin translation. This explanation is doubtless true as far as it goes, but perhaps slightly dis-

---

verny, "Avicenne et les médecins de Venise," p. 189. The remarks of Amatus Lusitanus, quoted in n. 20, above, may also be recalled here.

[91] Massa commissioned a translation of the life from Arabic into Italian from Marco Fadella, an interpreter for the Venetian merchant community in Damascus; see Vita, fol. 24.

[92] "Nescio litteras Arabes" and "sive modo ita stet littera Arabica sive non, ego id nescio quoniam ignarus sum." Da Monte, comm. Canon 1.2 (Venice, 1557), pp. 93, 247.

[93] I owe the point about opportunities for Venetians to acquire Arabic to Richard Palmer, in discussion at the conference on "Medicine in the Sixteenth Century," Cambridge, September 1983. Regarding Scaliger, see n. 24, above.

[94] "Ut enim nihil de Avicennae eloquentia, qui Arabice scripsit, decernere possimus, credendum tamen est, virum sublimi ingenio, politissimisque disciplinis ornatum, hac etiam in parte, quantum ferat idioma illud, non fuisse infelicem." Canon 1, ed. Graziolo (Venice, 1580), preface to the reader [b3ʳ].

[95] Ibid. [b3ᵛ–4ʳ]; D'Alverny, "Avicenne et les médecins de Venise," pp. 183–84.

ingenuous. Graziolo's version is not identical with that of Ramusio, as is shown by the notation of variant readings ascribed to the latter. However, a comparison of the opening of the chapter on humors in Graziolo's version and in the Latin translation of *Canon* 1.1 from the Hebrew by Jacob Mantino (Venice, *ca.* 1540) suggests that at least for this part of Graziolo's work Mantino was a major source.

If in their presentation of the text the Italian scholarly editors of the mid- and later sixteenth century were unable to go much beyond one or another combination of the work of Gerard of Cremona, Ramusio, Andrea Alpago, and Mantino, they displayed both learning and ingenuity in supplementing the text with other material. One variety of supplement that had earlier played an important role, namely commentary written before 1500, dropped out of *Canon* editions after the 1520s. Yet precedents for other forms of supplementary material that lent themselves to expansion and development were already in existence; for example the Venice edition of 1507, printed without commentary, contains a short life of Avicenna and a glossary of Arabic terms. Setting aside the purely complimentary dedications and the elaborate title pages that began to proliferate in printings of Avicenna, as of other authors, and the textual apparatus indicating variant readings that has already been referred to, the expanded supplementary material found in the editions with which we are concerned can be broadly classified as follows: biography of Avicenna; indices and glossaries; evaluation of the worth of Avicenna and of the *Canon*; citations of other authors; explanatory annotations or scholia. It is from the last three categories that the priorities of the editors can most readily be determined, but the development of the first two deserves to be briefly mentioned.

The history of the Latin biography of Avicenna is a subject that has yet to be fully studied. Prior to the sixteenth century, very little information about his life from Arabic sources appears to have been available in the Latin West. Moreover, several stories circulated that could have no counterpart in the authentic Arabic biographies of Avicenna.[96] Besides the famous—and extremely persistent—association of his name with Córdoba, it was, for example, variously claimed that Avicenna had corresponded with Saint Augustine and that he had been a contemporary of Averroes and had suffered at the latter's hands.[97] If

---

[96] For Arabic biographical material concerning Avicenna, see *The Life of Ibn Sina*, ed. and tr. William E. Gohlman (Albany, N.Y., 1974).

[97] The supposed letter of Avicenna to Saint Augustine is found in BAV, MS Vat. lat. 5108, fols. 107ᵛ–8ʳ, and Padua, Biblioteca Comunale, MS BP 1223, p. 160. The sense of the text is similar in both, with some slight variations in wording. I quote the Vatican manuscript. "Aicenna [*sic*] medicinae professor Beatissimo Augustino salutem dicit. Ap-

the origins of these assertions are unclear, the purpose of the last two seems fairly plain: both appear in different ways to be designed to guarantee Avicenna's suitability as an author for Christian readers. The story about Averroes must presumably date from no earlier than the 1260s, when Averroist ideas first came under attack in the West.[98] Both stories also appear to imply an awareness, and perhaps endorsement, of the Platonist element in Avicenna's thought.

Three different biographies of Avicenna appear in the various sixteenth-century Latin editions of the Canon; biographical information is also contained in a brief note by Andrea Alpago included in the 1527 and various subsequent editions.[99] The short life included in the Venice, 1507, and other early editions may possibly be based on an Arabic source, but contains little specific information other than medical detail about the cause of Avicenna's death. A slightly longer and purportedly more critical life was written by Franciscus Calphurnius of Vendôme, an associate of Champier, for the Champier and Rustico edition of 1522. The author stressed the uncertainty and inconsistency of available information about Avicenna, and firmly repudiated the fiction of his correspondence with Saint Augustine. However, this biography retained the tradition that Avicenna had lived in Córdoba (where he flourished "like a hyacinth among the nettles") and also asserted that he was a contemporary of Averroes. Calphurnius named Champier as his source for the story that Avicenna was poisoned by Averroes in a fit of jealousy.[100]

Alpago's biographical comments laid to rest Avicenna's supposed

---

paruisti compatriota noster homo admirabilis in universa terra altissimi ingenii subtilissimi intellectus [rerum] humanarum divinarumque scientia ac sapientia peritissimus. Dicam quod de te sentio. Parcat Plato parcat Socrates, parcant mundi sapientes, tu enim tantum possides sapientiam quantum humanae menti tribui potest. Epistolas tuas mihi saluteria documenta sonantes interim legam. Video quod ad sectam Crucifixi quem dei filium praedicant me trahere cupis. Non puto tecum posse errare. Saepe mihi scribe, et quid prima causa sublimi dei velit expectabo. Vale." Both manuscripts are fifteenth-century humanist literary miscellanies. An example of the story about Avicenna and Averroes follows shortly.

[98] The celebrated disputes at Paris of this period are summarized in David Knowles, The Evolution of Medieval Thought (New York, 1964), pp. 272ff.

[99] This note, headed De arabicorum nominum significatu, appears in various positions in most of the major editions after that of Venice, 1527. A brief account of Avicenna's life included in Canon 1.1, tr. Ledesma (Valencia, 1547–48), fols. 3ʳ–4ʳ, also denies Avicenna's association with Spain or Córdoba (on the grounds that plants mentioned in the Canon do not grow in Spain) and asserts that he was a citizen of Bochara in Persia, "ut Arabum ipsorum testantur historiae."

[100] Avicenne Cordube principis vita a Francisco Calphurnio vindocinensi declarata, in Canon (Lyon, 1522), fol. + 1ᵛ.

association with Córdoba. However, much more, and more authentic, information was provided in the well-known life of Avicenna by Nicolò Massa, which was printed for the first time in Paolo Alpago's second edition of the Canon (Venice, 1544). This life was actually a free Latin rendering of the biography Avicenna's pupil Abu Ubayd al-Juzjani, whose name was Latinized as Sorsanus.[101] Massa's work made available for the first time in the West a reasonably full account of Avicenna from a contemporary Arabic source. This Latin biography was reprinted in all the subsequent major editions of the complete Canon, with the exception of that published by Valgrisio in 1564. In the editions of 1562 and thereafter, Massa's work, originally dedicated to the papal physician Tommaso Cademusto, was updated by a new dedication to Cardinal Carlo Borromeo.

Hence, while Alpago and the subsequent sixteenth-century editors and revisers did not have access to the full range of Arabic biographical material about Avicenna, they abandoned the Western myths about him and supplied fuller and more accurate information than had been available before. The biographical material about Avicenna supplied in their editions of the Canon was superior to that which continued to be disseminated in the West in general works, such as, for example, the Bibliotheca universalis (first published in 1545) by the celebrated medical humanist and encyclopedist of nature Conrad Gesner. Gesner provided a fairly comprehensive account of Avicenna's writings and an evaluation of their work from the standpoint of medical humanism. He stressed Avicenna's status as a compiler rather than an original medical author, and his probable lack of personal experience of medical practice. Yet Gesner also repeated the stories about Avicenna's royal birth, association with Córdoba, and rivalry with Averroes, although admittedly in noncommittal language that evaded personal endorsement.[102]

A few more items of information about Avicenna were subsequently added by Plemp, who could draw upon a much wider body of learning about Moslem history and culture than was available to any of the sixteenth-century Italian scholars who worked on the Latin editions of the Canon: in the life of Avicenna prefaced to his own edition of the Canon,[103] Plemp announced that his intention was merely to supplement Massa's version of Sorsanus' biography. This he did by supplying a precise calculation of Avicenna's dates based on understanding of

---

[101] The Arabic life in question is edited and translated into English in The Life of Ibn Sina, ed. and tr. Gohlman.

[102] Bibliotheca universalis, sive catalogus scriptorum locupletissimus, in tribus linguis, Latina, Graeca, et Hebraica . . . authore Conrado Gesnero (Zurich, 1545), 1:110^r–11^r.

[103] Canon 1, 2, 4.1, tr. Plemp (Louvain, 1658), fol. 4^{r-v}.

the relationship between Moslem and Christian calendars; providing references to later Arabic accounts of Avicenna and to a modern work on Persian history, cited as the source for the information that Avicenna's native language was Persian although he always wrote in Arabic, and that he had written works that had not been translated into Latin; and indicating the way in which Avicenna had become the subject of Oriental as well as Western myth. Plemp's account of various sixteenth-century Western authors other than Alpago and Massa who had written on Avicenna's life shows not only the persistence of older Western myths about him, but also that the subject of the biography of Avicenna continued to stimulate the creative impulses of religious and regional apologists. Plemp attributed to Juan Mariana, S.J., the hypothesis that there had been two Avicennas, one living in Spain, the other in the East.[104] He added that there were those who maintained that the Oriental Avicenna had written the philosophical works. The Spanish one was responsible for the *Canon*, which, however, he had not composed but translated from a work of Isidore of Seville, of which all Latin exemplars were subsequently lost. The object of this imaginative exercise in historical reconstruction was presumably to sever the *Canon* from association with possibly heterodox philosophical works by a Moslem author, and to provide it with an impeccably Christian pedigree. Plemp took evident satisfaction in exposing the utter baselessness of this speculation, and indeed its total implausibility in terms of intellectual history.

If the development of Avicenna's biography over successive editions of the *Canon* in Latin is a history of expansion, modernization of form, and greater precision, the same can be said of the indexing of the work. In the Gerard of Cremona translation, the *Canon* includes a lengthy table of contents, adequate to locate the treatment of most topics in the bulky work, which is placed immediately after Avicenna's own preface. In addition, some early editions contain registers of the *quaestiones* discussed in the commentaries printed with the *Canon*.[105] Readers of

---

[104] I have been unable to find any such passage in either *Joannis Marianae . . . Historiae de rebus Hispaniae libri triginta* (The Hague, 1733), which mentions Avicenna as an outstanding savant said by some to have been a prince of Córdoba in Book 10, chap. 17, pp. 422–23, or in the vernacular version, *Historia general de España . . . por el Padre Mariana* (Madrid, 1852), 1:323. Possibly the story is in Mariana's other writings or in early editions of the *Historia* to which I have not had access. Mariana died in 1624.

[105] For example, *Tertius Canonis Avicenne cum amplissima Gentilis Fulginatis expositione* (Venice, 1522) opens with a *Tabula dubiorum . . . Gentilis*. Some separate editions of older commentaries contain subject indices to the commentaries; for example, *Jacobi Foroliviensis in primum Avicenne Canonem expositio* (Venice, 1518), and *Jacobi Foroliviensis . . . expositio et quaestiones in primum Canonem Avicennae* (Venice, 1547).

the edition prepared by Rinio had the convenience of an alphabetically arranged subject index. In the Basel edition of 1556, this is relatively spare, occupying sixteen folios. In 1557, Junta published a much more comprehensive and complicated index, seventy-six folios long, with numerous subheadings and cross-references, compiled by the physician Giulio Palamede;[106] this was reissued in 1562, and replaced the former index in the revised edition of Rinio's work published in the same year.[107] The indexing of the Costeo and Mongio editions was even more elaborate. Not only did those scholars provide an index to the text of the *Canon* exceeding Palamede's in length, they also supplied a separate index to their own annotations. In addition, in their second, revised edition Paolino's tables provided yet another guide to the whole work.[108] In most editions, too, separate indices of the simples in Book 2 were provided. That appearing in the Champier and Rustico edition of 1522 subsequently gave way to an index of Arabic names of substances compiled by Andrea Alpago (1527); in the editions prepared by Rinio, an index of Greco-Latin names for substances in Book 2 compiled by Rinio himself was also added.[109] Both of these indices or lists were expanded in the Costeo and Mongio editions. The main change as far as glossaries were concerned was, of course, the introduction of the important and well-known one compiled by Andrea Alpago.[110] Alpago's glossary, to which some additions were made by Rinio, appeared in all the major editions under discussion. However, the shorter, so-called "old" glossary, sometimes ascribed to Gerard of Cremona, also survived and continued to be printed alongside that of Alpago.

The evaluations of Avicenna prefaced to the various editions are of course rhetorical, but nonetheless revealing of the goals and preoccu-

[106] *Index in Avicennae libros nuper Venetiis editos . . . Julio Palamede Adriensi medico auctore* (Venice, 1557). In the BL copy it is bound with *Canon*, ed. Rinio (Venice, 1555).

[107] In *Canon*, ed. Rinio (Venice, 1562), Palamede's index is found with its own title page and separately foliated; the shorter index found in *Canon*, ed. Rinio (Basel, 1556), after *De syrupo acetoso* and before Alpago's glossary has been dropped. Palamede's index was again reissued by Junta in 1584, presumably to accompany the reissue of Rinio's edition of the *Canon* in 1582, with which the copy owned by NLM is bound.

[108] On the medieval antecedents of tables of this type, see Michael Evans, "The Geometry of the Mind," *Architectural Association Quarterly* 12 (1980), 32–55; also John E. Murdoch, *Album of Science: Antiquity and the Middle Ages* (New York, 1984), no. 36, p. 46, for a fourteenth-century medical example.

[109] It would be interesting to explore the possibility of a relationship between this list and the alphabetical index in the book of simples of the elder Rinio, printed in De Toni, "Il libro dei semplici" (1925), pp. 206–64; as noted, this manuscript was owned by the younger Rinio.

[110] On Alpago's glossary, see Lucchetta, *Alpago*, pp. 39–47.

pations of the different editors. The edition prepared by Champier and Rustico and published in 1522, just when bold criticism of the Arabs was becoming a shibboleth of modernism in medicine, includes prefatory material decidedly critical of Avicenna.[111] Champier set the tone of his "castigations and errata" in a brief preface addressed to Robert Coleburn, bishop of Ross, in which he explained Avicenna's importance for medicine as an interpreter of Galen, while deploring his membership in the "filthy and wicked Mohammedan sect." He then summarized the views on the soul of Avicenna, Algazel, and Averroes, condemning the last. Next follows discussion of seven supposed errors of Avicenna, all of them in the realm of philosophy, religion, and ethics, not medicine. Among the errors repudiated are the legitimacy of divorce and the view that all supposed miracles have a natural explanation. Then comes a set of *dubia* examining instances in which Avicenna appears to differ from Galen or other Greek medical authorities;[112] the topics relate to confusion or error in the names or attributes of medicinal plants and of diseases and in the prescription of treatment. Finally, ten instances in which Avicenna appeared to disagree with Dioscorides are identified as errors and discussed.

The issues of Avicenna's relationship to Greek medicine and of problems of pharmacological and botanical nomenclature, originally raised by critics of the Arabs, had now been introduced into an edition of the *Canon* itself. Subsequent Italian editors of the *Canon*, all of whom were principally concerned with defending not attacking Avicenna, were repeatedly to address these themes, although they usually avoided the religious issue also introduced by Champier. Overall, the Champier-Rustico edition seems something of an amalgam of conflicting intentions. The biography places Avicenna in a positive light; moreover, the claim that the text has been purified presumably indicates that the editors valued the work as a whole. Yet the message conveyed by the prefatory material seems to be that, on both religious and scientific grounds, the Christian physician should approach the *Canon* with a good deal of caution.

The brief dedication and preface placed by Paolo Alpago before his uncle's revision of the *Canon* are naturally chiefly concerned with An-

---

[111] *Canon*, ed. Champier and Rustico (Lyon, 1522), +2ʳ–[+10ʳ].

[112] Rustico's *castigationes* may be incorporated in some of the *dubia*, as some of them seem to parallel the subject matter of one of his other works. In particular, nos. 7, 8, 9, and 10 deal with *bubones, ignis persicus,* and *pruna,* conditions on which Rustico had discussed Avicenna's views in *Qui venenosa formidas apostemata et pestiferos paves bubones ecce dicta Avicene arabis de igne persico pruna vel carbone . . . ordinata, exposita, discussa Rustico medicine cultore,* printed with Baviero Baviera, *Consilia* (Pavia, 1521).

drea Alpago's accomplishment, the circumstances that charged Paolo with responsibility for publication, and his editorial procedures. Of Avicenna, Paolo asserted only that he had drawn on earlier Arabic and Greek writers, above all Galen, so skillfully that physicians still regarded him as their prince and used the *Canon* as a standard work of reference for both theory and practice.[113] The substantial and carefully reasoned defense of Avicenna supplied by Benedetto Rinio was therefore a novelty in an edition of the *Canon*. In a prefatory letter to his four sons, whom he urged always to have Avicenna in their hands, he expressed his astonishment at the temerity of those who "thirty years ago" (Rinio was presumably writing in 1555 or shortly before) attacked Avicenna. He attributed these attacks to a rage for all things Greek, while asserting that Greek, Latin, or barbarian origin should not prejudge a man. In defense of Avicenna, Rinio pointed out that none of the works of the major medical authors from Hippocrates to Haly Abbas was without some drawbacks. Avicenna's special merit was to have sifted the wheat from the chaff in the writings of his predecessors and to have presented the result aptly and harmoniously arranged. Consequently, reliance on the *Canon* was both labor- and time-saving. Furthermore, those who condemned Avicenna for drawing upon the work of his predecessors should be aware that Aristotle and Galen had unquestionably done the same thing. Rinio admitted that Avicenna's dependence on Arabic translations of Greek works meant that through the fault of the translators he had sometimes been misled or confused, especially about the names of plants and animals. These deficiencies had, however, largely been remedied by the work of Andrea Alpago. And in a few instances, Avicenna had supplied information about medicaments unknown to the Greeks.

Rinio called not only upon classical tradition and the modern work of Alpago, but also upon medieval sources in defending Avicenna. Possibly in indirect allusion to some of Champier's criticisms, he noted that Avicenna's merits as a philosopher had earned the approval of Albertus Magnus, Thomas Aquinas, and Duns Scotus, "lights of the whole world." Moreover, he pointed out that the long tradition of lecturing on the *Canon* in the Italian medical schools had produced the commentaries of "the great speculator Gentile, the clear expositor Giacomo, and the subtle disputant Dino."[114]

[113] Letter of dedication to Giorgio Cornelio, and "Paulus Alpago ad lectorem" (Canon, 1527).

[114] "Benedictus Rinius Fabricio, Scipioni, Alberto, et Claudio, filiis iucundissimis." *Canon*, ed. Rinio (Venice, 1555), +iii–[iv^v]. Aspects of this preface are discussed in d'Alverny, "Avicenne et les médecins de Venise," pp. 196–97.

In the following decade, Costeo and Mongio echoed some of the same themes. They, too, deplored the prevalence of scorn for the Arabs, while pointing out that no one had yet produced a work that surpassed the *Canon* in organization, comprehensiveness, generally accurate presentation of Greek medicine, and range of medicaments.[115] They took the war into the enemy's camp with the assertion that the Arabs were disliked by those who had entered medicine without any study of dialectic and philosophy and were therefore incapable of appreciating the weighty and recondite statements of Arab authors (by contrast "the Greeks, indeed, with their suavity in words and copious effusion of speech are not difficult to understand").[116] And in Costeo's preface to Book 4 the argument culminates in a diatribe against the "Galenici," who act "as if it were a sin to add anything to Galen's writings or as if it were a virtue to know nothing he did not know."[117] This, he said, was certainly quite unlike the behavior of any men of real distinction in any branch of science, and certainly unlike Galen and Aristotle, who had never hesitated to criticize their predecessors.

Around 1580, Graziolo elected a historical approach. His preface opens with a brisk summary of the transmission of knowledge from the Hebrews to the Egyptians to the Greeks to the Latins, the devastating effects of the barbarian invasions, and the rebirth of learning in Italy (dated by references to the flight of Greek scholars from Constantinople and the invention of printing).[118] Among the arts and sciences that were as a result "recalled to their sources" and "restored to light" was medicine. This conventional historiography was used to make the point that the arts, far from being confined to the Greeks, had arisen among barbarians (the ancient Egyptians!) and had been further developed by other peoples after Greek ingenuity had grown old. Among the latter were the Arabs, who had not merely acquired but added to

[115] Preface to Book 1, Costeo to Paterno; to Book 2, Mongio and Costeo to Cortusio, *Canon* (Venice, 1564).

[116] "Eget Avicennae, eget Arabum doctrina acri, solerti, et accurata plerunque lectione; quam ii, qui ad medicinam nullo vel dialectices, vel philosophiae studio initiati se se contulere, non satis assequi possunt; proptereaque huic hominum generi soli placent Graeci medici, displicent modis omnibus Arabes; Graeci quidem verborum suavitate, et effusa dicendi copia intellectu non difficiles; Arabes vero sententiarum gravitate, et recondita quadam brevitate non faciles." Preface to *Canon* 3, Mongio and Costeo to Sanmichele, *Canon* (Venice, 1564).

[117] "Verum quia Galenus id non scripserit, non audere aliquid proferre confiteantur, quasi piaculum sit ad Galeni scripta quidquam adijcere; aut nihil scire fas fit quod is non norit. . . . At vero non ita Galenus. . . . Non ita quicunque in omni scientiarum genere illustres unquam fuere." Ibid., preface to *Canon* 4, Costeo to Modegnano.

[118] "Andreas Gratiolus lectori." *Canon* 1, tr. Graziolo (Venice, 1580), b^r–c^v.

Greek learning, especially in mathematics (algebra), astronomy, astrology, and medicine. Graziolo also repeated some of the familiar themes: Avicenna's fidelity to Greek medical authors and skill in presenting their ideas; the outmoded character of disdain for Avicenna; and the faults of the *recentiores*, who wanted to destroy medicine rather than teach and study it and who were ignorant not only of Avicenna but also of Hippocrates and Galen. In hazarding the opinion that a man of such genius as Avicenna must have been a polished and elegant writer in his own language and, as a consequence, stressing the stylistic defects of Gerard of Cremona, Graziolo may have been echoing G. B. Da Monte,[119] although he was doubtless also insinuating the merits on which he thought his own version should be judged.

Although it added little new in substance, the preface written by Fabio Paolino for the edition of 1595 was markedly more elegant in style than those of his predecessors.[120] Indeed, it may be that Paolino's principal contribution to the edition was to lend Avicenna's cause the support of a classical scholar of some reputation. Only a few points need be noted here. Paolino, like Costeo and unlike Rinio and Graziolo, admitted the existence of contemporaries, as well as of an earlier generation of medical teachers, who discouraged their students from reading the *Canon*. His account of the origins of hostility to Avicenna and the *Canon* among the medical humanists shows a fairly balanced historical perspective. An ardent enthusiast of Greek letters, Paolino was unable to dismiss earlier critics of Avicenna as cavalierly as Costeo had done. Instead, he asserted that although these critics had indeed included men of great erudition, their opinions were not based on close study of the *Canon* but were, rather, part of the polemic in which they engaged to foster the goals of a new medical sect that had arisen in their own time. This sect, called by its supporters the Galenic, had as its program the union of sound medical teaching with elegance of expression. In the resultant polarization of the medical community, those who valued the substance of learning alone and were suspicious of rhetorical embellishments were stigmatized by the Galenic faction as "Avicennan" or "barbarous." In reality, Paolino thought, the quarrel was more about translators than about medical content: since Arabic was much more linguistically distant from Latin than was Greek, it was scarcely surprising that translators from Arabic had committed barbarisms in Latin. In Paolino's view, it would have been preferable if Avicenna's critics, instead of casting slurs on a great writer, had learned Arabic and

[119] For Da Monte's remarks on the subject, see the following chapter.
[120] "Fabius Paulinus medicus medicinae studiosis," *Canon* (Venice, 1595), 1:[a6^{r-v}].

translated him in good Latin style. This, Paolino had reason to think, would soon be done.

The provision of a systematic, precise, and comprehensive set of references to other, chiefly Greek, medical authors was an important and novel feature of the major *Canon* editions produced in Italy in the second half of the sixteenth century. It was a contribution made possible by the achievements of mid-sixteenth-century medical humanism. Scholastic commentators had, of course, long since drawn attention to passages in the *Canon* where Avicenna appeared to differ from or be supported by Galen, Aristotle, or other ancient authors. The objective of such commentators was, however, the identification and elucidation of separate medical or philosophical problems, not the systematic comparison of entire texts, a task for which, in any case, they had inadequate facilities. Some of the late fifteenth- and early sixteenth-century critics of the *Canon* had, as we have seen, supported their arguments by pulling out instances in which Avicenna differed from Galen, Dioscorides, or other ancient medical authors, but such accounts were incomplete as well as polemical in intent. It was the accessibility of the Renaissance collected editions of Galen's works in Greek or new Latin translation, with their accompanying apparatus, and the examples of the goals and methodology of Renaissance Greek scholarship that made systematic confrontation of the Latin text of the *Canon* with the sources of Greek medicine both imaginable and technically feasible. As already noted, the Aldine editio *princeps* of Galen's works in Greek appeared in 1525; the first edition of the collection of his *Opera* in humanist Latin translation published by Junta appeared in 1541–42; and the indexing of Galen's works was undertaken by Antonio Musa Brasavola (1500–1555).

Benedetto Rinio, in his *Canon* edition of 1555, was the first to attempt to provide a comprehensive system of references, which could be used not only to demonstrate the extent of Avicenna's dependence on Greek authorities and the great number of instances in which he could be shown, even from the available Latin versions of the *Canon*, to have reported Galenic ideas accurately, but also the way in which Galen's teachings were reordered, abbreviated, and clarified (or oversimplified) in the *Canon*. Rinio did not confine himself to providing references to works of Galen, but also included other Greek authors (notably Dioscorides in Book 2), a few other Arabic authors, and cross-references within the *Canon*. Some indication of the scope of his endeavor and how much of his editorial effort it must have absorbed can perhaps be gained from the information that for the brief *Canon* 1.1 alone (excluding the anatomical chapters), Rinio provided multiple citations of more than thirty separate works of Galen. Of these, the most frequently cited was the lengthy *De usu partium* to which Rinio referred over forty times. A check of the references to the three works most frequently cited by Rinio in *Canon* 1.1—*De usu partium*, *De temperamentis*, and *De naturalibus facultatibus*—reveals him as thorough and careful in seeking out parallels (and therefore presumed sources). He also noticed instances where Galen could be cited in opposition, but naturally in the physiological survey contained in *Canon* 1.1 instances of agreement are far more numerous.

Costeo, Mongio, and Graziolo also gave considerable attention to the citation of ancient, and especially Galenic, sources, although they did not confine their own annotations to this in the way that Rinio had. Instead, they wove the references into broader and more general *annotationes* and scholia to the text. Only the most salient features of the latter, illustrated by a few examples drawn from their treatment of *Canon* 1.1, can be indicated here. Costeo's own description of the objectives of his annotations seems to apply as well to Graziolo's scholia: the collection and citation of relevant passages from philosophers and physicians, the exposition of controversies, demonstration of the closeness of Avicenna's agreement with Hippocrates and Galen, and elimination of the objections of both ancients and *recentiores*.[121] Despite their relative brevity and somewhat episodic nature, the philosophical, medical, and bibliographical disquisitions in which these aims are realized have more in common with both the earlier and the contemporary tradition of Latin commentary on the *Canon* than with, say, the medical and philological scholia supplied by Plemp, let alone the mainly philological treatment by Kirsten.

But although a good many of the issues discussed by the sixteenth-century Italian editors ultimately derive from differences between the teaching of Aristotle and Galen that had been the topics of *quaestiones* discussed by Latin physicians since the thirteenth century—for example, the origin of the nerves, the existence and powers of the so-called female sperm, the identity or nonidentity of *complexio* or *temperamentum* with substantial form[122]—little trace of dependence on medieval treatments remains. Neither the form of the scholastic *quaestio* nor citations of Latin commentators on the *Canon* can easily be found. Instead, in both form and content, the closest relation is with the most recent commentaries on the *Canon*. Like those commentaries, the an-

---

[121] Preface to *Canon* 1, Costeo to Paterno (Venice, 1564).

[122] These topics are discussed in Costeo and Mongio's annotations to *Canon* 1.1 (Venice, 1595), 1:33, 34, 13–14. For discussions of the same topics by late thirteenth- and early fourteenth-century Italian physicians, see Siraisi, *Alderotti*, pp. 321, 342, 338–39.

notations and scholia by Costeo, Mongio, and Graziolo are replete with allusions to controversy and bibliography dating from the middle years of the sixteenth century. Thus, Graziolo's treatment of the nature of *complexio* or *temperamentum* is directed against the views of Jean Fernel (1497–1558) and supported by arguments based on the recently edited and translated *De mixtione* of Alexander of Aphrodisias (see Chapter 7).[123] Similarly, it seems likely that Costeo's diatribe against those who identify *temperamentum* with substantial form is directed against G. D. Da Monte (who is not named), who had endorsed that view in his commentary on *Canon* 1.1 written in the early 1540s.[124] Costeo and Mongio introduced a paean of praise to sixteenth-century botanists into their annotations on Book 2, while simultaneously avowing Avicenna's work on this subject to be superior to that of any earlier writers, noting that he often differed from Dioscorides, and disclaiming any intention to provide detailed analysis or correction of Avicenna's contribution to botanical or pharmacological knowledge.[125] In these and other instances, the evident goal was not the continuance of an older tradition of scholastic exposition, but the reactive defense of Avicenna against the adverse criticisms of *recentiores* of the previous generation, and the demonstration that much of his work was indeed defensible in the light of Greek and some modern, that is, mid-sixteenth century, medical learning.

To the seventeenth-century northern European Arabists who worked on the *Canon* the method and goals of their Italian predecessors seemed worthy only of disdain. Of the efforts of "the very learned Costeo," Peter Kirsten remarked dryly, "He would have done better, in my opinion, if he had sought to restore this author from Arabic sources, rather than setting himself the task of restoring him from Galen." Welsch simply noted that Costeo was "extremely ignorant of all oriental languages." Of Graziolo, Plemp commented, "He called himself a translator . . . but he was utterly ignorant of the Arabic language; nor did he follow the words or content of the author, but took the sense from the commentators, often badly. Sometimes he inserted entire sentences from Galen."[126]

Such procedures could scarcely fail to arouse the indignation and

---

[123] *Canon* 1, tr. Graziolo (Venice, 1580), fols. 13ᵛ–14ʳ.

[124] *Canon*, ed. Costeo and Mongio (Venice, 1595), 1:13–14.   [125] Ibid., 1:259–60.

[126] "Doctissimus Ioannes Costaeus, in sumtuosa sua hujus Canonis editione praestiterit, qui mea opinione, melius fecisset se ex fontibus Arabicis hunc authorem restituere voluisset, quam quod sibi proposerat eum ex Galeno restituere." *Canon* 2, ed. Kirsten (Breslau, 1609), p. 131. And: "Ille [Costaeus] vero leviculis quibusdam totus occupetur, et linguarum orientalium omnium ignarissimus." Welsch (1674), fol. b1ᵛ. And: "An-

contempt of men who had devoted themselves to the study of the *Canon* as an Arabic text. The goal of the editions thus disdained was the different one of restoring the reputation of the *Canon* as a functional Latin medical textbook. In hindsight, this objective appears chimerical, not only because of the forthcoming revolution in physiology. The medical defenders of the *Canon* in sixteenth-century Europe valued the work essentially for its Galenic doctrines and pharmacological compendia. But the fundamental humanist contention that Galen is best studied from Galen is hard to gainsay. And to arrive at a satisfactory understanding of the possible range of meanings underlying Arabo-Latin botanical and pharmacological terminology would call for an investment of effort likely to be greater than any medical results would justify. Unquestionably, however, the approach adopted by Rinio, Graziolo, and Costeo and his partners was that most likely to secure the position of the *Canon* in their own milieu. One may speculate that the display of Greek learning and awareness of recent concerns in their elaborate editions helped to provide intellectual justification for the assignment of sections of the bare Gerard of Cremona text to students for a good many years to come.

The study of the *Canon* was thus at least in part perpetuated not by traditionalism but by efforts at modernization. The Italian editors of the *Canon* did not seek to preserve the traditions of medieval scholastic medicine unchanged; moreover, the reduction to a trickle of the stream of printed editions of early commentaries on the *Canon* in about the 1520s suggests that such an endeavor would have had little chance of success. But the form taken by their efforts to modernize the study of the *Canon* was in another sense backward-looking, in that it was largely shaped by developments, progressive in their day, that had occurred between about 1490 and 1530. In those years, the enthusiasm for Galen and for Greek medicine was at its height; attacks on Arabs and scholastics were mainly on the grounds of their inadequacy in transmitting Greek medicine; and, also, the work of Alpago and Mantino on the text, fundamental to the endeavors of subsequent Italian medical

---

dreas Gratiolus Salodianus librum primum integrum nobis latiniorem dedit, adjectis scholiis Hippocratis et Galeni praecipue loca commonstrantibus. Vocat se interpretem nihil minus quam interpres existens: Arabicae quippe linguae prorsus nesciens fuit; nec sequitur authoris verba aut contextum, sed ex commentatoribus sensum hausit, saepe male. Aliquando Galeni integras periodos inseruit. Ea non sunt interpretis." *Canon,* ed. Plemp (Louvain, 1658), fol. §3ʳ. Plemp and Welsch were also somewhat critical of Kirsten's grasp of Arabic, although in milder terms; see ibid. and *Canon* 4.3.2.21–22, ed. and tr. Welsch (Augsburg, 1674) c2ᵛ. On the development of Renaissance ideas about the task of the *interpres,* see Glyn P. Norton, *The Ideology and Language of Translation in Renaissance France and Their Humanist Antecedents* (Geneva, 1984).

editors and revisers, appeared. The intellectual patrimony, even when they reacted against it, of the Italian scholars who devoted themselves to revising the *Canon* after 1550 was the medical humanism of the early part of the century.

In the context of sixteenth-century medical teaching, the reassertion of Avicenna's usefulness as a summarizer and rearranger of Galen could appear as a reasonable position. Moreover, the effort to enhance the usefulness of the *Canon* for teaching in itself involved a loosening of established patterns of thought. The scholars who edited or revised the *Canon* accepted the need to find explicit justification for the continued study of Avicenna, did much to clarify Avicenna's relationship to Galen, and used improved editorial techniques to highlight inconsistencies and obscurities within the text. It seems likely that their editions facilitated an evaluation of the merits and defects of the one-time "prince of physicians" that was more detached than had hitherto been possible.

6

Commentators and Commentaries

The output of commentary is probably the single most satisfactory measure of the actual nature, extent, and duration of the uses of the *Canon* in western European medical schools after 1500. While, as we have seen, the printing history of editions of the *Canon* in Latin also offers a good deal of information, ambitious new editions do not necessarily reflect the daily realities of teaching (even though, as noted, annotations and scholia included in some of the sixteenth-century editions discussed in the last chapter were certainly related to current pedagogic practice). University documents are, of course, an indispensable source of information about curricula; but with rare, if important, exceptions they usually provide information only about formal requirements that may not always have been other than nominally observed. However, there also survives a fairly substantial body of material, in manuscript and print, that records or derives closely from the actual teaching of the *Canon* in faculties of medicine between the sixteenth and the early eighteenth century.

It is to these notes, outlines, *lectiones*, and commentaries, produced not in connection with the preparation of new editions but in the course of routine teaching, that one must turn for a somewhat closer view of Avicenna in the Renaissance classroom. Such material is the subject of the remainder of this book. What follows is a general survey of these productions, with reference to their place in the larger body of Renaissance medical commentary and their geographical and chronological distribution, together with some account of leading commentators and the ways in which they approached the text. Discussion of some of the philosophical and scientific content is reserved for later chapters.

More than sixty expositions of the *Canon* written after 1500 and about evenly divided between manuscript and printed items are listed in Appendix 2. These works are the result of lectures on the *Canon* itself, and are therefore to be distinguished from various contemporary works (some of which were mentioned in Chapter 4) that drew upon Avicenna as a medical authority to expound a particular subject or a book other than the *Canon*. The works listed in Appendix 2 range from brief notes or outlines, to sets of lectures fully written out in manuscript, to formal commentaries reproduced in handsome printed volumes. The presentation of such diverse kinds of material within a single category reflects the historical reality that almost all the items are more or less closely linked to university teaching. The printed commentaries may stand at a slightly greater distance from the classroom than some of the manuscript material, but the great majority of them were the work of university professors, and they rather frequently bear such obvious traces of school origin as division into numbered *lectiones*, references to the previous day's lecture, and so on. Yet the division between script and print also merits attention, not only because valid questions may be raised about possible differences in objectives and audience between manuscript and printed works, but also because commentary on the *Canon* has a place in the broader picture of the vast output of Renaissance printed commentary on texts in all fields.

To take up the latter point first, the large extent to which commentary as a genre flourished in the Renaissance and early modern period is now becoming well known.[1] Retention in university curricula of traditional authoritative texts and of the practice of teaching by means of lectures on those texts would doubtless in itself have been sufficient to ensure the continued production of some commentaries. But in addition, the philological interests of the humanists; new translations of long-known Greek works; the diffusion of hitherto unknown or neglected literary, historical, philosophical, and scientific classical texts; the birth of rigorous classical scholarship,[2] the formation of new educational or religious institutions;[3] and the biblical and patristic scholarship of the era of the Reformation—all of these called for the continued growth and development of exposition of texts, and hence of commentary production in a wide variety of different disciplines. Within this vast amount of material, Latin commentary on the *Canon* obviously occupies a very modest space indeed. Yet the context may

---

[1] See Buck and Herding, *Der Kommentar in der Renaissance*, and Lohr, "Renaissance Latin Aristotle Commentaries." The inclusion of Renaissance commentaries in *CTC* is also revealing further the extent of this material as successive volumes appear. In the opinion of Cesare Vasoli, "La storia delle nuove edizioni, traduzioni e commenti usciti durante il Quattrocento e il Cinquecento dalla penna di maestri umanisti o, comunque, di forma e di 'tecnica' umanistica potrebbe quindi costituire, da sola, un grosso capitolo di una futura recensione delle 'fonti' scientifiche di questi secoli." Cesare Vasoli, "La cultura dei secoli XIV–XVI," *Atti del primo convegno internazionale di recognizione delle fonti per la storia della scienza italiana: i secoli XIV–XVI*, ed. Carlo Maccagni. Domus Galileiana, Pisa. Pubblicazioni di storia della scienza (Florence, 1967), sezione 5, vol. 1, p. 47.

[2] Grafton, *Scaliger*, is illuminating on the history of the development of various forms of literary and philological commentary on classical texts over the course of the fifteenth and sixteenth centuries.

[3] For example, the schools of the Society of Jesus, for which the celebrated Coimbra commentaries on Aristotle were written; see Lohr, *Renaissance Quarterly* 28 (1975), 717–719.

perhaps serve as a useful reminder that, in the period under discussion, an author's decision to adopt the commentary form does not in itself convey any information about his approach and point of view; and in particular, such a decision in no way necessarily reflects any especially reactionary or backward-looking tendencies on his part. Sixteenth-century exposition of texts often departed widely from earlier scholastic commentary in both content and form; and even those authors who in their commentaries continued the practice of arguing *quaestiones* on traditional topics in scholastic format did not necessarily always do so with traditional goals or opinions in mind. These remarks apply even to commentaries on works by authors often thought of as symbols of scholastic conservatism. Recent studies have, for example, brought out the varied standpoints of fifteenth- to seventeenth-century commentators on works of the prototypical "school" author, Aristotle; these ranged from philological study of the Greek text, to Counter-Reformation Catholic theology, to wholly secular natural philosophy.[4]

Turning to commentaries on medical texts, we may note that these continued to appear, mostly on Hippocratic and Galenic works, throughout the sixteenth and much of the seventeenth century. Until we have for the major ancient medical authors catalogues comparable to Charles Lohr's invaluable survey of Renaissance Aristotle commentaries, it will remain impossible to arrive at any accurate assessment of the extent and significance of Renaissance medical commentary, but there can be no doubt that the output was large. Furthermore, it seems clear that a good deal of this literature was inspired not merely by the continued use in university faculties of medicine of traditional textbooks of Greek or Arabic origin in their medieval Latin translations, but also by the interest of medical humanists in securing a fresh approach to Greek medicine. Greek medical works unknown, or little known, in the Middle Ages were supplied with commentary (there are, for example, fourteen sixteenth-century Latin expositions of Paulus Aegineta);[5] and the publication of the Greek text or of humanist Latin translations of works long studied in earlier Latin versions were also productive of new expositions. Indeed, Greek medicine itself incorporated an impressive and authoritative body of commentary in the shape of Galen's own commentaries on Hippocrates, which played a large part in shaping the entire Hippocratic tradition.[6] Certainly, Renaissance editors and translators did not neglect this aspect of Galen's

---

[4] Charles B. Schmitt, *Aristotle and the Renaissance* (Cambridge, Mass., and London, 1983), passim; and Lohr, *Studies in the Renaissance* 21 (1974), 228–32.

[5] Rice, "Paulus Aegineta," pp. 145–47, 176–89.

[6] Wesley D. Smith, *The Hippocratic Tradition* (Ithaca, N.Y., 1979), pp. 123–76.

work. The few commentaries by Galen available in Latin during the Middle Ages were all retranslated; a considerably larger number of such expositions was translated for the first time; and Galen's commentaries appeared in numerous printings, both separately and in collected editions of his works. If the number of Renaissance editions is any criterion, Galen's commentary on the Hippocratic *Aphorisms* stood third in popularity among his works, being exceeded in number of impressions only by the *Ars medica*, used as a textbook in almost all university faculties of medicine, and the useful *De differentiis febrium*.[7]

Most medical commentary was no doubt devoted to the exposition of works of Greek origin. The principal Arabic medical authors other than Avicenna who continued to be studied were Rasis and Mesue; their works, along with fourteenth- and fifteenth-century commentaries on them, were reprinted a number of times in the first half of the sixteenth century. But new expositions of these authors seem to have been restricted to a small group of commentaries on the *Almansor* of Rasis.[8] Among Arabic medical authors, therefore, Avicenna probably attracted much the largest body of Latin commentary written after 1500, but there is no doubt that the total number of commentaries on various works of Galen and Hippocrates, not to mention other Greek medical writers, greatly exceeded that of commentaries on the *Canon*.

Commentaries on works of Arabic origin are not necessarily to be distinguished by type from those on the Greeks. If one were to attempt the classification of Renaissance medical commentaries (an imprudent enterprise, given the present state of knowledge of this body of writing), the main division, in this as in other branches of learning, probably lies between school commentaries on works used as textbooks and scholarly endeavors to establish the original meaning of recently introduced or less studied texts.[9] Commentaries on the *Canon* belong, al-

---

[7] Durling, "Census," pp. 243 and 294–95, nos. 149–60.

[8] Commentaries on Rasis are listed in H. Otto Illgen, *Die abendländischen Rhazes-Kommentatoren des XIV bis XVII Jahrhunderts* (Leipzig, 1921). A good idea of the extent of sixteenth-century printing relating to Rasis and Mesue can be gained from *A Catalogue of Sixteenth-Century Printed Books in the National Library of Medicine*, comp. Richard J. Durling (Bethesda, Md., 1967). The collection of the NLM includes at least ten editions of works of Rasis that appeared between 1500 and 1544; there are also a number of editions of commentaries written before 1500, most notably that of Marco Gatinaria, with thirteen editions between 1500 and 1575. Sixteenth-century authors of some note who wrote on Rasis included Leonardo Giacchini, Giambatista Da Monte, and, of course, Vesalius.

[9] Anthony Grafton, "On the Scholarship of Politian and Its Context," *Journal of the Warburg and Courtauld Institutes* 40 (1977), delineates such a difference between genres among Renaissance commentaries on classical literary texts. The same author's "Teacher, Text and Pupil" presents detailed examples of the way in which school lec-

most without exception, to the former category, but so do many commentaries on, for example, the Galenic *Ars medica*. The salient features of expositions of both the *Canon* and the *Ars* tend to be an emphasis on discussion of the subject matter in general and major authors' views on it, a disposition to channel commentary into the well-worn grooves of traditional problems or *quaestiones*, and a loose structure easily allowing for the interpolation of material more or less unrelated to the base text. Moreover, these features are common both to traditional scholastic medical commentary as practiced in the fourteenth and fifteenth centuries, and also to sixteenth-century productions marked by abandonment of highly structured syllogistic arguments and by reliance chiefly upon ancient or recent, not medieval, authors.

Thus, for example, the discussions of resolutive and compositive method and of whether or not there is a neutral state between health and sickness, discussions that were staples of lectures on the *Ars*, do not seem much different in character from the topics taken up in commentary on the opening sections of *Canon* 1.1—indeed, identical *quaestiones* were often discussed in commentaries on both texts. And commentators on the *Ars* allowed themselves just as much freedom to interpolate material in accordance with the demands of current controversy, pedagogical tradition, or their own whims as their colleagues who expounded the *Canon*. To take only one example, the commentary on the *Ars* by Giovanni Argenterio, a noted neoteric with a reputation for unconventional medical ideas (and a critic of teaching by commentary), incorporates a substantial section on the elements, with frequent citations of Aristotle and treatment of such subjects as the rainbow and falling stars. This certainly goes well beyond anything called for by the brief remark in the text about the constitution of the body from hot, wet, cold, and dry. In the same commentary, Argenterio also devoted much attention to refuting the views of two of his contemporaries: Giambatista Da Monte (on whether medicine is an art or a science) and Matteo Corti (on the forms of the elements).[10]

---

tures on Roman poets (to an audience considerably younger and more unformed than medical students) were used as a vehicle of general instruction.

[10] *Joannis Argenterii . . . Operum in tres tomos divisorum volumen primum* (Venice, 1592), pp. 106–13 (physics of matter, natural phenomena involving the elements; discussion of the elements in human bodies begins on p. 113). At p. 106: "At quoniam ut diximus ex elementis similares partes fieri tradit Galenus nec tamen hoc loco explicat quomodo id fiat, operae pretium esse duco hoc loco disputationem instituere de elementis paulo diligentiorem, ut philosophis non satis bene institutis, aut medicis etiam rudioribus, qui haec nostra legere cupient, consulamus."

Argenterio's dislike of teaching by commentary is noted in Lonie, "Fever Pathology," p. 20. Regarding Renaissance discussions of resolutive and compositive method based on

One area where one might expect to find significant difference between commentary on Greek and on Arabic texts is of course that of philology. Obviously, given the relative state of knowledge among Western medical authors of the Greek and Arabic languages, texts of Greek origin offered a good deal more scope for close philological commentary. Yet such an emphasis is by no means always present in Renaissance commentaries on Greek medical works. Thus the text of the *Ars* accompanying Argenterio's commentary is printed in both Greek and Latin, but the commentary pays little attention to the niceties of the Greek text. Argenterio was, no doubt, more interested in medical ideas than in Greek authors as such; the picture is somewhat different when one turns to the commentary on the Hippocratic *Aphorisms* by Oddo Oddi, who enjoyed considerable renown as a Galenist. Oddi's commentary is sharply focused on the Hippocratic text, and on supporting or interpretive passages of Galen; yet even Oddi disclaimed any intention of embarking on an exposition of the entire vocabulary of the *Aphorisms*, remarking that the language of Hippocrates was a matter for the grammarian rather than the physician.[11]

Finally, the example of Oddo Oddi, just cited, may serve as a reminder that the authors of commentaries on the *Canon* were themselves in many, probably most, instances also the authors of commentaries on Greek medical works included in the standard university curriculum. Given the requirements of their teaching positions, such a combination was, of course, scarcely to be avoided. While the same author might certainly approach the exposition of different works differently—the enthusiasm manifested by Capodivacca for lecturing on the *Aphorisms* was less evident when he undertook *Canon* 4.1[12]—the con-

---

the *Ars*, see, most recently, Daniela Mugnai Carrara, "Una polemica umanistico-scolastica circa l'interpretazione delle tre dottrine ordinate di Galeno," *Annali dell'Istituto e Museo di Storia della Scienza di Firenze* 8 (1983), 31–57.

[11] ". . . constituimus taediosam quoque nominum interpraetationem evitare, neque enim nomina omnia exponenda sunt, ut recte Galenus in expositione linguarum Hippocratis sentit, id enim grammaticae peritiae, non medicae artis munus est." *Oddo de Oddis . . . in primam Aphorismorum Hippocratis sectionem elaboratissima et lucidissima expositio* (Padua, 1564), fols. 1ᵛ–2ʳ.

[12] ". . . statim ad ipsos *Aphorismos* interpretandos accedamus. Neque mihi elaborandum est, ut vos inflammatos reddam. Video enim vos satis superque ardentes. . . . Vos enim liberos, moratos, atque maxime idoneos conspicio. Accedit etiam quod vos incredibili vestra humanitate me ad hanc sedem elevastis; et ob id me utilitati vestrae paratissimum semper audietis. Et ideo audacter ac hilari etiam animo propositam rem aggrediar." *Hieronymi Capivaccei . . . In primum Aphorismorum Hippocratis librum doctissima et dilucidissima explanatio, in scholis per ordinarias lectiones tradita*, p. 23, printed with his *Tractatus de foetus formatione* (Venice, 1599). Capodivacca's propensity to cultivate good relations with students has already been noted in Chapter 4, above.

ception of the task of commentary was unlikely to be radically transformed between one set of lectures and the other. In sum, while the commentaries on the *Canon* are far from representative of the whole range of Renaissance medical commentary, they are neither isolated nor idiosyncratic.

Whatever may be the case in general, where expositions of the *Canon* are concerned it is extremely hard to evaluate possible differences in intent and effect between manuscript and printed works. In the first place, one whole area in which the impact of printing upon the dissemination of scientific information requires particularly close attention is simply not present in most of these commentaries, since as a rule they are not illustrated and contain little or nothing in the way of tables, diagrams, or mathematical notation. The one major exception to this generalization—the illustrations of scientific instruments designed by the author found in the several editions of Santorio Santorio's commentary on *Canon* 1.1—is deservedly famous in part just because it is so uncharacteristic of the genre.[13] The chief general comment inspired by the physical appearance of mid- and later sixteenth- and seventeenth-century printed commentaries on the *Canon* is that the format often gives an impression of modernity—by the use of such devices as small page size, italic type, and so on—that is sometimes, but not always, justified by the contents.[14]

When one comes to consider the content, it is impossible to reach any general conclusions about the amount of editing or revision normally likely to intervene between a teacher's original lecture and his printed commentary, or indeed between the original lecture and a surviving manuscript copy. In a number of instances, sets of manuscript lectures and printed editions closely resemble one another in degree of polish and thoroughness of treatment. But there are few cases in which the survival of both a manuscript and an edition of the same work permits direct comparison, and even in such cases the process of transformation of the written to the printed text is not always easy to follow. For example, some of Giambatista Da Monte's lectures on *Canon* 1.1 survive in two versions in the same manuscript. It is unclear whether

[13] Thus, the broad claims for the revolutionary impact of precisely reproducible illustrations made in Elizabeth L. Eisenstein, *The Printing Press as an Agent of Change* (Cambridge, 1979), 2:566–74, have little relevance as far as commentaries on the *Canon* or much of the other academic medical writing published in the sixteenth century is concerned. Regarding Santorio's instruments, see further below.

[14] For example, the Venice, 1557, edition of Da Monte, comm. *Canon* 1.1 is presented in such a format (the choice of Da Monte's posthumous editor or publisher); regarding the mix of traditional and innovative material in this work, see below and Part IV.

these represent lectures given in different years, or the collation of two copies (by two different student *reportatores?*) of the same set. Nor can it easily be determined how the two sets were used to produce the printed version.[15] Similarly, Bernardino Paterno's treatment of *Canon* 1.1 appears to differ in manuscript and printed versions.[16] But Paterno must have lectured on *Canon* 1.1 a minimum of ten times during his fifty-year teaching career; and the edition was prepared for publication several years after his death by one of his former pupils.[17] Hence, one cannot say whether the differences between the manuscript of his lectures given in the academic year 1578–79 and the edition of 1596 are due to Paterno's own revisions over the years or to the editorial activities of Bernardino Gaio.

Nor is it any easier to arrive at conclusions about the probable readership of these editions. Presumably, the fact of printing indicates that a commentary was considered (at any rate by its author or editor and its publisher) to be potentially of interest to and hence salable among a circle wider than that of the author's own students. Certainly, printing indicates that at the date and place of publication authorship of a commentary on Avicenna could still add to, or at any rate not substantially detract from, the prestige of a learned physician (although we may note that a few of these works were published under titles—*De febribus, Dis-*

---

[15] Verona, Biblioteca Civica, MS 1507 (Biadego 580). A set of seventy-three numbered lectures headed (fol. 1ʳ) "Excellentissimi Domini Johannes Baptistae Montani Veronensis in primum primi Avicennae doctissima interpretatio" occupies fols. 1ʳ–124ᵛ. On fol. 126ʳ another set of lectures on the same text begins, the first being numbered 62. The first lecture no. 62 begins (fol. 107) "Cum in superioribus lectionibus"; the second lecture no. 62 begins (fol. 126) "*Nutriens masticatione. Iam vidisti in precedenti capitulo*" (the lemma is the incipit of *Canon* 1.1.4.2). The second incipit appears to match that in the printed Da Monte, comm. *Canon* 1.1 (Venice, 1554), fol. 236ʳ.

[16] A comparison of the introductory remarks on *complexio* (lemma: "*complexio est qualitas*") as they appear in Paterno, comm. *Canon* 1.1, lecture 12, WL MS 602 (unnumbered folios), and in Paterno, comm. *Canon* 1.1 (Venice, 1596), fol. 27ʳ⁻ᵛ, reveals that, while the same points are made—Avicenna first laid out general *theoremata* about *complexio* and then proceeded to specific varieties; Da Monte was critical of Avicenna's apparent departure from Galen's definition—the wording of the two versions is different. WL MS 602 is a notebook containing several sets of Paterno's lectures, apparently compiled by a student.

[17] Paterno held the first chair in theory at Padua from 1563 until his death in 1592; however, he had previously held a lesser chair in theory at Padua in 1536–37, and subsequently taught at Pavia and Pisa (see Palmer, *Studio of Venice*, p. 98). The claim in the title of his comm. *Canon* 1.1 (Venice, 1596) that he had taught medicine "totos quinquaginta annos" therefore seems amply justified. During the thirty years he spent at Padua he would presumably have been teaching *Canon* 1.1 every third year. For Gaio's contribution to the edition see his preface in Paterno, comm. *Canon* 1.1 (Venice, 1596), fol. 2ʳ⁻ᵛ.

quisitiones physiologicae[18]—that do not stress their status as commentaries).

On the whole, as one might expect, there seems to have been a tendency to select for printing commentaries by men of distinction, at least as measured by output of other works and fame among contemporaries, but there are surprising exceptions to this generalization. For example, the extensive lectures on *Canon* 1.1 by Matteo Corti, who enjoyed considerable reputation in his day, seem never to have been printed.[19] In several cases, commentaries first appeared in print posthumously, either in separate editions that owed their existence to the filial piety of the author's pupils (as in Paterno's case), or in the case of men of larger renown, as part of editions of their collected works (as happened with Girolamo Cardano). Such editions can scarcely be regarded as evidence for any great demand for the individual commentary in question, although they attest to the reputation of the author.

A surer sign of a public for particular commentaries is presumably their appearance in second or subsequent separate editions. It is therefore worth remarking that several sixteenth- and seventeenth-century commentaries on the *Canon* achieved this distinction; others appeared in editions beyond the first as part of an author's collected works. Other evidence for an audience for these commentaries beyond the author's own pupils comes from the inclusion of excerpts from them in later commonplace books. Thus, the humanist and churchman André Dudith, in retirement at Paskow after his break with the Roman church and the end of his diplomatic career, occupied some of his time with medical studies, which led him, in 1577, to copy a set of excerpts from printed medical books, including seventy-five folios from the second edition of Giambatista Da Monte's commentary on *Canon* 1.1, published at Venice in 1557. Similarly, substantial excerpts from Santorio Santorio's commentary on *Canon* 1.1, first published at Venice in 1625 or 1626, were copied by J. H. Marmi into his commonplace book in 1716. Moreover, the frequency with which Renaissance commentators on the *Canon* discussed the way their recent predecessors had expounded the same text suggests that some among these works (notably

---

[18] See Massaria, comm. *Canon* 4.1 (Book 7 of his *Practica medica*, Trèves, 1607), and Costeo, comm. *Canon* 1.1 (Bologna, 1589). In neither these nor other works with variant titles was any effort made to conceal their status as commentaries, so that the titles may be taken as simply additional explanation of the subject matter. The practice was an old one; for example, Dino del Garbo's early fourteenth-century commentary on *Canon* 1.4 is referred to in both manuscripts and printed editions as his *Dilucidatorium totius practice*.

[19] At any rate, no such commentary is listed in Vicenzo Bianchi, *Le opere a stampa di Matthaeus Curtius* (Pavia, n.d.), nor have I succeeded in locating an edition.

the, in some respects, original treatment by Da Monte) were valued not just as crutches for earnest students, but as contributions to medical discourse of interest in their own right.[20] A natural assumption would be that printed editions reached a wider audience than manuscripts. This may well be the case, but it should be noted that manuscripts could still serve as channels for the transmission of medical knowledge and ideas in the sixteenth century, as the long essays on scientific topics exchanged by physicians under the guise of personal letters testify. Doubtless in some cases, the act of writing out a set of academic lectures in full reflected the intention of author or copyist to proceed to publication; but it is also apparent that on occasion medical students in the sixteenth century continued a practice of their medieval predecessors and made manuscript *reportationes* of lectures for circulation among themselves. Yet awareness of the probable deficiencies of such *reportationes* was in itself, as Da Monte noted, a reason for professors to welcome, and indeed seek out, any opportunity to print their commentaries.[21] On balance, it seems evident that the ap-

[20] Examples of second or subsequent editions of commentaries published as separate works: Da Monte, comm. *Canon* 1.1; Santorio, comm. *Canon* 1.1; Betti, comm. *Canon* 1.4; Stefano, comm. *Canon* 4.1; Da Monte, comm. *Canon* 1.4 (see Appendix 2). Examples of second or subsequent editions as part of an author's collected works: Capodivacca, comm. *Canon* 4.1; Santorio, comm. *Canon* 1.1. The two commonplace books referred to are Paris, Bibliothèque Nationale MS lat. 7084, where the excerpts from "Joh. Bapt. Montani lectionibus in primi lib. Can. Avic. pr. Fen" occupy fols. 74ʳ–148ᵛ, with, at fol. 71ʳ, "Pascovie, Andr. Dudith 18 Xbr 1577" (the lectures excerpted include some of those in which Da Monte vigorously attacked Avicenna's ideas on humors); and WL MS 3453, Marmi, J. H., Commonplace books, vol. 9. Dudith's medical interests at Pascow are described in Pierre Costil, *André Dudith, humaniste hongrois, 1533–1589, Sa vie, son oeuvre et ses manuscrits grecs* (Paris, 1935), p. 172. Various instances of citation of Renaissance commentators by their successors will be noted in the course of this chapter; to them may be added the frequent references to Da Monte found in an anonymous seventeenth-century commentary on *Canon* 1.1, Perugia, Biblioteca Comunale Augusta, MS conv. sopp. 978 (M 1), e.g., pp. 58, 89, 140, 156, 167.

[21] A number of medical letter collections were printed, following the success of the influential and widely circulated *Epistolae medicinales* of Manardo (see Chapter 3, n. 95, above). Others remain in manuscript.

An example of the work of student reporters of lectures is provided by the lectures on *Canon* 1.1 of Matteo Corti contained in Siena, Biblioteca Comunale, MS C IX 11, which were copied in 1537–38 (fols. 74, 106ᵛ). The set is made up of lectures given in 1529 (fol. 6ʳ), noted down by Giustiniano Finetto (Sinetto?) (fol. 7ʳ), supplemented by lectures given by Corti in 1527 obtained from Girolamo Stefanelli (fol. 90ᵛ). (Stefanelli was teaching philosophy at Padua in the 1540s; see Palmer, *Studio*, p. 110.) Of his commentary on *Canon* 1.2 Da Monte remarked: "Speramus ea commentaria, si deo placuerit, nos esse aedituros, non quidem gloriae captandae gratia, a qua semper fuimus alieni, sed ut ingenue fatear, erit aeditionis causa, quod video divulgari disseminarique a meis auditoribus ea, quae me legente transcribunt, quae Dii boni ita conscribuntur, ut cum mihi quan-

pearance in print of a sequence of new expositions in modern format by contemporary professors of medicine holding senior positions in major universities must, at least in the academic circles with which those professors were connected, have preserved and probably expanded a readership for commentaries on the *Canon*; furthermore, it seems likely that changing printing styles were themselves an essential ingredient in the continuing acceptability of such commentaries. Hence, the printing industry, which, up to the 1520s, played an important part in perpetuating and expanding the audience for fourteenth- and fifteenth-century scholastic medical commentaries, thereafter was equally crucial in securing a readership for contemporary expositions of Avicenna's medieval text.[22]

Only in Italy and the Iberian peninsula do new lectures and commentaries based on medical school courses on the *Canon* appear to have been committed to writing in any number after about 1520. And of the works included in Appendix 2, the great majority were the product of Italian universities. Thus, although the list of lectures or commentaries remaining in manuscript could perhaps be extended by a more systematic search of Iberian libraries than was undertaken for the present work, it seems clear that Italian universities maintained their historic predominance in the output of *Canon* commentary; this was certainly the case as far as printed works were concerned. The commentaries written in the Italian schools fit into a pattern with the sequence of editions of the text of the *Canon* published in Italy in the same period and with the impression of various well informed contemporaries that serious attention to Avicenna was peculiarly characteristic of Italian medical teaching. Hence it is to the characteristics of the commentaries written in Italy that the following discussion is principally directed.

The commentaries of Italian provenance are by no means equally distributed, either as regards chronology, or portion of the *Canon* expounded, or institution of origin. Chronologically, most of the expo-

---

doque offeruntur, non amplius ut mea recognoscam, ita sunt corrupta, contaminata, et infeliciter explicata." Da Monte, comm. *Canon* 1.4 (Venice, 1556), fol. 51ʳ. Unfortunately, Da Monte did not survive long enough to see any of his commentaries through the press himself.

[22] A few pre-sixteenth-century commentaries on parts of the *Canon* pertaining to *practica* continued to appear in new editions after the 1520s, including Dino del Garbo on sections of Book 4 (*Dinus in chirurgia*, Venice, 1536 and 1544), Giovanni Arcolano on *Canon* 4.1 (*De febribus*, Padua, 1685), and Biagio Astario, also on fevers. Astario's commentary was printed with M. Gatinaria, *De remediis morborum*, in editions of Venice, 1575, Paris, 1540, and Lyon, 1556; a chapter from it was reprinted, presumably for the last time, in Christian Gottfried Gruner, *De variolis et morbillis fragmenta medicorum Arabistarum* (Jena, 1790), pp. 73–85.

sitions are clustered between about the 1540s and the 1580s, although at least ten were composed, and a few others reissued, after 1620. Among the parts of the *Canon* used in teaching, Book 1, Fen 1, was by far the most frequent subject of written exposition, accounting for about half the items. It was followed by Book 4, Fen 1 (fevers), on which about ten sets of lectures or commentaries have been located, and by Book 1, Fen 4 (general therapy), with four items. No more than three treatments have been located of any other single portion of the *Canon*. In terms of institutional distribution, the most salient feature is the predominance of Padua: almost half the items listed come from Padua, which was followed in productivity, at some distance, by Pavia, then Bologna (see Appendix 2). The different levels of output reflect the conditions described in a previous chapter: the relative sizes and general levels of scholarly and scientific activity at different institutions, and variations of emphasis in statutory curricula, which tended to be most traditional in the oldest established institutions. These considerations serve at least partially to explain the fact that to the various achievements of the Paduan medical school between the time of Vesalius and that of Harvey must be added the rather dubious distinction of leadership in production of commentaries on the *Canon*.

In type, the commentaries may be divided into three main groups. The first of these comprises expositions produced between about the 1520s and the 1540s, and consists of the work of men whose views were formed at the height of the controversy over the Arabs and at a time when enthusiasm for every aspect of Greek medicine, and concomitant hostility to Latin medical scholasticism, were still innovative forces in medical thought. Meanwhile, the rather rapid sequence of publications containing the work of Alpago and Mantino could reasonably be perceived as holding out the promise that linguistic studies would lead to the restoration of Avicenna's own tarnished reputation. Commentators in this group, while widely divergent in their opinions, tended to take the task of reevaluating Avicenna and his earlier Latin interpreters very seriously, and could on occasion be strongly critical of both.

For the commentators in the second group, writing between the 1550s and the 1620s and more or less contemporary with the various text editions of Rinio, Costeo and Mongio, and Graziolo, the controversy over the Arabs was no longer a particularly pressing issue. In this period, the most frequently studied portions of the *Canon* were often simply accepted as useful, if unremarkable, introductory handbooks to certain parts of Galenic medicine, still the reigning orthodoxy.

Finally, over the course of the mid- and later seventeenth century the gradual dilution, breakdown, and ultimate replacement of aspects of Aristotelian natural philosophy and of the entire system of Galenic physiology combined with the decline of the north Italian universities to reduce much of the traditional teaching based on Avicenna to a cursory and pro forma exercise. Some lecturers, however, used the assigned text of Avicenna to designate the general topics to be taught, and then drew most of their actual subject matter from recent scientific and medical writings, which either ignored or contradicted not only the medieval but also, increasingly, the ancient past. Let us examine some examples from each of these categories.

Paduan Commentaries from the 1520s to the 1540s: Matteo Corti, Oddo Oddi, Giambatista Da Monte

Within the space of little more than fifteen years, between 1528 and the mid-1540s, three leading professors at Padua wrote substantial commentaries on portions of the *Canon*. In different ways, the commentaries of Corti, Oddi, and Da Monte all seem designed to contribute to the modernization of the teaching of *theoria*; but given the intellectual and institutional setting in which their work was produced, it is small wonder that their approach to this endeavor was highly ambiguous and eclectic. For the task of commenting on the *Canon* was probably never more difficult or more controversial than at the time when Corti, Oddi, and Da Monte wrote.

A glimpse of the strong passions apt to be aroused at Padua in those years by the subject of Avicenna, especially considered as a guide to practical treatment, can be found in the prefatory material to two rival commentaries on a portion of the surgical material in *Canon* 4. Gian Filippo Ingrassia, who had received his medical degree at Padua in 1537 and later taught at Naples, introduced his work with a stinging attack on those who still would hear no criticism of Avicenna and the Arabs and their older Latin followers, characterizing such people as afflicted with the incurable disease of stupidity and grunting like pigs in their attempt to gain nourishment from indigestible acorns.[23] In 1543, Mariano Santo, a practitioner in Venice, expended equal vehemence in his

---

[23] Ingrassia, *De tumoribus* (comm. *Canon* 4.3.1) (Naples, 1553), dedicatory epistle, fols. + ii^r–iii^r. Ingrassia (ca. 1510–80) taught anatomy and *practica* at Naples from 1544; in 1556 he went to Palermo as *protomedico*. An admirer of Vesalius, he is remembered for his anatomical studies. On him, see *DSB*, 7:16–17. The immediate reference is to disputes at Naples, but Ingrassia's ideas were shaped at Padua. On the position of *protomedico*, a state official supervising medical practitioners, see Palmer, "Physicians and the State."

187

dedicatory letter addressed to the Riformatori of the University of Padua in denouncing the literary rather than scientific interests, the arrogance, the ignorance of Arabic, and the lack of practical experience of the "galenistici," who, as he saw it, dominated academic instruction. For Santo, the defense of Avicenna was part of a broader attack on the exaltation of verbal over manual skills in medicine.[24] The *Canon* for him was the tool of the working practitioner, rather than the symbol of the inadequacy of older Latin medicine that it was for so many of his contemporaries.

Corti's long and successful career included teaching positions at Pavia, Bologna, and Pisa, as well as at Padua, and appointment as personal physician to Pope Clement VII (with ultimately fatal results for the pope, according to Girolamo Cardano).[25] His interest in the reevaluation of scholastic medical teaching was manifested as early as 1518, when he, along with Pietro Antonio Rustico, who was soon to be Symphorien Champier's collaborator in the revised edition of the *Canon* published in 1522, was one of a group of professors at Pavia to whom Champier dedicated his revised and corrected edition of Giovanni Arcolano's commentary on *Canon* 4.1. Champier's letter of dedication reveals that not only the *Canon* itself, but also the older tradition of commentary aroused ambiguous response in humanist circles. It explains that while all right-thinking physicians studied Hippocrates and

[24] Santo, comm. *Canon* (4.3, portions) (Venice, 1543), dedicatory epistle. Santo was a successful surgeon and lithotomist who also held a degree in medicine. On him, see *Biogr. Lex.*, 2nd ed. (Berlin-Vienna, 1932), 4:81–82. The opening words of his preface (Santo, fol. 1ʳ) are "Et si diu mecum ipse de medicina ratiocinaturus, quid potissimum esset in ea auspicandum foelici sidere cogitassem, de manuali tamen medicina, et ipsius laudibus, et doctrina, et utilitate incipiendum non ab re fore mihi cogitanti succurrit, tanquam de primaria partium medicinae, nomine, atque auxilio sanctissimae trinitatis locuturo." The themes of praise of manual skill and experience in medicine, and hostility to the *ficta* and chimera of an academic and verbal medicine are brought together in his concluding epistle (ibid., fol. 313ʳ) to Francesco Frigimelica, professor of theory and practice at Padua.

[25] As regards Corti's biography, writings, and intellectual position, Lynn Thorndike, *History of Magic and Experimental Science* (New York, 1941), 5:324–26, where references to most of the earlier published accounts of Corti are collected, and Aldo Scapini, *L'archiatra mediceo e pontificio Matteo Corti (secolo XVI) e il suo Commento all'Anatomia di Mondino di Liuzzi*, Scientia Veterum, no. 142 (Pisa, 1970), pp. 6–14 (noting Cardano's opinion on p. 9), are superseded by Vivian Nutton, " 'Qui magni Galeni doctrinam in re medica primus revocavit'; Matteo Corti und der Galenismus im medizinischen Unterricht der Renaissance," paper delivered to the Heidelberger Tagung der Senatskommission der DFG für Humanismusforschung, September 1985. The account of Corti's views that follows was written before I had access to Nutton's paper, but reaches much the same conclusions. Nutton establishes Corti's death date as 1544. See also *DBI*, 29:795–97.

Galen and rejected the barbarous Latin style, methodology of *quaestiones*, and absence of worthwhile philosophical and medical content in such scholastic authors as Arcolano, Pietro d'Abano, Giacomo da Forlì, and so on, nonetheless their works had a certain usefulness for beginning students, for mental relaxation(!), as aids to memory, and when composing medical works.[26]

Corti's own rejection of the recent past went a good deal further, if one may judge by his well-known commentary on the *Anatomia* of Mondino, an exposition largely devoted to acerbic criticism of Mondino for his failures to understand, his oversimplifications of, and his disagreements with Galen.[27] In the present context, Corti's commentary on Mondino is of interest as a possible model for the use of the commentary as a vehicle of attack on the commented-upon author by Da Monte, and to a lesser extent Oddo, or Marco, Oddi. Yet in that work Corti seems for the most part to have confined his criticisms to Mondino himself; where Arabic authors were concerned, he displayed a concordist tendency and attempted to reconcile them with Galen.[28] However, in the lectures on the first four *doctrinae* of *Canon* 1.1 that he delivered as first professor of theory at Padua in 1528–29,[29] Corti turned to the problem of arriving at an accurate estimate of Avicenna's actual contribution to Latin medicine. That this interest continued to develop for the rest of his career is perhaps suggested by the information that in old age he attempted—apparently unsuccessfully, or too late for any use—to learn Arabic.[30] (Although occasional references to

[26] *Joannis Herculani Veronensis expositio perutilis in primam fen quarti Canonis Avicenne una cum adnotamentis prestantissimi viri domini Symphoriani Champerii* (Lyon, 1518). The dedication is on fol. [1ᵛ].

[27] An Italian translation of the commentary is contained in Scapini, *L'archiatra mediceo*. As Scapini remarkˢ on p. 16, "La prima impressione che, almeno superficialmente, si trae dopo la lettura del Commento di Matteo Corti all'Anatomia di Mondino e che, ancor più che di commento, di una filippica contra l'Anatomia di Mondino . . . oppure un ottimista potrebbe definire quest'opera soltanto un lungo meraviglioso inno a Galeno."

[28] For example, in Scapini's translation, "Tuttavia il parere di Avicenna puo accordarsi con Galeni, se si intenda che gli intestini sono involuti affinche il cibo non esca facilmente dall'essere vivente; e infatti Galeno non negherebbe cio, ma non si deve dire, come Mondino, affinche il cibo rimanga più a lungo negli intestini." Ibid., p. 89.

[29] Corti, comm. *Canon* 1.1, Bologna, Biblioteca del Archiginnasio, MS A 922, contains an end note saying the lectures were given in 1528. Corti, comm. *Canon* 1.1, Biblioteca Comunale, Siena, MS C IX, 11, dates the exposition 1529 (fol. 6ʳ); this set of lectures breaks off in *Doctrina* 3 (complexions) on fol. 90ʳ, and is supplemented for part of *Doctrina* 4 (humors) by seventeen lectures given by Corti in 1527. Since the opening portions of both commentaries appear to be the same, I take it they are (except for the portion identified as coming from 1527) two copies of the same set of lectures given in the academic year 1528–29.

[30] "Curtius in ultima senecta operam Arabicae linguae praestare decreverat, ut Hasen

189

the "littera nova"[31] show that he was familiar with Alpago's emendations to the Latin text of the *Canon*, no signs of any knowledge of Arabic appear in, at any rate, the first twenty of the lectures that he gave in 1528–29.)

Corti introduced his lectures on *Canon* 1.1 by remarking that some teachers insisted that their pupils first study and imitate Avicenna, reserving Galen for later, optional, reading; others thought that primary emphasis should be given to the study of Galen; and yet others held that both authors should be studied together. Corti aligned himself with the last group, while pointing out that effective simultaneous use of both authors was impossible unless the students knew how the subject matter of various sections of the *Canon* corresponded to that of various books of Galen.[32] He then proceeded to devote most of his first three lectures to supplying this information and providing a general comparison of the two authors and an evaluation of their respective contributions to different branches of medicine. Time after time, his conclusions favored Galen. For example, he excused the prolixity often complained of in Galen with the explanation that Galen had needed to devote much space to the refutation of the ancient medical sects in order to establish the superiority of rational medicine, something Avicenna had been able to take for granted.[33] He expressed the opinion that for many parts of medicine Galen's treatment was much clearer and better than Avicenna's and that it was greatly to be regretted that not all Galen's works were available.[34] When he came to individual branches of medicine, Corti both gave pride of place to anatomy and stressed the striking superiority in scope and detail of Galen's contribution to it;[35] here as in many other important areas (notably complexions and pulse) Avicenna had done no more than provide an efficient summary of Galen's teaching.[36]

---

in fonte videret." Cardano, comm. *Canon* 1.1, 1563, proem, in his *Opera* (Lyon 1663), 9:460.

[31] Corti, comm. *Canon* 1.1, Siena, Biblioteca Comunale, MS C IX 11, fol. 16ᵛ.

[32] "Id quod melius esset, esset ambos simul legere et imitari: et hoc non est possibile fieri a scholaribus nisi prius sciant quod sunt capitula et loca Galeni correspondentia Avicennae, et ideo hoc declarabo." Ibid., fol. 7ʳ.

[33] Ibid.

[34] "Primo declarabo multas esse partes medicinae longe clarius, et perfectius a Galeno quam ab Avicenna traditas esse [*sic*], et utinam haberemus omnes libros Galeni." Ibid., fol. 8ᵛ.

[35] "Septem sunt de quibus medicina, et tota medicina, tractat: Prima est anatomia. . . ." Ibid., fol. 7ᵛ. " . . . modus quo tradidit Galenus anatomiam est clarior." Ibid., fol. 8ᵛ. On Corti as an anatomical lecturer and his association with Vesalius, see Adelmann, *Malpighi*, 1:91.

[36] Corti, comm. *Canon* 1.1, Siena, Biblioteca Comunale, MS C IX 11, fol. 8ᵛ.

Corti also cast doubt on the supposed usefulness of the *Canon* as a handy work of reference for the practicing physician by pointing out that Avicenna's account of any particular subject often required supplementing from other sources, that it was often necessary to look in several different sections of the *Canon* in order to assemble everything Avicenna had to say on a particular subject, and that it was no more difficult to look things up in a Galenic work than in the *Canon*.[37] Corti assured his listeners that on topics on which Avicenna had simply summarized Galen they would reach understanding more easily if they read Galen's own text; when Avicenna interpreted Galen, however, the Arab author aided understanding. Although, ideally, students should read both authors, if they were only able to consult one of them, that one should be Galen.[38]

In the body of his commentary Corti seems to have had two main objectives: the first, and probably most important, was to provide detailed citations of relevant passages in Galen's works to substantiate and fill out his general comments in the proem about the relationship between the subject matter of the different parts of the *Canon* and various books by Galen. But he also announced that he would "follow the order of Jacobus both in questions and in raising *dubia* on the text."[39] His procedure seems to have been to take the sequence and subjects of *quaestiones* and *dubia* from Giacomo da Forlì, while repeatedly and vigorously disagreeing with that author's conclusions. Thus, these lectures serve as a commentary on Giacomo da Forlì as well as on Avicenna, and to that extent recall their author's similar treatment of Mondino de' Liuzzi.[40]

---

[37] "Licet communiter creditur quod Avicenna in unico capitulo dicit quo ad curam fieret, tamen non est verum: et oportet habere omnes 5 libros Canonis pro curatione." Ibid., fol. 10[r].

[38] "Dico ergo quod melius est videre ambos, et qui volunt solum unum videre . . . melius est ut videat [*sic*] Galenum." Ibid., fol. 10[v].

[39] "Nos in legendo textum Avicennae servabimus ordinem Jacobi, et in quaestionibus, et in movendo dubitationes super textum: et decidemus ut veritas est." Ibid., fol. 12[r].

[40] Corti criticized Giacomo for an excessive attention to philosophy and theology—"non est inculcanda theologia in medicina" (Siena, C IX 11, fol. 15[r])—as well as on numerous medical topics, among them the question of whether there is a neutral state between health and sickness (fol. 21[v]), and the definition of various kinds of *spiritus* (fol. 24[r-v]). The element of novelty in Corti's criticisms of earlier Latin medical authors can easily be overstated, since the debates in which fourteenth- and fifteenth-century physicians themselves engaged led them on occasion to criticize each other with almost equal vigor; see, e.g., the controversy recorded in Tommaso del Garbo, *Summa medicinalis* (Venice, 1506), fols. 96[r]–99[r]. Nonetheless, it is clear both that Corti had a substantial and detailed knowledge of fourteenth- and early fifteenth-century medical writers, and that his attack was more sweeping and wholesale than the expressions of differences of opinion among these authors themselves.

Corti's approach to the *Canon* appeared sufficiently radical to arouse the opposition of those of his colleagues who, in his words, "thought the teaching of Avicenna different from that of Galen." According to Corti's own account, earlier in his teaching career, while he was at Pavia, he had already been pursued by accusations that he did not understand Avicenna and indeed had not even read the *Canon*. More recently at Padua, there had been complaints that he was not practiced in lecturing on the *Canon* and that his lectures were fruitless and confused.[41] In reality, Corti seems to have been using the techniques of commentary in a conscious endeavor to induce students to approach the *Canon* (and early Latin commentaries on it) in a spirit of critical detachment that bordered on outright hostility. This becomes clear from the preface of his undated lectures on Book 2 of the Hippocratic *Aphorisms*. There, Corti divided medical teachers into two groups, not three, as in the preface to the lectures on the *Canon*: there were those older men who thought it impossible to provide therapy without the Arabs and therefore urged them upon students; and there were those who thought Hippocrates and Galen the only true *medici* and the Arabs merely inferior transmitters and interpreters. He then added: "And I certainly don't see what use it would be to you to have and to read them [the Arabs], since there is nothing good in them that is not set forth more safely and more clearly by Hippocrates and Galen; for I showed you last year that nothing is said by Avicenna that is not present more clearly and better in Galen."[42]

It seems likely that the commentary of Oddo Oddi was originally based on lectures given while he held the second chair in *theoria* between 1535 and 1543,[43] although he was still working on it after

---

[41] According to a note in a different hand at the end of Bologna, Archiginnasio MS A 922, which has been printed in Carlo Lucchesi, "Manoscritti della Biblioteca Comunale dell'Archiginnasio di Bologna contenuti opere di lettori dello Studio di Padova," *Studi e memorie per la storia dell'Università di Bologna* 7 (1922), 46–47: "non enim defuerunt qui dicerent quod, cum in Avicena non sim bene exercitatus, lectiones nostras non multum profuturas esse, existimantes doctrinam Avicenae diversam a doctrina Galeni."

[42] Paris, Bibliothèque Nationale, MS lat. 6852, containing Corti's seventy-one lectures on *Aphorisms* 2 (fols. 1^r–162^r) and his sixty-nine lectures on fevers (fols. 1^r–104^r, 2nd ser.): "et certe non video quod utilitas vobis sit habere et legere illos [Arabes] cum nihil boni sit apud illos quod non habeatur tutius et clarius ab Hippocrate et Galeni. Ostendi nam ego vobis anno praeterito quod nihil fore ab Avicenna dictum est quod non habeatur clarius et melius apud Galenum. Non tamen inficias eo quod in artem experimentandi reperiantur multa apud Arabes quae non fuerunt experta apud vel Hippocratem, sicuti et apud nos sunt in usu multa multaque experta nostro tempore sunt quae nec tempore Graecorum nec Arabum cognita fuere, quia ars experimentandi adhuc non est completa" (fol. 1^r, 1st ser.).

[43] On Oddo Oddi, see Bertolaso, "Ricerche d'archivio" (1959–60), pp. 23–24; To-

1547[44] and it was unfinished at his death in 1558 (it was subsequently completed and edited for publication by his son Marco).[45] Certainly in some respects it looked like both a continuation of and a response to Corti's work. Oddo was, as we have seen, a noted Galenist and in his preface he (or perhaps Marco) was openly and sharply critical of Avicenna, accusing him of introducing confusion and obscurity into Galen's own clear thought.[46] Furthermore, although in the body of his work much of the time he treated Avicenna with nominal respect, this was apt to be achieved through a procedure of deducing Avicenna's "real" opinion by consulting Galen.[47] In addition, Oddo Oddi had a long-standing interest in the problem of securing a better Latin text of the *Canon* (he was on the academic committee that approved Alpago's work and he encouraged Graziolo many years later); he based his exposition on Alpago's text, which he claimed to be in general use, and rather frequently compared the latter's renderings with those of Gerard of Cremona and Jacob Mantino.[48] Yet Oddo also filled his pages with detailed examinations of the views of his predecessors on particular topics, usually citing them in order to disagree: fourteenth-century scholastics such as Tommaso del Garbo and Gentile da Foligno and older contemporaries such as Marcantonio Zimara and Corti are treated in much the same way.[49] The refutation of Corti's views seems indeed in some passages to be a major objective of the work, so that one

masini, *Patavini illustrium virorum elogia*, pp. 46–47, whence we learn that he was called "the soul of Galen"; and *Biogr. Lex.*, 4:403.

[44] Since it contains references to *Canon* I.1, tr. Mantino, published in that year (see Appendix 1); see Oddi, comm. *Canon* I.1 (Venice, 1575), p. 28. The edition prints both the text of the Alpago version (headed "Tr. Bellu.") and that of Mantino ("Tr. Mant."), but this, of course, may have been a decision of Marco Oddi or the publisher.

[45] Marco's dedicatory epistle explains the circumstances; see ibid., sig. [A3v]–[A4r]. N. C. Papadopoli, *Historia Gymnasii Patavini* (Venice, 1726), 1:313, gives the date of Oddo's death as 1558; J. Facciolati, *Fasti Gymnasii Patavini* (Padua, 1757), vol. 2, gives the date as 1563 on p. 343 and 1559 on p. 348. Marco himself became first extraordinary professor of *theoria* in 1578, transferring to the position of first extraordinary professor of *practica* in 1583. In the commentary on *Canon* I.1 (Venice, 1575), the end of Oddo's work is noted on p. 372 (in the middle of *doctrina* 5, on the members), the rest being by Marco (who may also have supplied the preface, or parts of it).

[46] Ibid., pp. 1, 7–9.

[47] See, for example, ibid., pp. 155–56: "Ego autem responderem ex Galeno, quod medicina ad actum deducitur, quia a calore nostra calefit . . . et haec videtur esse vera Avicennae opinio."

[48] Ibid., p. 3, and see n. 44, above.

[49] See, e.g., ibid. pp. 118–25, discussing the views of Tommaso del Garbo—which Oddi appears to have studied in some detail—on whether or not there could be a *complexio* equal *ad pondus*.

is tempted to wonder if Oddo Oddi was not among those who accused Corti of not understanding Avicenna.

Considerably more complex was the attitude toward Avicenna of Giambatista Da Monte, who held the first ordinary professorship of *practica* at Padua from 1540 and moved to the first ordinary chair of *theoria* in 1543. Nineteenth- and twentieth-century historians of medicine have frequently taken note of Da Monte's efforts to revitalize the teaching of *practica*, exemplified by his role in the founding of the Paduan botanic garden and his practice of giving his students clinical instruction in a hospital,[50] while attention has also been drawn to the significance of his writings on method.[51] What chiefly characterized Da Monte as a modern in the eyes of some of his contemporaries, however, was probably his commitment to Greek medical learning in its Renaissance forms. Da Monte, who had been a pupil of Leoniceno, helped prepare the celebrated edition of Galen's *Opera* in new Latin dress published by the Junta press in Venice in 1541–42.[52] As Fracastoro elegantly put it just before announcing his own differences with Da Monte: "If I may speak as a Pythagorean, the soul of Galen seems to have migrated" into Da Monte.[53] Yet Da Monte was known as a modern in still another sense; he acquired a reputation as a critic of Galen on some points, so that, for example, Capodivacca habitually grouped together "Montanus and the moderns" and faulted them for boldly differing from Galen.[54] Certainly, Da Monte took an active part in current medical debate, announcing himself an admirer of Vesalius[55] and engaging in controversy with Fracastoro.

[50] For Da Monte's career, see, in addition to Bertolaso, "Ricerche d'archivio" (1959–60), pp. 23–24, G. Cervetto, *Di Giambatista da Monte e della medicina italiana nel secolo XVI* (Verona, 1839), and Facciolati, *Fasti*, 2:331, 343, 386; also Bylebyl, "School of Padua," pp. 346–49, and Bylebyl ["Early Clinical Teaching at Padua"], in *A Celebration of Medical History*, ed. Lloyd G. Stevenson (Baltimore, 1982), pp. 204–7.

[51] See William P. D. Wightman, "Quid sit methodus? 'Method' in Sixteenth-Century Medical Teaching and Discovery," *Journal of the History of Medicine and Allied Sciences* 19 (1964), 360–76; and Wear, "Galen in the Renaissance," pp. 242–45.

[52] The Junta edition of Galen's *Opera* went into at least eight editions in the sixteenth and early seventeenth centuries. I have consulted *Galeni Opera ex sexta Juntarum editione* (Venice, 1586), in which Da Monte's preface, explaining his responsibility for the ordering of the works of Galen in the sequence adopted for this edition appears at vol. 1, sig. [A8ʳ]–B2ʳ.

[53] For Fracastoro's comment, see *Hieronymi Fracastorii De contagione et contagiosis morbis et eorum curatione, libri III*, ed. and tr. W. C. Wright (New York and London, 1930), 2.3, pp. 76–78.

[54] See Capodivacca, *Opera omnia* (Frankfurt, 1603), pp. 369, 421, 425, 435, and numerous other locations.

[55] Da Monte, comm. *Canon* 1.2 (Venice, 1557), p. 45: "Vesalius lumen totius artis anatomicae"; see also Nutton, "Vesalius, Montanus."

As already noted, Da Monte's apparent desire to extend the practice of lecturing on the *Canon* at Padua was connected with his ideas about the proper organization of medical education. Yet his evident belief that *Canon* 1 could be made to play a useful part in the medical curriculum is certainly not to be equated with unquestioning acceptance either of scholastic tradition or of Avicenna himself. Instead, Da Monte's commentaries are, like that of Corti, consciously detached from earlier tradition in some respects, although the severance is by no means complete. Thus, in the preface to his commentary on *Canon* 1.1, Da Monte showed his awareness of contemporary criticisms of the *quaestio* method, but disavowed any intention to abandon it completely. In a somewhat ambiguous formulation, he announced that he would discuss "pertinent" questions, while dismissing "vain" ones.[56] A reading of the subject index of Da Monte's commentary immediately reveals elements of a register of *quaestiones* such as often accompanied fourteenth- or fifteenth-century scholastic commentaries in manuscript and subsequently in printed editions. Over fifty of the entries in this index are in fact the titles of questions beginning "whether" ("An" or "Utrum"). The impression of continuity is strengthened by a comparison of these question titles with the titles of forty-six questions of *Canon* 1.1 written by Giacomo da Forlì before 1414.[57] In fact, at least half the questions listed in Da Monte's index had earlier been taken up in one form or another by medical authors going back to Taddeo Alderotti and his pupils at the end of the thirteenth and beginning of the fourteenth century and, in some instances, beyond.[58]

Although such a comparison is a salutary reminder of the strength of academic tradition, it is also somewhat misleading. As we shall see, access to a wider range of ancient materials, new philosophical interests, and new scientific developments meant that old questions came to be viewed in a different focus and new topics were added. Furthermore, although the practice of isolating *quaestiones* for discussion was not

[56] "Quaestiones igitur omnes vanas praetermittam, vanas dico, quoniam quaestiones quae pertinent ad rem non sunt praetermittandae. . . . Tractabo autem sicut docuerunt Aristoteles et sui boni expositores, et Averroes, et Galenus, solvendo scilicet difficultates per naturam rerum, et non per ambagam implicationem." Da Monte, comm. *Canon* 1.1 (Venice, 1554), fol. 1ʳ. He was presumably objecting to some of the typical features of scholastic medical commentary as it had developed in the hands of such authors as Giacomo da Forlì and Ugo Benzi.

[57] *Jacobi Forliviensis medici singularis expositio et quaestiones in primum Canonem Avicennae* (Venice, 1547); the *quaestiones* occupy fols. 188ʳ–225ᵛ. This is one of very few commentaries on a theoretical portion of the *Canon* to be reprinted after the 1520s.

[58] On the history of medical question literature, see Brian Lawn, *The Salernitan Questions* (Oxford, 1963), and idem, *The Prose Salernitan Questions* (London, 1979); also Siraisi, *Alderotti*, chap. 8 and Appendix 1.

abandoned entirely, Da Monte and other mid-sixteenth-century commentators on the *Canon* did to a considerable extent discard or modify
the typical structure of scholastic disputation, with its list of arguments
pro and contra, objections, and resolution, in favor of a less rigid, more
essaylike treatment.

Like Corti, Da Monte evidently was fairly familiar with the writings
of the principal scholastic authors, whom he termed *moderni*, and like
Corti he had a generally low opinion of them. In his commentary on
Canon 1.1 such authors are cited by name infrequently, and usually
only to disagree. Evidently, a conscious effort was made to derive citations chiefly from Greek authors, although Averroes is singled out
from among the Arabs for fairly frequent citation and respectful handling (see Chapter 7). Thus, Da Monte engaged in a long discussion of
medicinal qualities and how these are brought from potentiality to actuality when a medicine is applied or ingested.[59] This topic, under the
title "the reduction of medicine to act" was a favorite in the late thir-
teenth- and fourteenth-century Italian medical schools. Tommaso del
Garbo devoted a treatise to it, and Gentile da Foligno discussed it in a
quaestio in which he reviewed the opinions of eleven Italian medical authors beginning with Taddeo Alderotti.[60] One could read Da Monte's
discussion without realizing that the subject had ever been raised by
anyone other than Galen, Avicenna himself, and Averroes. But for
long sections of Da Monte's commentary on *Canon* 1.2 exposition of
Avicenna's text takes second place to analysis of views of Pietro
d'Abano, Giacomo da Forlì, and other scholastic medical authors, who
are denounced with a vigor reminiscent of Corti's treatment of Mondino.[61] On one occasion, Da Monte informed his students that the
Venetian authorities ought to pay him a double salary, since he had the
dual tasks of eradicating belief in the false teachings of the *moderni* and
inculcating correct views.[62]

[59] Da Monte, comm. *Canon* 1.1 (Venice, 1554), fols. 78ʳ–88ᵛ.

[60] Tommaso's treatise is printed with his *Summa medicinalis* (Venice, 1506); Gentile's
quaestio is printed in *Quaestiones et tractatus extravagantes clarissimi domini Gentilis de Fulgineo* (Venice, 1520), q. 46, fols. 63ʳ–65ᵛ.

[61] For example, Da Monte, comm. *Canon* 1.2 (Venice, 1557), pp. 65–74, an announced
digression on the concepts of *causa, dispositio,* and *accidens* as they relate to disease, which
reviews the opinions of Pietro d'Abano ("Conciliatorem, qui profitetur se conciliare
homines; vir magnus certe, sed nunquam vidi hominem magis confusum quam in hoc
negocio," p. 70) and Giacomo da Forlì ("Jacobus Forliviensis in eodem paragrapho affirmat et negat, et ideo vidi omnes confusissimos in hac materia," ibid.).

[62] "Et certe isti domini Veneti deberent solvere me duplo pretio quoniam duplicem la-
borem sustineo, primo quidem ad removendas falsas opiniones, quas acquiritis ab istis

In his approach to pedagogy, too, Da Monte mixed traditional with innovative elements. Various indications—the constant use of the second person plural, a somewhat condescending tone, and frequent repetitions and summaries to drive his points home—all reinforce the impression that he perceived his task of lecturing on the various parts of the *Canon* as teaching at an introductory level. Just as much as any of his scholastic predecessors, Da Monte, who like so many others before him had taught philosophy before he taught medicine, evidently believed that discussion of philosophical issues had a proper place in elementary medical instruction and assumed that his hearers would have had some philosophical preparation. Thus, discussion of Avicenna's chapter on the elements, a subject rather indirectly connected with medicine, occupies a larger proportion of Da Monte's commentary on *Canon* 1.1 than it does in that of Gentile da Foligno.[63] Nor was Da Monte any readier than his predecessors to multiply examples drawn from clinical experience in a discussion of general principles, although he laid stress upon the clinical usefulness of a knowledge of such relatively abstract concepts as the theory of temperament. Possibly responding to what he perceived as a desire on the part of his students to move on to more practical or more innovative aspects of contemporary medical teaching, he stressed the practical value of speculative discourse about the humors even for the understanding of anatomy: "For without this knowledge you cannot know the fabric of the human body [*fabrica humani corporis*—surely a Vesalian echo], because they [the humors] are the immediate components from which the essence of the parts of the body is constituted, and when we talk about the parts of the body without knowledge of humors, we are talking in air, as they say."[64]

---

doctoribus, et etiam authoribus modernis, secundo vero ad introducendas veras sententias, in animos vestros." Ibid., p. 137.

[63] Discussion of *Doctrina* 2, on the elements, occupies fols. 23^v–54^r of Da Monte, comm. *Canon* 1.1 (Venice, 1554), out of a total of 258 fols. The same section occupies fols. 9^r–10^r of Gentile, comm. *Canon* 1 (Pavia, 1510), out of a total of 73 fols. devoted to *Canon* 1.1.

[64] ". . . pulcherrima speculatio, et utilissima, est speculatio de humoribus quod autem ita sit patet, nam sine hac cognitione non potestis cognoscere fabricam humani corporis, quia sunt elementa proxima, ex quibus constat essentia membrorum et, quando loquimur de membris sine cognitione humorum, loquimur in aere, ut dicunt." Da Monte, comm. *Canon* 1.1 (Venice, 1554), fol. 141^v. Medieval and Renaissance medical authors sometimes used the term *elementa* for constituent parts of the human body; see, for example, the discussion of whether or not semen can properly be termed an element of the human body in Isaac, *De elementis*, in *Omnia opera Ysaac* (Lyon, 1515), fol. 5^{r-v}. The adjective *proxima* distinguished elements in the sense of bodily parts from the more remote

Although the progress of anatomical studies may have lessened student interest in discussions of medical *theoria*, Da Monte was compensated by advantages unknown to medical commentators of the late Middle Ages and early Renaissance. As noted, he was able to assume that his audience knew at least a little Greek. Furthermore, he made some use of printed materials for class distribution; on one occasion, he apologized to the students for not being able to give out the tables of diseases that he had promised, explaining that he had been too busy to get them to the printer on time.[65]

Most of the time, Da Monte's attitude toward Avicenna as a medical authority combined by then conventional themes of criticism with a measure of apparently sincere, if modified, esteem. Thus, in his preface to *Canon* 1.1 he demoted Avicenna from his traditional place as "prince of physicians" with the remark that the expression should be used only in the sense that in medicine Hippocrates was the emperor, Galen the king, and Avicenna the prince. Defending the utility of the *Canon* as "real and not imaginary," he attributed this utility to Avicenna's role as Galen's vicar and to his ability to assemble and organize material from different sources. These remarks were not pro forma, since he incorporated somewhat similar observations in his preface to the Junta Galen.[66] For Da Monte, as for Corti, the identification of Avicenna's borrowings from and differences with Galen was a fairly major goal. But Da Monte also held that Avicenna had in many respects been a

---

four elements, of which the human body, like all other material things, was held to be ultimately composed.

[65] Da Monte, comm. *Canon* 1.2 (Venice, 1557), p. 206.

[66] Da Monte, comm. *Canon* 1 (Venice, 1554), fols. 1ʳ–2ᵛ; at 2ᵛ: "haec utilitas non est imaginosa, sed vera. Videtis enim, tot praeclaros medicos fuisse versatos duntaxat in doctrina Avicennae sine Galeni lectione, neque ego possum comparare Avicennam cum aliquo Graeco alio, quam cum Galeno, fuit enim verus Galeni vicarius." Further praise for Avicenna's ability to organize a comprehensive account of medicine, proceeding from the general to the particular, is found on p. 12, where, in line with the views on method that he expressed elsewhere (see Wightman, "Quid sit methodus?"), Da Monte distinguished between methodology appropriate for teaching and methodology appropriate for scientific investigation, and praised Avicenna for the former: "respondendum est ad quaesitum, quo ordine sit usus Avicennae. Utitur nam compositivo, qui est aptior ad docendum, nam resolutivus magis est aptus ad inveniendum, quam ad docendum, et ita non convenit rudis, et incipientibus discere." On Renaissance discussions of method, among which Da Monte's remarks in this passage must be included, see, in addition to Neal W. Gilbert, *Renaissance Concepts of Method* (New York, 1960), and in a context more specifically medical, William F. Edwards, "Niccolò Leoniceno and the Origins of Humanist Discussion of Method," in *Philosophy and Humanism: Renaissance Essays in Honor of Paul Oskar Kristeller*, ed. Edward P. Mahoney (New York, 1976), pp. 283–305; Mugnai Carrara, "Una polemica umanistico-scolastica"; and Wear, "Galen in the Renaissance," pp. 238–45. For Da Monte's remarks in the preface to Galen, see n. 52, above.

more faithful follower of Galen than the fashionable Greek medical authors, Aetius, Paulus of Aegina, and Oribasius.[67] Other scattered remarks strengthen the impression of a certain detachment in regard to the competing schools of medical opinion. Da Monte observed, for instance, that Manardo was wrong to claim that Avicenna had not understood Greek views on *pituita*, since the opinion Manardo reprehended could be found in an (unnamed) Greek source. In another passage, defending an opinion of Aristotle against Galen, he characterized Galen as malign, and his arguments on the point at issue as frivolous.[68]

Awareness that problems presented by Avicenna's text might be in part the result of language difficulties also played a somewhat more significant part in Da Monte's commentaries than they had in that of Corti, although he seems to have been less interested in comparing different Latin versions than were the two Oddi. Da Monte based his exposition on Alpago's emended text, with which he appears to have been reasonably satisfied. If his occasional remarks about the "barbarism" of Gerard of Cremona's translation were conventional enough, much less usual were his repeated allusions to the limitations imposed by his own ignorance of Arabic and the assurance he gave his readers that Avicenna was in Arabic a most polished and eloquent author, who was held to be as much a master of style in his own language as were Cicero and Boccaccio in Latin and Italian, respectively.[69] Moreover, as

[67] After noting that the passage of the *Canon* under discussion contained "multa falsa" and blaming this on the form in which the texts reached Avicenna, Da Monte added: "Avicenna fuit divinissimus sequens Galenum, et rectissime commodissimeque transcribens ab eo, ita quod certe est omnibus praeferendus qui transcripserunt ab ipso Galeno, est enim primus certe post ipsum Galenum. Habetis quidem Graecos illos transcribentes a Galeno, sed certe nihil sunt apud Avicennam. Hic est divinissimus, habetis Aetium, habetis Paulum Aeginetam, habetis Oribasium, sed non sunt comparandi Avicennae. Aetius, Paulusque sunt paedagogi, certe nihil aliud sunt; Oribasius modo melior, est enim vir non contemnendus, certe nihil aliud sunt; Oribasius modo melior, est enim vir non contemnendus, licet Avicenna melius transcripserit a Galeno." Da Monte, comm. *Canon* 1.2 (Venice, 1557), p. 190.

[68] Da Monte, comm. *Canon* 1.1 (Venice, 1554), fol. 224ʳ, for the remark about Manardo. The attack on Galen's view is in the extra chapter (also attributed to Da Monte) added to the second edition, Da Monte, comm. *Canon* 1.1 (Venice, 1557), p. 605. Da Monte had studied at Ferrara under Leoniceno (ibid., p. 253), and was a friend of Manardo, who addressed *Epistolae medicinales*, 2.1 (Basel, 1540), pp. 299–302, to him.

[69] "Avicenna est elegantissimus in sua lingua, ut nullus Arabum, est eloquentissimus et utitur maxima proprietate loquendi, sicut mihi retulit D. Diegus Orator illius Imperatoris, quod in publicis scholis Avicenna propter linguae ornatum, sicut apud nos Cicero et Boccacius apud nostros vulgares praelegitur." Da Monte, comm. *Canon* 1.2 (Venice, 1557), p. 35. Da Monte's informant was Diego Hurtardo de Mendoza (1506–75), a poet and humanist as well as a diplomat, and the owner of a large library; his interests are said to have included "letras griegas, latinas y arabes"; see Angel González Palencia and

one might expect, given his own familiarity with the problems of translating Galen, he was sensitive to the possibility not only that Gerard might have misrepresented Avicenna but that Avicenna himself might have misunderstood Galenic texts because of problems in translation. On some occasions he quoted a word or two in Greek to demonstrate Avicenna's misunderstanding, although such instances are not especially numerous. Da Monte's more usual attitude toward Avicenna's differences with Galen is, however, summed up in the remark "I would not say that Avicenna does not understand Galen, but rather that he speaks from his own opinion against Galen."[70]

Yet on certain issues, Da Monte treated Avicenna's opinions and interpretations with sustained and contemptuous hostility. The section on humors in his commentary on *Canon* I.1 is a striking case in point. Of Avicenna's assertion that good humors all become part of the body as it is nourished, he protested: "Is not milk a humor that is good and intended by nature? Semen, too; is it not a good humor and intended by nature? But into what part of the body are these absorbed, since they are excretions? For since they are excreted they are not produced on account of the nourishment of the body but are useful excretions for other purposes. . . . And Gentile da Foligno and the others saw these difficulties, but they so admired Avicenna that they didn't dare to carp. But Plato is a friend and Socrates is a friend; but a better friend is truth."[71] On the same general topic, we subsequently learn that Gentile da Foligno defended Avicenna by telling a lie; that some of Avicenna's views on various kinds of humidity in the body are "totally false"; and that "Avicenna is far both from Galen and from the truth of the thing itself." The passage ends with the exhortation: "And so you have the classification and opinion of Galen, which is very true, and that of Av-

---

Eugenio Mele, *Vida y obras de Don Diego Hurtado de Mendoza*, 3 vols. (Madrid, 1941–43) 1:253–307, with the remark quoted at p. 282.

[70] Ibid., p. 93, and "ego non dixerim Avicen. non intelligere Galenum. Sed potius loqui ex propria intentione contra Galenum." Da Monte, comm. *Canon* I.1 (Venice, 1554), fol. 156ᵛ.

[71] "Praeterea lac nonne est humor bonus et intentus a natura? Sic semen nonne est humor bonus, intentus a natura? Sub quo igitur membro continebuntur ista, quae sunt excrementa? Nam quae excernuntur extra nec sunt propter nutrimentum corporis, sed sunt excrementa utilia propter alius usus. Et ita divisio mala est neque potest excusari. Et viderunt Gentilis et alii has difficultates, sed ita admirabantur Avic. ut non auderent carpere. Sed amicus Plato, et Socrates, magis tamen amica veritas." Ibid., fol. 153ʳ. The "amicus Plato" tag was of course a commonplace; see Henry Guerlac, "Amicus Plato and Other Friends," *Journal of the History of Ideas* 39 (1978), 627–33, where it is noted (p. 631) that one late sixteenth-century edition of the *Adages* of Erasmus (expanded after his death) ascribed the saying to Galen.

icenna, of which you have seen how much it is in error. And if anyone subsequently prefers to eat acorns rather than bread, he should choose what he prefers. For he has acorns and he has bread."[72] In another passage, Da Monte jocularly distinguished between Avicenna's venial and his mortal sins in misinterpreting Galen.[73] Still later, summarizing his lecture on Avicenna's views on the humor *pituita*, he declared: "Now you have seen all the distinctions of *pituita* that are taught by Avicenna, and you have heard them faithfully expounded by us; but I don't think any one of you is of such divine ingenuity that he can say he has learned anything from Avicenna."[74]

After perusing Da Monte's diatribe against Avicenna's views on humors, the reader feels disposed to echo a rhetorical question posed by Da Monte at the beginning of the section on bile: "Someone may say here 'Why are you expounding a book that you attack so vigorously?' " Da Monte's response was: "In the first place, I am not attacking the whole book, but only those things in it that seem to me reprehensible; besides, I am not doing anything new. For Galen never wrote better commentaries than on books that he reprehended."[75] For Da Monte, as for Matteo Corti, the goal of commentary was not, as it had been for most of their predecessors, the exposition of an authoritative text with the ultimate goal of reconciling differences of scientific opinion. Rather, for these two authors, as for a lesser extent for Oddo Oddi, the objective had become the critical evaluation of the commented text, judged on the one hand by its faithfulness to its Greek sources and on the other by its usefulness in conveying what was conceived to be correct and currently needed information. A secondary, but important goal was the detachment of readers from reliance upon earlier Latin interpreters of Avicenna's work.

---

[72] "Et ita habetis divisionem et sententiam Galeni, quae est verissima, et illam quae est Avicennae, quae quantum peccet vidistis. Et si quis velit postea magis vesci glandibus quam pane, eligat quod vult. Habet enim panem, et habet glandes." Da Monte, comm. *Canon* I.I (Venice, 1554), fol. 157ʳ. Also ibid., fols. 154ʳ, 154ᵛ for the other remarks cited.

[73] Ibid., fol. 173ʳ. See also Chapter 8, below.

[74] "Iam vidistis omnes differentias pituitae quae docentur ab Avicenna; et audivistis eas, a nobis fideliter declaratas, sed non arbitror quemquam ex vobis esse tam divini ingenii qui possit dicere se ab Avicenna aliquid didicisse. Audiatis modo ut discatis veras divisiones pituitae in quibus erraverit Avicenna." Ibid., fol. 179ᵛ.

[75] "Hic dicat quis: Cur exponis tu librum quem vituperas? Primum quidem ego non vitupero librum totum, sed ea tantum quae mihi videntur reprehendenda. Praeterea non facio rem novam. Nam Galenus nullibi facit meliores commentationes quam in libros quos repraehendit, sicut in librum *Prorrheticorum*, et in librum *De natura humana*." Ibid., fols. 190ᵛ–91ʳ.

Yet despite their generally humanist and Galenist orientation, these authors did not (or at any rate not in these works) advocate either the abandonment of teaching by commentary or the exclusion of Avicenna from the curriculum. On the contrary, Da Monte apparently wished to extend the role of the *Canon*. Doubtless such practical considerations as the lack of an equivalent respected text covering the same ground as *Canon* 1.1 and the difficulty of challenging an entrenched curricular tradition played some part here. Nonetheless, although their respect for Avicenna as a medical author seems on the whole to have been less than that held by those who worked on the text of the *Canon* in the same period—for example, Miguel Jeronimo Ledesma of Valencia[76]—their initiation of modern commentary implied a determination to salvage, not reject, the work.

Commentaries from the 1550s to the 1620s

For an idea of the approaches to Avicenna suggested to their pupils by professors at Padua, Bologna, and Pavia in the second half of the sixteenth century, we may turn to seven extended expositions by the holders of senior professorships. Two of the seven authors were mildly critical of Avicenna. Vettor Trincavella, lecturing on *Canon* 4.1 at Padua in 1553, two years after his appointment as first ordinary professor of *practica*, remarked that Avicenna had lost some of his authority owing to recently improved knowledge of Greek medicine, but not to the point where he should be condemned. Lecturing on the same text a generation later, Alessandro Massaria characterized Avicenna as more obscure and difficult than Galen, and assigned his students Galenic books to read alongside the *Canon*.[77] (When Massaria was appointed to the first ordinary chair in *practica* at Padua in 1587, he described his colleagues as divided into Galenists, Arabists, and *moderni* who followed Fernel and Argenterio; aligning himself with the first group, he pointed out the superiority of the Greeks to the Arabs, but reserved his severest denunciations for the moderns who differed from and slighted Hippocrates, Aristotle, and Galen.)[78]

Two others allied a strong defense of Avicenna with denunciation of his critics, although from somewhat different standpoints. Antonio

---

[76] Ledesma's own commentary is essentially a set of annotations to his version of the text, and does not appear directly to record a set of university lectures.

[77] Trincavella, *Opera*, 3 vols. in 2 (Venice, 1599), 3:1; Massaria, *De febribus* (comm. *Canon* 4.1), in his *Practica medica* (Treves, 1607), p. 314. Massaria was appointed to the first ordinary chair in *practica* at Padua in 1587 and died in 1598.

[78] Riccobono, *De Gymnasio patavino*, fols. 71r, 99r.

Maria Betti (d. 1562) was an octogenarian who had been teaching for forty years, most of them at Bologna, when he published his commentary on *Canon* 1.4 in 1560. Presumably his ideas, hardened by the passage of time, had been formed at the beginning of the century, when criticism of the Arabs was only just beginning to get under way. It is not surprising, therefore, to find him among the few authors who openly defended the *Canon* on grounds of simple conservatism, although he also added a rider stressing Avicenna's agreement with Galen. In Betti's eyes, sheer impudence and audacity, joined to a thirst for novelty for its own sake, were responsible for the present generation's repudiation of an author "received in all the schools for so many centuries."[79]

At about the same time, however, Girolamo Cardano, perhaps more accurately, perceived the denigration of Avicenna as having already taken on the characteristics of received, and unexamined, tradition. Cardano, who is today better remembered as a mathematician, a gambler, an eclectic natural philosopher, and the author of a remarkable autobiography, was also a professor of medicine at the University of Pavia and, subsequently, Bologna; in the judgment of a historian of the former institution he was the most distinguished member of its medical faculty in the sixteenth century.[80] In his usual combative tone, Cardano prefaced the lectures he gave on *Canon* 1.1 at Pavia in 1561 with the assertion that the best of the moderns, among them Da Monte, Mattioli, and Vesalius, thought Avicenna equal or preferable to all the Greeks except Hippocrates—a statement of which the kindest thing that can be said is that it is an exaggeration; that Avicenna knew many books of Galen subsequently lost; and that Galen was guilty of lack of skill or experience (*imperitia*), speaking ill of others, tedious prolixity, and impious opinions, none of which could be ascribed to Avicenna. Even more pugnacious and idiosyncratic was the defense of Avicenna that Cardano prefaced to the same set of lectures when he gave them again at Bologna in 1563.[81] It included a scathing attack on what Cardano conceived to be the rhetorical inanities of medical humanists

[79] Betti, comm. *Canon* 1.4 (Bologna, 1560), *iia^{r-v}: ". . . audacia pro sapientia utantur. . . . Verumenimvero, etsi late patet hoc vitium, et est in multis, neminem tamen adeo impudentem, adeo cerebrosum fore credidissem, qui Avicennae doctrinam, tot iam seculis ab omnibus Academiis receptam, communi pene omnium gentium consensu approbatam reijcere, ac repudiare auderet. Novi tamen quidam, hac nostri aetate, Asculapii extiterunt . . . ," and so on.

[80] Pietro Vaccari, *Storia della Università di Pavia* (Pavia, 1957), p. 136 For Cardano's career, see *DSB* 3:64-67.

[81] Cardano's two prefaces precede his comm. *Canon* 1.1 in his *Opera* (1663), 9:455-61.

("further from the discipline of Galen in their practice than from the doctrine of the Arabs in their language") and a spirited defense of the Islamic contribution to the "solid disciplines," especially astronomy and mathematics.

However, Cardano, like the rest of this group of commentators, showed no signs of knowledge of Arabic or of the Arabic text of the *Canon*. Cardano added that real Galenic scholars appreciated the worth of Avicenna, this time invoking the names of Matteo Corti and Da Monte. With what seems reckless disregard for the conventional pieties, whether religious or humanistic, Cardano also pointed out that neither Hellenism nor Christianity guaranteed superiority in philosophy and science ("were not the gymnosophists among the Indians thought to be the wisest of all philosophers?"), and that it was irrational to criticize Avicenna for having been a Moslem, when Galen had worshipped idols.[82] Cardano's second preface bears comparison with the introductory letter to "students of good arts and lovers of truth and true wisdom" that Nicolò Massa wrote especially for the second edition of his *Epistolae medicinales*, published in 1558.[83] Massa, too, deplored the importation of rhetorical values into philosophy, science, and medicine, and the consequent neglect of Avicenna. However, unlike Cardano he provided his comments with an impeccably orthodox context by paralleling the case of Avicenna with that of Thomas Aquinas, whom he considered to be suffering equally from unmerited neglect.

The three remaining commentators all wrote in the last third of the

---

[82] "At o viri egregii, quod ad provinciam attinet, demiror quin etiam legem obieceritis cum Mahumetanus sit, sed deterior in hac parte Galenus, qui etiam idola coluit. Sit Arabs, sit Gallus vel Italus, numquid apud Deum, aut Musas, aut sapientes, deteriore in conditione habendus est? Nonne apud Indos Gymnosophistae omnium Philosophorum sapientissimi extiterint? . . . Quot pulchra ingenia in brevi tempore floruerunt inter Arabes? . . . Non est certamen in rhetorica, o viri fucati, sed in solida disciplina quae ingenio, sedulitate, ordine, scientia rerum atque utilitate humani generis constat. Video nos cum contemptu Arabum etiam philosophiam et dialecticam et mathematicam omnes bonas artes neglexisse. Garulos in sermone, ambitiosos in conversatione, infelices in medendo, magis re alienos a Galeni disciplina quam verbis ab Arabum doctrina. . . . Nonne Curtius atque Montanus, qui vere duo lumina in Galeni doctrina nostris temporibus fuere, maxime Principis doctrinam probarunt. Montanus etiam in praefatione in Galenum, ubi minus conveniebat, nostrum Hasen paulo minus Galeno praetulit, certe coaequavit." Ibid., pp. 459–60.

[83] *Nicolai Massae Epistolarum medicinalium tomus alter* (Venice, 1558), A[r]–[Aiv[v]]. The letter "Ad bonarum artium studiosos ac veritati[s] et verae sapientiae amatores" is dated 1556; the first edition of Massa's *epistolae* appeared Venice, 1550. Some of his epistles are also included in *Epistolae medicinales diversorum authorum* (Lyon, 1556), but this letter is not among them.

century, and all espoused a generally favorable attitude toward the *Canon*, never even mentioning that it had been subjected to criticism. Capodivacca (on *Canon* 4.1, at Padua, between 1564 and 1589, perhaps 1579–80)[84] and Costeo (on *Canon* 1.1, at Bologna, 1589)[85] praised Avicenna's adherence to Galen, while Paterno provided his readers with orientation only toward the subject matter, not toward book or author, in the preface to his exposition of *Canon* 1.1 (at Padua, probably between 1578 and 1592).[86] Paterno and Costeo were, of course, staunch defenders of the *Canon*, who, as we have seen, shared a long-standing interest in improving the presentation of the text. By the time their commentaries were written, replies to Avicenna's critics had appeared in the various text editions prepared by Rinio, Graziolo, and Costeo himself. Conceivably, therefore, Costeo and Paterno felt that Avicenna's opponents had already been disposed of; but it seems more probable that they took advantage of diminishing interest in the controversy to present Avicenna to students as an author who had never been controversial.

In the body of their commentaries, moreover, Costeo and Paterno were seldom critical of Avicenna; rather, they implicitly endorsed the contemporary relevance of passages of the *Canon* by explaining and enlarging upon them in the light of the views of classical philosophical and medical authors and with reference to modern controversies. In so doing, they almost completely detached Avicenna from the older Latin scholastic medical tradition. As we have seen, Matteo Corti and even Da Monte on occasion had paid considerable attention to scholastic commentators on Avicenna, often with a view to refuting them. Among the group of writers under discussion, Betti's pages are filled with informed and frequently approving summaries of the views of Dino del Garbo, Jacques Despars, and other similar writers, while Cardano cited scholastic medical authors from time to time, not always in a hostile sense. By contrast, Costeo and Paterno very seldom mentioned writers of this kind.

Moreover, Costeo was responsive to contemporary trends in medi-

---

[84] Capodivacca, *Practica*, Book 6: *De febribus* (comm. *Canon* 4.1) in his *Opera* (Frankfurt, 1603), pp. 814–19. The preface in the printed edition is different from that in Capodivacca, comm. *Canon* 4.1, Siena, Biblioteca Comunale, MS C IX 18, a. 1579.

[85] Costeo, *Disq. phys.* (Bologna, 1589), letter of dedication to Bernardino Paterno, begins "Quum medicae disciplinae statum intueor, Paterne, aetatis nostrae splendor, eius quidem semina iecisse Hippocratem, excoluisse ad uberrimam frugem deduxisse Galenum; delegisse autem et in unum quasi horreum ex omni antiquitate meliores fructus collegisse Avicennam plane intelligo."

[86] Paterno, comm. *Canon* 1.1 (Venice, 1596), fols. 1ʳ–2ᵛ. This preface does not appear to be present in Paterno, comm. *Canon* 1.1, WL MS 602 a. 1578.

cal education. The extensive natural philosophical content in his commentary shows that he did not reject the aspects of traditional medical *theoria* that seem to have engendered impatience on the part of some of those primarily concerned with practically useful professional training. Yet the title of his work suggests that he intended to provide an adequate survey of current physiological concerns, an impression confirmed by his expansion of the discussion of anatomy and addition of a section on *spiritus*. And his assertion that *Canon* 1 encompassed all the five classical divisions of medicine[87] suggests that he may have shared Da Monte's desire to use commentary on the *Canon* as a vehicle for reinvigorating the medical curriculum.

A more far-reaching effort to infuse new life into the teaching of *theoria*—or at any rate into that part of it consisting of the exposition of *Canon* 1.1—seems to have been made by Santorio Santorio, who held the position of first ordinary professor of *theoria* at Padua from 1611 until 1624.[88] In Santorio, the chair, which had stood vacant since the death of Augenio in 1603,[89] acquired an occupant who was both an experienced medical practitioner and a scientific innovator of some consequence. Educated at Padua, where he was a pupil of Paterno and Zabarella, he spent a number of years in practice in eastern Europe, before returning to Venice in 1599. There he combined a prosperous medical practice among a distinguished clientele with contacts with the circle of intellectual Venetian aristocrats around Galileo. In 1602, Santorio published a book on diagnosis and treatment, *Methodi vitandorum errorum omnium qui in arte medica contingunt*, from which it is clear that he had already begun to develop the quantitative and iatrophysical approach to medicine for which he subsequently became well known.[90]

Santorio's scientific work consisted chiefly of efforts to introduce

---

[87] Costeo, *Disq. phys.* (Bologna, 1589), p. 2, on the five parts of medicine and *Canon* 1; for Costeo's treatment of anatomy and *spiritus*, see Chapter 8, below.

[88] Regarding Santorio's career, writings, and scientific contribution, see M. D. Grmek, "Santorio, Santorio," *DSB*, 12:101–4; M. D. Grmek, *L'introduction de l'expérience quantitative dans les sciences biologiques*, Conférence donnée au Palais de la Découverte le 7 Avril, 1962 (Paris, 1962); M. D. Grmek, *Santorio Santorio i Njegovi aparati i instrumenti* (Zagreb, [1952], with English summary on pp. 79–82); L. S. Ettari and M. Procopio, *Santorio Santorio: La vita e le opere*, Monografie dei "Quaderni della Nutrizione," no. 4, Istituto Nazionale della Nutrizione, Città Universitaria, Roma (Rome, n.d.); Modestino del Gaizo, "Ricerche storiche intorno a Santorio Santorio ed alla medicina statica," *Resoconto della R. Accademia Medico-Chirurgica di Napoli* (1889); and Arcadio Capello, *De vita clarissimi viri Sanctorii Sanctorii* (Venice, 1750).

[89] Bertolaso "Ricerche d'Archivio" (1959–60), p. 23.

[90] *DSB*, 12:101. One of Santorio's patients was Paolo Sarpi. Santorio's relationship with Galileo himself was not close, although Santorio sent Galileo a copy of *De statica medicina* in 1615; see Ettari and Procopio, *Santorio*, p. 45.

quantification, measurement, and experimental method in general into physiology. Essentially, he believed that the changes in the balance of humors, in temperament, or in the nonnaturals postulated by Hippocratic-Galenic physiological and pathological theory as responsible for alterations in health must produce physically measurable consequences. The physician would therefore be aided in his work by a more precise knowledge of variations in the body's heat, respiration, retention of nutrients, and exudation of "insensible perspiration" through the skin.[91] Accordingly, Santorio devoted a good deal of attention to the design of instruments to measure these and other variables; he is best remembered today for his contribution to the invention of the thermometer, but his "thermoscope" was only one of many medical instruments he devised.[92] In his own lifetime, and for a century thereafter, Santorio was chiefly celebrated as the author of *De statica medicina*, a little book first published in 1614 in which he presented his ideas about the importance for health of a proper balance between ingestion and excretion (including the excretion of insensible perspiration), and described his own experiments, extending over many years, in monitoring the variations in this balance in himself. *De statica medicina* is said to have subsequently gone into some forty editions; it was also translated into various modern European languages and several times accompanied by commentary.[93]

When Santorio succeeded to the first chair in theory at Padua he was a man of fifty with well-formed and to some extent original scientific interests who had spent most of his adult life in medical practice. The contrast with his own teacher and penultimate predecessor in the same position, Bernardino Paterno, who spent fifty years teaching *theoria* "according to the ancient discipline,"[94] could hardly be more striking. While Santorio doubtless owed his appointment to the representations of his influential friends,[95] the willingness of the Riformatori dello Stu-

---

[91] Grmek, "Introduction," pp. 16–17.

[92] On Santorio's instruments of measurement, Grmek, *L'introduction*, pp. 20–26. On the relationship between Santorio's work on heat-measuring devices and that of Galileo, see W. Knowles Middleton, *A History of the Thermometer and Its Use in Meteorology* (Baltimore, 1966), pp. 5–14. Santorio's original device was a thermoscope designed to show changes in heat; subsequently, he added some form of scale to permit measurement. There seems little point in pursuing further the claims that have been made for priority on behalf of either Galileo or Santorio as regards the thermoscope or thermometer; the question is fully discussed by Middleton.

[93] *DSB*, 12:104. I have consulted *Ars Sanctorii Sanctorii Justinopolitani . . . De statica medicina aphorismorum . . .* (Leipzig, [1626]).

[94] See the title of his commentary in Appendix 2.

[95] *DSB*, 12:102.

dio to accept him surely also implies a readiness on their part to try a new approach to the teaching of *theoria*. By the time Santorio was appointed, the traditional curriculum in this subject had not only been reduced to the position of an introductory survey, but was also the target of objections that, even as a survey, it did not constitute a well-designed overview of the whole of medicine. Santorio himself rehearsed and answered objections of this kind in an oration he delivered at the university in 1612, observing that "at first sight" lectures on *Canon* 1.1, the *Aphorisms*, and the *Techne* seemed useless, because the content of the first pertained more to philosophy than to medicine and the other two were only partial in their coverage; in reality, however, the natural scientific and physiological generalities of *Canon* 1.1 pertained both to philosophy (from the standpoint of contemplation) and to medicine (from the standpoint of operation).[96]

Although the last statement echoed an ancient truism,[97] Santorio interpreted it in an unprecedented way. His own commentary, based on lectures he gave at Padua and revised for publication shortly after he left the professorship in 1624,[98] is characterized by a remarkable mixture of approaches. In important ways, the work is fairly conventional. In it, Santorio seldom rejected any major Galenic tenet. He appears to have approached the task of expounding the *Canon* just as seriously as Costeo and Paterno had done; like them he was seldom critical of Avicenna as a medical author, although he showed a fair amount of interest in discussing the implications of differences between the Alpago and Mantino versions of the Latin text of *Canon* 1.1. And from time to time he attempted to solve real or supposed differences between Aristotle, Galen, Avicenna, and Averroes by scholastic reconciliation.[99] He also drew fairly heavily on his sixteenth-century predecessors, for example

---

[96] "Quidquid autem potest de his omnibus enunciari, illud est, quod primo aspectu videtur supervacanea et inutilis horum librorum interpretatio, quia prima fen qui agit de corporis humani structura, de elementis, temperamentis, humoribus, spiritibus, et innato calido, de animae facultatibus, de functionibus et similibus, pertinere videtur ad philosophum naturalem, non ad medicum. . . . Delegerunt enim primam fen primi libri Avicennae, quae continet phisiologiam, quam philosophus ad contemplationem, medicus vero ad operationem referre debet." *Oratio a Sanctorio Sanctorio habita in Archilyceo Patavino dum ipse primarium theoricae medicinae explicandae munus auspicaretur anno salutis 1612*, printed with Capello, *Vita*, pp. xix–xxiv, at p. xxiii.

[97] See Siraisi, *Alderotti*, pp. 118–19, for examples of discussions of the relation of philosophy or natural science, medical *theoria*, and medical *practica* emanating from Bologna in the thirteenth and early fourteenth centuries.

[98] The following discussion is based on the edition of Venice, 1646.

[99] For example, on whether there is a neutral state between sickness and health, as Galen had asserted (a difference between Galen and Aristotle repeatedly discussed since

examining in turn the views of Da Monte, Paterno, Corti, and Costeo on Avicenna's method (whether definitive, resolutive, or compositive).[100] In this and a number of other passages Santorio used the format of the scholastic *quaestio*, a fact to which the reader's attention is drawn by an *index quaestionum* at the beginning of the volume. Furthermore, he showed himself a good deal readier than either Costeo or Paterno to cite medieval scholastic authors, both medical and philosophical or theological.[101] Moreover, although he strongly denied that medicine was in any way subordinated to philosophy, he showed no disinclination to discuss questions of current philosophical or scientific interest that were of slight or questionable relevance to medicine.[102]

In other respects, Santorio followed patterns of innovation already established by Da Monte and Costeo, improving the adequacy of *Canon* 1.1 as a survey of physiology by providing expanded coverage of areas of contemporary interest. Thus, he included a defense of the place of anatomical studies in medicine and devoted considerable attention to the topics of the heart, blood, and arteries.[103]

However, yet other aspects of the work represent bold new departures from the entire previous tradition of commentary on *Canon* 1.1. Santorio perceived his own approach to teaching *theoria* as sufficiently

---

the thirteenth century): "Nos communissima distinctione conciliamus Galenum cum Aristotele." Ibid., col. 58.

[100] Ibid., cols. 13–19. Again the topic was one that had been of concern to physicians since the early fourteenth century. Santorio's references to Corti are of some interest. As noted earlier, I have been unable to find any trace of a printed version of Corti's commentary on *Canon* 1.1. But it seems improbable that Santorio would have consulted it in manuscript.

[101] For example, see cols. 39–44 (Pietro d'Abano and Torrigiano), 202, 214–15 (Tommaso del Garbo), 250–51 (Dino del Garbo), 269 (Jacques Despars), 614, 667 (Ugo Benzi), 698 (Taddeo Alderotti), and many other examples. Most of these citations involve some discussion of the views of the authors named. They are often, though by no means always, disagreed with, but the tone adopted toward them is in general neither hostile nor condescending. Disagreement with predecessors was standard methodology among scholastic physicians. Citations of ancient and sixteenth-century medical authors are, however, more numerous, and the discussion of their views is usually more extensive. The views of Thomas Aquinas are mentioned or discussed in cols. 103 (influence of the heavenly bodies on terrestrial affairs) and 232 (*complexio*). The opinions of Aquinas, Egidio Colonna, Gregory of Rimini, Henry of Ghent, and Duns Scotus are all mentioned in col. 124. Theologians and philosophers are usually referred to with regard to philosophical rather than strictly theological issues, and questions of orthodoxy or heresy seem not as a rule to be raised.

[102] *Quaestio* 13: "An medicina sit subalternata philosophia." Ibid., cols. 140–41. See Chapter 7, below.

[103] Ibid., cols. 143–45; 860–61, 877–86. See Chapter 8, below.

novel to distinguish him from all his predecessors, both medieval and sixteenth-century, whom he characterized as having sought to explain the subject in the light of the teachings of Hippocrates and Galen while making little or no effort to confirm theory by evidence drawn from *practica*. He stressed, by contrast, that his own teaching of *theoria* at Padua relied habitually and extensively on "experimenta . . . instrumenta, et statica ars."[104] Given the famous example of Santorio's attempt to establish his physiological theories on an experimental basis by controlled and repeated measurement of daily fluctuations in his own weight, we may believe that he meant "experiment" in something like the modern sense, although the experiments he used in teaching were presumably demonstrative rather than investigative in purpose. The *statica ars* was of course his own theory of physiological balance. He further asserted his belief that theory could not be understood unless it was corroborated by *practica* and that it was his goal to demonstrate precise applications of theory to "the curative part of medicine."[105]

But the most notable manifestation in this commentary of Santorio's novel method of teaching *theoria* is, of course, the famous series of illustrations and explanations of the scientific instruments that he had devised. These descriptions and illustrations are closely related to the passages of text and commentary in which they appear (for examples, see Part IV). Since the instruments are about evenly divided between measuring devices of various kinds and therapeutic equipment, they serve Santorio's announced purposes of establishing physiological *theoria* upon a basis of physical demonstration and of enlisting *theoria* in the service of therapy. These two goals become one in the case of instruments intended to measure physiological change in ways that

---

[104] "Theorici celebres, tum antiqui tum moderni, qui ante me omne studium in theorica posuerunt, conati sunt in suis commentariis rationibus et auctoritatibus Hippocratis et Galeni hanc medicinae partem explicare, et recte quidem; sed de ipsa confirmanda a posteriori per ipsam practicam vel nihil, vel parum dixerunt. . . . Ego quoque . . . dico quod et sanatio, et experimenta, necnon etiam instrumenta, et statica ars quae omnia longo usu et periclitatione adinveni hanc medicam philosophiam reddere possint claram et manifestam. Quae instrumenta et statica experimenta in Patavino Gymnasio theoricam ordinariam primae sedis diu profitens auditoribus, quorum erat magnus ad publicas et privatas lectiones concursus, ostendi." Ibid., preface *ad lectorem*.

[105] "Sicuti practica non intelligitur nisi confirmetur per ipsam theoricam, tanquam a priori, et per demonstrationem propter quid, sic theorica nisi corroboretur per ipsam practicam, tanquam a posteriori et per demonstrationem quia, minimi percepi potest. Nostra igitur intentio est . . . haec duo docere: primum, theoricam ipsam; secundum cui parti medicinae curatricis vel conservatricis dicta theorica inserviat." Ibid., col. 3.

would be directly useful to the medical practitioner—the thermoscope being an obvious example. There is no way of knowing whether the balance between scholastic elements, features derived from the tradition of *Canon* commentary as it had developed since the 1520s, and actual innovation was the same in Santorio's original lectures as in his published commentary. If we may believe Santorio's own account of the crowds who flocked to his lectures on *Canon* 1.1, his approach to *theoria* was warmly welcomed by the students (although he ended his career at Padua on very bad terms with the German Nation).[106] Yet he does not seem to have engendered any lasting revival of the teaching of *theoria*. Instead, the first ordinary professorship in that subject at Padua was unoccupied for a number of years later in the seventeenth century,[107] and Santorio's was the last full scale commentary on *Canon* 1.1 by an Italian professor of medicine to be published in or shortly after the author's lifetime.

Santorio's treatment of *Canon* 1.1 stands in sharp contrast to the preoccupations of two of his contemporaries in Spain, who were also engaged in reshaping the tradition of scholastic medical commentary to suit their own ends. Pedro Garcia Carrero's *disputationes* on *Canon* 1.1, published in 1611,[108] are entirely scholastic in their approach, seem in many sections to be as much concerned with theological as physiological issues, and rest upon scriptural and theological as well as medical authorities. Among the questions discussed is whether, if Christ had lived to old age, he could have died of natural causes (to which, in Garcia Carrero's opinion, the answer was no).[109] The main objective of the *disputationes* on *Canon* 1.1 published in 1624 by Antonio Ponce Santa Cruz, professor of medicine at Valladolid and physician to Philip IV, seems to have been to defend views of Thomas Aquinas that the author considered to have been impugned by the humanist reevaluation of Avicenna.[110] Ponce Santa Cruz's approach is summed up in one of his chapter titles: "The Nature of Temperament, According to the View

---

[106] See *Acta*, ed. Rossetti, pp. 147–49.

[107] Bertolaso, "Ricerche d'archivio" (1959–60), p. 23.

[108] Garcia Carrerro, *Disputationes medicae* (Comm. *Canon* 1.1) (Alcalá de Henares, 1611). The work was reprinted in Bordeaux, 1628.

[109] Ibid., p. 544. My examination of this commentary has been cursory.

[110] Ponce Santa Cruz, *Disputationes* on *Canon* 1.1, in his *Opuscula medica* (Madrid, 1624), pp. 1–305. On the permeation of natural philosophy by religious apologetic in late sixteenth-century Spain, a development that provided the intellectual context for the commentaries of Garcia Carrero and Ponce Santa Cruz, see Giancarlo Zanier, "Il *De sacra philosophia* (1587) di Francisco Vallés," in his *Medicina e filosofia tra '500 e '600* (Milan, 1983), pp. 20–38. (However, Ponce Santa Cruz himself attacked Vallés for criticizing Avicenna; see *Disputationes*, p. 167.)

of Avicenna and St. Thomas and against Fernel."[111] On the long-debated question of the elements in a mixture, he remarked: "Our conclusion is as follows: It is impossible that the elements should remain *formaliter* in a mixture. I have said 'impossible' because they are the words of St. Thomas, whom we follow in everything."[112] Naturally, this author had little use for the sixteenth-century Italian commentators on the *Canon*, Da Monte, and Paterno (especially Da Monte), who were among the principal targets of his attack.[113] Ponce Santa Cruz displayed the same interest in physiologico-theological questions as Garcia Carrero, speculating on the possibility of Christ's old age, sickness, and death and inquiring into the physiological nature of his bloody sweat and whether it would have coagulated.[114] In case readers should overlook this aspect of the work, their attention was drawn to it by the inclusion in the front matter of a list of the scriptural passages expounded.

At least one reader in Italy attentively studied the commentaries of both Santorio and Ponce Santa Cruz. This was Carolus Vallesius (Charles Valois), a native of Bordeaux, who taught at the University of Rome from 1656 until his death in 1689.[115] Vallesius' own lectures on *Canon* 1.1, which survive in manuscript, show that he knew a fairly wide range of sixteenth- and early seventeenth-century medical authors, although he may have become familiar with some of them via Santorio.[116] Like Santorio, he showed little interest in criticism of Avicenna of the older humanistic variety. His citations of fourteenth- and fifteenth-century scholastic medical authors were probably fewer than Santorio's, even if he did claim that the circulation of the blood had

---

[111] Ponce Santa Cruz, *Disputationes* 3.3, p. 14.

[112] "Nostra conclusio talis est: Impossibile est, quod elementa maneant formaliter in mixto. Dixi: Impossibile; quia sunt verba S. Thomae, quem in omnibus secuti sumus." Ibid., p. 7.

[113] See, e.g., ibid., pp. 5, 134, 147–61, 164, 166–67, 174.

[114] Ibid., pp. 116–18, 135.

[115] See J. Carafa, *De professoribus gymnasii romani* (Rome, 1751), 2:369, and Filippo Maria Renazzi, *Storia dell'Università degli Studi di Roma detta comunemente La Sapienza* (Rome, 1805), 3:189.

[116] Vallesius, comm. *Canon* 1.1, Rome, Biblioteca Lancisiana, MS 127, fols. 299ʳ–413ᵛ. A notebook with many insertions and loose pages; however, the commentary may have been intended ultimately for publication, as a complimentary preface about Innocent XI and the Sapienza is included. In it Vallesius described himself as expounding "institutiones medicas ex aureo *Canone* Avicennae." Owing to the restricted opening hours of the Biblioteca Lancisiana and the absence of microfilming facilities, my study of this commentary was hasty and superficial. Some of the medical authors cited by Vallesius include Santorio (fol. 328ʳ), Da Monte (ibid.), Riolan (fol. 355ʳ), Sennert (fol. 398ʳ) and Fernel (ibid.).

been known to Gentile da Foligno.[117] But he also shared Ponce Santa Cruz's theological preoccupations, although in a manner that would presumably have dismayed that author, since he held that both Ponce Santa Cruz and Avicenna had expressed heretical opinions. Thus, Ponce Santa Cruz had been heretical when he said God added air and fire when He made man out of the dust of the earth, since one should not add to Scripture; instead, the other elements entered man by transmutation. Also heretical was Avicenna's definition of temperament, presumably because of materialist implications, and the view that an initial endowment of a fixed amount of innate heat, gradually consumed over time, limited human life to a fixed span (since the length of human life is in the hands of God). Vallesius' tendency to worry over possible heretical implications of physiological theories contained in or derived from the *Canon* does not seem to have come from the earlier tradition of *Canon* commentary in Italy. Although he was less imbued with neo-Thomist learning than Garcia Carrero and Ponce Santa Cruz, his exposition, like theirs, had drifted into the orbit of Counter-Reformation religiosity. By contrast, although the ideological commitments and external pressures of the Counter-Reformation certainly touched the academic medical community everywhere in Italy, even in the Veneto, commentaries on the *Canon* produced in north Italian universities between the mid-sixteenth and the early seventeenth century seldom introduced religious topics.[118] Whatever their limitations in other respects, medical commentaries written at Padua, Pavia, and Bologna remained tools of secular professional education.

After 1625: The Decline of Commentary

The production of published commentaries, and indeed of fully transcribed handwritten lectures, tapered off sharply in the middle years of the seventeenth century. Presumably by that time the gulf between Avicenna and the scientific views of the moderns was so wide that the kind of interweaving of Avicenna's presentation with contemporary concerns successfully practiced by Costeo and Santorio was ceasing to be feasible. The nadir of commentary may have been reached in the so-called *ratiocinationes* on *Canon* I.I written (in a handsome, perhaps pre-

[117] "Gentilis docet pituita iterum ad hepar excurrere ac transmitti ut in sanguinem a principio haematoseo transmutetur nec enim vitium primae coctionis in secunda emendatur, nec secunda in tertia, quae opinio constituta sanguinis circulatione magis efflorescit." In the margin: "ergo circulatio cognita a Gentili." Ibid., fol. 373ʳ.

[118] Ibid., fols. 337ʳ, 360ʳ. Much information about the impact of the Counter-Reformation on intellectual life in the Veneto is contained in Grendler, *Roman Inquisition.*

sentation, copy) at Rome by Matteo Naldi (d. 1682) and dedicated to Cardinal Francesco Barberini; Naldi's is a purely rhetorical piece that seems to have no real philosophical or physiological content of any kind whatsoever—even the most conservative.[119]

The few minor publications based on the *Canon* that appeared from Italian presses in the middle years of the seventeenth century reflect the intellectual situation just described. They include paraphrases, designed to simplify the Latin text for students, of *Canon* 4.1 (fevers) and 3.9 (diseases of the throat) by Giovanni Stefano, prior of the Venetian College of Physicians,[120] and a work on fevers "ad Avicennae ordinem" by Sebastiano Scarabicio, who was appointed to one of the lectureships on *Canon* 3 at Padua in 1644.[121] Scarabicio, who was a pupil of Cremonini,[122] prefaced his mainly practical work on diagnosis and treatment with a theoretical consideration of the concepts of innate and complexional heat. When Charles Patin, son of Guy Patin, William Harvey's opponent at Paris, was appointed to one of the lectureships at Padua on *Canon* 3 in 1676, he delivered and subsequently published a laudatory oration on Avicenna.[123] It is mainly biographical and historical, and shows that Patin had taken the trouble to familiarize himself with the work on the *Canon* of Da Monte (cited for his remark about Avicenna's eloquence in his own language), Plemp, and Welsch; he was also able to allude to the versions of Ramusio, Mantino, Cinqarbres, Rinio, Graziolo, Kirsten, and Vattier.[124] His knowledge of the northern European editors and translators may perhaps be attributed to his French background. Patin stressed Avicenna's vast erudition, quoting, with apology for the comparison of the profane with the sacred, an apothegm of Plemp's to the effect that the relative stature of Hippocrates, Galen, and Avicenna was the same as that of the Bible, Saint Augustine, and Saint Thomas Aquinas. However, to err is human, and Avicenna had made a few mistakes, wrongly ascribing a cer-

[119] Biblioteca Apostolica Vaticana, MS Barberini lat. 269.

[120] Stefano, *Paraphrasis, Canon* 4.1 (Venice, 1646); reprinted in his *Opera* (Venice, 1653), pp. 242–96, a volume that also contains his *Paraphrasis, Canon* 3.9, at pp. 88–233.

[121] Scarabicio, *De ortu ignis febriferi historia* (comm. *Canon* 4.1) (Padua, 1655). A biography of Scarabicio is to be found in Charles Patin, *Lyceum patavinum sive icones et vitae professorum Patavii, MDCLXXXII publice docentium* (Padua, 1682), pp. 20–23.

[122] Ibid., p. 4. Cremonini's ideas on innate heat were one of his areas of difference with the Galenists.

[123] Charles Patin, *De Avicenna oratio habita in Archi-Lycaeo Patavino, die x Novembris, 1676* (Padua, 1678), pp. 27–32.

[124] Ibid., pp. 27, 28, 30, 31. Mantinus is miscalled "Mutinus." Patin pronounced Plemp's version the best; he did not allude to that of Costeo and Mongio, which was probably by this time the complete edition most widely used at Padua.

tain opinion to Hippocrates and confusing some plant species and attributes. These failings had led to Avicenna being neglected and held in contempt by Fuchs and others, although valuable information could be drawn from the *Canon* if it was read with caution. The one area in which, in Patin's opinion, Avicenna had gone seriously astray was in his polypharmacy.[125]

Whereas Patin proudly published his oration on Avicenna, the lectures on *Canon* 1.1 written out a generation later by the young Morgagni remained in manuscript (as their author perhaps intended) until brought to light by the diligence of his twentieth-century editor.[126] For Morgagni, the traditional curriculum assigned to him as professor of *theoria* at Padua was objectionable not only because of its obsolete scientific content and the no longer defensible distinction between *theoria* and *practica*, but also because the three separate books—(*Canon* 1.1, *Aphorisms*, and *Ars*—collectively provided no systematic and well-ordered overview of the five parts of medicine.[127] By the age of Boerhaave, the provision of a comprehensive and well-ordered survey of medicine for beginners, a preoccupation of some Italian medical teachers since Da Monte's time, had become a central concern of medical education. Morgagni therefore proposed to use his lectures on *Canon* 1.1 for a general introduction to the whole subject, and to teach physiology; to teach pathology, semiotics, hygiene, and therapy when he lectured on the *Aphorisms*; and to use the occasion of his lectures on the *Ars* to draw the whole together and to discuss method.[128] His goal of presenting the student with an overview of the entire discipline was thus quite similar to that espoused by Boerhaave at Leiden in the same period.

Hence, Morgagni's seventy-seven full-length lectures on the text of Gerard of Cremona's translation of *Canon* 1.1 are to a very large extent a textbook of late seventeenth- and early eighteenth-century physiology. But Morgagni's purpose was not only to ensure that his students became, as he said, "well versed in the opinions of the *recentiores*," but also that they should have some knowledge of the old system (still,

---

[125] Ibid., pp. 30–32. Another of Patin's orations showed partial acceptance of new ideas in physiology only if they could be reconciled with the ancients, viz. *Circulationem sanguinis a veteribus cognitam fuisse, Oratio habita in Archi-Lycaeo Patavino, Die iii Novembris MDCLXXXV* (Padua, 1685).

[126] Morgagni, comm. *Canon* 1.1, in his *Opera postuma*, ed. Pazzini, vols. 4–6.

[127] "Erant qui dictitarent, non venire [to Padua] propterea quia unum integrum ut opus erat systema medicum non audirent, non unum, quia alia alio anno traderentur et multa repeterentur, non integrum quia vel per saltus, vel ex una tantum parte libri explicarentur." Ibid., 4:6.

[128] Ibid., 4:5.

after all, needed for their examinations, such as they were) and, above all, of the differences between the two.[129] Morgagni consistently used the commentary framework to instruct his hearers in the nature and scope of these differences and to emphasize the superiority of the moderns. With the partial exception of the treatment of *Doctrina* 3 on complexion theory,[130] the stress on recent science runs through most of the work. Avicenna's statement in *Doctrina* 1 that the *medicus* should take general scientific principles from those learned in natural science or philosophy led Morgagni to remind his listeners that much of Aristotelian biology must be rejected.[131] *Doctrina* 3, on the elements, produced not only a revised list of elements—salt, sulfur, earth, air, and water—and a discussion of seventeenth-century chemistry, but also an account of the views of Copernicus, Galileo, and Descartes on cosmology (on religious grounds Morgagni affirmed his own adherence to the Tychonic system).[132] Above all, the fifty-nine lectures on the specifically physiological *doctrinae* (4, 5, and 6—humors, members, and faculties) are largely given over to systematic and detailed exposition of recent work in such areas as the origin, composition, and circulation of the blood; the lymphatic system; digestion; reproduction; and embryology—all with reference to the work of Leeuwenhoek, Van Helmont, Willis, Lower, Malpighi, Borelli, and numerous other seventeenth-century figures.[133] Moreover, the new is expounded in much more detail than the old; for example, the copious stream of citations of Galen, so typical of sixteenth- and seventeenth-century commentaries on the *Canon*, has been reduced to a trickle.

However, introductory lectures provide a rather favorable account of Avicenna as a historical figure, as well as a well-informed survey of the Latin *fortuna* of the *Canon*, with due attention to the scholastic commentators. Morgagni hailed Giacomo da Forlì as a fellow townsman,

---

[129] "Expositare doctrinae causas iuxta veterum systema propono, ne veterum dogmata ignoretis. . . . Eiusdem doctrinae causas iuxta recentiorum experimenta et systemata examino, ut recentiorum sententias calleatis. . . . Ratione et experientia ducibus quid ego sentiam propono." Ibid., 4:6. Complaints that the formal examination system at Padua had become a farce were heard as early as 1672 (AAUP, 722, document of 26 February 1672).

[130] Morgagni rejected both Aristotelian element theory and the idea of the four primary qualities (ibid., 4:140); nonetheless, he included a good deal of discussion along traditional lines, drawing heavily on Santorio for this part of the work. Topics discussed include, for example, the ancient problems of whether *complexio* itself constitutes a fifth quality (4:105–6) and whether the *complexio* of boys or youths is hotter (4:235–39).

[131] Ibid., 4:50.

[132] Ibid., 4:60–64; 76.

[133] Ibid., 4:264ff.; and vols. 5 and 6, passim.

but remarked, in words characteristic of the spirit of his whole commentary, that he had no intention of expounding opinions that Avicenna and his early commentators would be the first to change if they were still alive.[134] Quite a few citations of Giacomo and occasional allusions to other scholastic authors are in fact scattered through Morgagni's work; but it seems likely that for these, as for some of his introductory material, he relied on Santorio's commentary, which he knew well and cited frequently. The early lectures, before the strictly physiological sections, are ornamented with a generous display of classical learning in the shape of quotations from the poets and allusions to philosophical authors, so that Morgagni may have treated them as a rhetorical exercise. But there is very little of anything that could be classed as philosophical discussion. With these lectures a more than 400-year-old tradition of Latin commentary on the *Canon* may be said to have come to a close.

[134] "Nemo a me expectabit, ut opinor, ut omnes ipsius Avicennae, nedum harum enarrationum sententias, easque imprimis quas illi, ut tuear, erant sinceri, si nunc viverent, primi omnium mutarent." Ibid., 4:17.

PART IV

Canon 1.1 and the Teaching of Medical Theory at Padua and Bologna

7

Philosophy and Science in a Medical Milieu

Renaissance commentaries on the *Canon* consist at least as much of general exposition of the topics covered as of detailed exegesis of Avicenna's text. And although long-used textbooks such as the *Canon* acquired over the centuries a roster of traditionally discussed issues that successive commentators were likely to take up, commentators also exercised great freedom in introducing material of current interest to themselves and their contemporaries. Hence, investigation of the philosophical and scientific content of six published commentaries on *Canon* 1.1 and one on *Canon* 1.2 written at Bologna or Padua yields a good deal of information about the scope and assumptions of introductory medical teaching in those schools.[1]

One effect of the use of *Canon* 1.1 as a textbook was to ensure the presence of some specific instruction in philosophy and general science within the introductory medical curriculum. While methodology, material, and assumptions drawn from natural philosophy permeated large areas of the entire medical curriculum of the medieval and Renaissance universities, the first two *doctrinae* of *Canon* 1.1 cover specifically philosophical and physical subject matter, namely epistemology and the theory of the elements. It is unlikely that lectures on these *doctrinae* were ever philosophically inclined physicians' main or only source of the learning on such subjects. Both pragmatic requirements of professional preparation and Avicenna's own remarks on the proper relation of natural philosophy to medicine suggest that the attention given to the former within university medical courses tended to be limited in scope and depth. Most of the philosophical instruction obtained by those who became academically trained physicians was probably acquired either before they began their medical studies, and not neces-

---

[1] Da Monte, comm. *Canon* 1.1 (Venice, 1554); comm. *Canon* 1.2 (Venice, 1557); Oddi, comm. *Canon* 1.1 (Venice, 1575); Paterno, comm. *Canon* 1.1 (Venice, 1596); Costeo, *Disq. phys.*; Santorio, comm. *Canon* 1.1 (Venice, 1646); Cardano, *Opera* (Lyon, 1663), 9:453–567. For the probable dates and circumstances of composition of these commentaries and or the lectures on which they were based, see Chapter 6, above.

sarily in the same school where the latter took place,[2] or in courses in philosophy undertaken simultaneously with them. However, the presence of philosophical or scientific instruction within the medical curriculum served both to reinforce the notion that philosophical learning was an appropriate accomplishment, or adornment, for the fully trained physician and to provide an opportunity for those professors of medicine who adhered to this ideal to mold students in their own image.

General endorsement for the idea that philosophical studies were a necessary preliminary to the training of the *optimus medicus* and the belief that the two disciplines of philosophy and medicine enjoyed a special relationship continued to be widespread in the Italian university milieu throughout the sixteenth century.[3] Moreover, the traditional institutional and intellectual links between medical and philosophical faculties[4] were not yet broken, although perhaps somewhat weakened over the course of the century. The leading philosophers associated with Bologna and Padua in the early part of the sixteenth century, Achillini (d. 1512), Nifo (d. 1532), and M. A. Zimara (d. before 1537), all held medical as well as arts degrees and taught medicine as well as philosophy; Pomponazzi (d. 1525) also acquired a medical doctorate, although he never taught medicine.[5] The leading Aristotelian philosophers of the late sixteenth and early seventeenth century in Italy—Zabarella (d. 1589) and Cremonini (d. 1631)—seem not to have obtained medical degrees or to have taught medicine, but Zabarella responded to the medical interests of many of his students and Cremonini defended Aristotelian views on innate heat and the role of the heart, subjects of medical significance, against the Galenists. Furthermore, leading physicians, up to and including William Harvey, continued to pay attention to Aristotle.[6] Hence, the sixteenth-century teachers of medi-

---

[2] Palmer, *Studio of Venice*, pp. 14–17, summarizes the situation as regards students of Italian origin; Bylebyl, "School of Padua," p. 351, regarding the earlier studies of transalpine medical students at Padua.

[3] Schmitt, "Aristotle among the Physicians."

[4] Siraisi, *Arts and Sciences*, pp. 22–30, and *Alderotti*, pp. 18–24, summarize the earlier history of this association at Padua and Bologna, respectively.

[5] See Lohr, "Renaissance Latin Aristotle Commentaries," *Studies in the Renaissance* 21 (1974), 236–37; *Renaissance Quarterly* 32 (1979), 532–33; 35 (1982), 245; 33 (1980), 645.

[6] At any rate, no medical studies are mentioned in the biographies of Zabarella and Cremonini supplied by Lohr, in *Renaissance Quarterly* 28 (1975), 728, and 35 (1982), 233. Cremonini studied law in addition to philosophy. For Cremonini's controversies with the Galenists, see Charles B. Schmitt, "Cesare Cremonini: un aristotelico al tempo di Galilei," reprinted in his *Aristotelian Tradition*, pp. 3–21 (original pagination); and Bylebyl, "School of Padua," pp. 363–65 (stressing Cremonini's scorn for anatomy). Fortunio

cal *theoria* who were obligated to lecture on *Canon* 1.1 inhabited a milieu in which philosophy was a flourishing discipline in its own right and in which generally positive assertions about the relationship of medicine with philosophy were both traditional and commonplace.

Nevertheless, sixteenth-century Italian universities also produced many medical teachers and students and academically trained practitioners of medicine who had little or no serious interest in philosophy or in any scientific discipline other than medicine and such related fields as anatomy, botany, and pharmacology.[7] Moreover, in considering physicians' attitudes toward the relationship between medicine and philosophy, a distinction needs to be made between, first, the general assumption that medical students should have had some preliminary instruction in philosophy; second, interest in specific aspects of Aristotelianism of direct relevance to physiology (for example, Aristotle's views on the heart); and third, readiness to introduce discussions of such subjects as cosmology or the theory of tides into courses on medical *theoria*. There is evidence that by the 1540s the question of whether material that was not of direct relevance to medical practice had any place within an introductory university medical curriculum had already emerged as an issue. We have already noted Da Monte's complaints that many medical students, in haste to proceed to *practica*, and some of their teachers thought *theoria* as a whole worthy of only cursory and reluctant attention. This attitude had become even more marked by the 1580s and 1590s. Hostility to material of such peripheral relevance to medicine as the contents of the first two *doctrinae* of *Canon* 1.1 was likely to be even stronger than to the physiological generalities of the last four. We have also seen that from the late sixteenth century justifications of the continued assignment of *Canon* 1.1 tended to treat the work primarily as an introductory manual of physiology, one of the five classic divisions of medicine.

Hence, although none of the authors of the six commentaries on *Canon* 1.1 reviewed in this chapter eliminated or significantly reduced in length (proportionate to the length of his commentary as a whole)

Liceti (d. 1657) combined medicine and philosophy in his career in the traditional manner, as he had taught philosophy for some forty years before becoming first professor of medical *theoria* at Padua in 1645; see Lohr, in *Renaissance Quarterly* 31 (1978), 540–41. Regarding Harvey and Aristotle, see Walter Pagel, *William Harvey's Biological Ideas* (Basel and New York, 1967), and Walter Pagel, "William Harvey Revisited: Part 1," *History of Science* 8 (1969), 1–17.

[7] Bylebyl, "School of Padua," passim; for the suggestion that by the early seventeenth century "anatomy had, to a significant degree, displaced Aristotelian natural philosophy from its traditional position as the basis for medicine at Padua," see ibid., p. 364.

the exposition of the philosophical *Doctrinae* 1 and 2, they differed among themselves in their estimation of the value of the subject matter of these *doctrinae* in medical education. Three of the six (Da Monte, Cardano, and Costeo) clearly had no reservations about the value of philosophical and general scientific material in a course on medical *theoria*, since they used the vehicle of commentary for long expositions of their own philosophical views or surveys of current areas of debate in natural science. Santorio, too, incorporated fairly lengthy discussions of nonmedical scientific topics, although he expressed reservations about the propriety of doing so. By contrast, Paterno alone among them objected strongly to this way of proceeding. It seems indeed as if among most of these teachers of medical *theoria* the long-established belief that medical education required a grounding in natural philosophy survived, but was gradually reformulated as the idea that medical students should command at least superficial information about current developments or controversies in sciences other than medicine. Belief in the value of the latter kind of instruction was especially likely to affect lectures on *Doctrina* 2 because its subject matter, the elements, offered one of the few opportunities for such teaching within the formal medical curriculum at Bologna and Padua. Thus, the emphasis on speculative natural philosophy in a medical context that characterizes Da Monte's commentary on *Doctrina* 2, written in the 1540s, gave way in that of Costeo, composed some forty-five years later, to surveys of alternative cosmologies and theories of matter.

The practice of using lectures on *Doctrina* 2 to provide a modicum of "general science" instruction for medical students perhaps culminated in the teaching of Lorenzo Bacchetto at Padua in the 1680s, which apparently ranged over a wide area of seventeenth-century contributions to physical science. It looks as if professors of medicine who used their lectures on *Canon* 1.1.2 in this way did not have much confidence in the adequacy of their students' premedical philosophical or scientific instruction, perhaps because it had in many cases been received elsewhere, and were trying to fill what they perceived as a need.[8] As far as relevance to the professional training of physicians was concerned, however, Bacchetto's modern approach to science was open to the same objections as the philosophical disquisitions of older commentators; neither was very useful for medical practice. Moreover, the intellectual limitations and professional priorities of the teachers of medical *theoria*, as well as the realities of teaching an introductory survey to an

---

[8] Probably more remains to be learned about the actual content of instruction in natural philosophy in sixteenth- and seventeenth-century universities. There is a useful comparative overview of some Italian developments in Dooley, "Science Teaching," pp. 115–25.

at least partially reluctant audience, continued to entail a restricted treatment of philosophical and scientific issues. Yet, except for Paterno, the authors of sixteenth- and early seventeenth-century commentaries on *Canon* 1.1 published in Italy evidently regarded themselves as having a serious responsibility to provide some philosophical and general scientific, as well as medical, education for their students.

In so doing, they mingled traditional scholastic content with material new to this context and derived from contemporary philosophical eclecticism or scientific innovation. But no matter what the proportion of innovation, all the commentaries continued to transmit patterns of thought that remained in fundamental ways characteristic of scholastic Aristotelianism. Thus, for example, none of the authors found it possible to discuss the subject of mixtures (in *Doctrina* 3 on *complexio* or temperament) without introducing the ideas of substantial form and elementary qualities.[9]

How much impact the courses in medical *theoria* on which these commentaries are presumably based had on those who took them probably depended more on the individual lecturer than anything else. Whatever the complaints of students about the irrelevance of general philosophy and science to medicine, those who were fortunate enough to hear Da Monte, Santorio, or even Costeo were exposed to fairly substantial and reasonably up-to-date philosophical or scientific teaching. Cardano's idiosyncrasies appear more muted and the level of discussion more elementary in his commentary on the *Canon* than in some of his other writings, but his exposition drew on many of his wide scientific interests. Certainly the parts of Oddi's commentary given over to the two philosophical *doctrinae* seem more routine than the later, physiological sections. But it is only for the generations of students obliged to study the *Canon* under Bernardino Paterno that one feels true sympathy; Paterno's enthusiasm for the *Canon* was not, alas, matched by the ability to lend depth or interest to its exposition. Seldom can a eulogist have been wider of the mark than the preacher at Paterno's funeral in 1592 who delivered himself of the opinion that as Pergamum celebrated Galen, Cos Hippocrates, and Córdoba Avicenna, so the University of Padua would for all time number Paterno among its most shining lights.[10]

[9] Da Monte, comm. *Canon* 1.1 (Venice, 1554), fols. 57ᵛ–61; Oddo, comm. *Canon* 1.1 (Venice, 1575), pp. 99–115; Cardano, *Opera* (Lyon 1663), 9:507–8; Costeo *Disq. phys.*, p. 105; Paterno, comm. *Canon* 1.1 (Venice, 1596), fol. 84ᵛ; Santorio, comm. *Canon* 1.1 (Venice, 1646), cols. 254–60. Many more instances of this kind of language could be cited.

[10] "Extollet profecto celeberrimum suum . . . Pergamus [*sic*] Galenum, clarissimum suum Cohos Hippocratem . . . celebratissimum suum Corduba Avicennam, Gymna-

Four topics seem especially suited to provide an idea of the kind of philosophical and scientific indoctrination given in courses on medical *theoria* based on *Canon* 1.1: treatments of the standard introductory themes of the kind of knowledge offered by medicine and its relation to the other arts and sciences; discussions of the four elements; passages in which the commentators took up such topics as astral influences and qualities, occult causes, and so on; and expressions of opinion about the relationship between the medical concept of *complexio* and the human soul. From this restricted range of subjects one can learn something of the criteria for scientific knowledge adopted by these medical professors; their handling of subject matter pertaining to general physical science; their attitudes toward the whole complex of beliefs pertaining to astrology and occult causes; and their treatment of an issue involving a high degree of philosophical abstraction as well as potential theological sensitivity.

The Nature of Medical Knowledge

In placing discussions of the nature of medical knowledge and the place of medicine among the arts and sciences at the beginning of their commentaries on *Canon* 1.1 our sixteenth-century authors were perpetuating one of the most durable features of the scholastic medical tradition as it evolved in the north Italian *studia*. From the thirteenth century on, not only in commentaries on the *Canon* of Avicenna but also in a wide range of other general works on medicine, one finds treatment after treatment of such *quaestiones* as whether medicine is an art or a science, whether medicine is subalternated to (that is, derives its principles from) natural philosophy; and whether medicine is divided into theory and practice. In these discussions, the basic understanding of terms is Aristotelian. *Scientia* is usually assumed to offer certain knowledge about universal truths arrived at by demonstration (that is, syllogistic reasoning) from generally accepted principles, and to be pursued for the sake of truth. Different *scientiae* are distinguished by their subject matter. Natural philosophy is a *scientia* that has as its subject mobile bodies, but may not in fact offer the same certitude of demonstration as mathematics. And *ars* is a rationally organized and transmitted body of knowledge or skill resulting in a product (not necessarily a material one). Hence the topics discussed under the *quaestio* heads just listed included whether medicine offers any certain knowledge, whether med-

---

sium quippe Patavinum Paternum augustissimum his nemini secundum in omne aevum merito ornabit, praedicabit, celebrabit." A. F. Raphael, *In funere Bernardini Paterni . . . Oratio* (Padua, 1592), fol. 6ᵛ.

icine or any part of it proceeds by demonstration, whether any part of medicine resembles the mechanical arts, whether medicine is in fact a unified field of knowledge, the role of empirically acquired experience of particulars or individuals in medicine, and more.[11]

In the period in which medicine was emerging as a university discipline (roughly the thirteenth to the first part of the fourteenth century) such discussions were stimulated by the recognition that ancient and Arab medical authors yielded different and apparently conflicting definitions of medicine—for example, the most famous of all Hippocratic aphorisms termed medicine an art, while the *Canon* opened with the statement that it was a science—and by the varying place of medicine in twelfth-century schemes of classifications of the arts and sciences.[12] In addition, the notion, propagated by the *Canon*, that the concept of specific form could be used to explain idiosyncratic properties of particular substances and hence to supplement the explanatory system of Galenic rational (i.e., complexional) medicine probably also confirmed the legitimacy of the presence in medicine of irreducible elements of the particular (and indeed the folkloristic), which could not easily be conceived as involving art, in the sense of a rationally ordered body of knowledge, let alone speculative science.[13]

Meanwhile, the growing familiarity with Aristotle's definitions of various types of knowledge and the influence of thirteenth-century philosophical discussions of those definitions led to an investigation of how they might be applied to medicine.[14] The need to explore and where possible reconcile differences between philosophical and medical authorities gave rise to interest in the subject of method, that is, in

---

[11] Aristotle's own explanations of *episteme*, *techne*, and related concepts are to be found principally in *Posterior Analytics*, 1, 71a1–89b20; *Metaphysics* 1.1–2, 980b21–983a23; *Nicomachean Ethics*, 6.3–11, 1139b14–43b14 (I do not here address the question of the internal consistency between these and other Aristotelian passages). For examples of late thirteenth- and early fourteenth-century medical *quaestiones* discussing these issues, see Siraisi, *Alderotti*, pp. 118–37, 314–17.

[12] For comparison of, and references to, various definitions of medicine by Greek and Arabic medical writers, see Ottosson, *Scholastic Medicine*, pp. 68–74. Regarding medieval views, see n. 9 to Chapter 2.

[13] See Michael R. McVaugh's introduction to Arnald of Villanova's *Aphorismi de gradibus* in his *Opera medica omnia*, vol. 2.

[14] The *Posterior Analytics* was no doubt a main source of thirteenth-century interest in Aristotle's theory of demonstration, especially when accompanied by the commentary of Robert Grosseteste, written in the 1220s. On Grosseteste's influential exposition, see Alistair C. Crombie, *Robert Grosseteste and the Origins of Experimental Science* (Oxford, 1953); William A. Wallace, *Causality and Scientific Explanation* (Ann Arbor, 1972), 1:28–47; and Steven P. Marrone, *William of Auvergne and Robert Grosseteste* (Princeton, 1983), pp. 157–286, presenting somewhat different points of view.

establishing how the Aristotelian distinction of knowledge *quia* and knowledge *propter quid* should be understood in relation to the Galenic differentiation of resolutive, compositive, and definitive methods of learning. As various scholars have demonstrated, method retained its vitality as a subject of medical, as well as philosophical, debate from the days of Pietro d'Abano to those of Giambatista Da Monte, although it is doubtful whether those debates had as much influence on the evolution of ideas about scientific procedure as was once supposed.[15] In addition, during the fourteenth century the influence of philosophical and logical inquiry into the process of cognition and the possibility of direct intuitive knowledge of particulars also provided some stimulus for further discussions by physicians on the nature of knowledge.[16]

In such discussions, the number of different formulations regarding the place of *scientia* and *ars*, *theoria* and *practica*, certitude and conjecture, universal and particular, in medical knowledge was limited only by the verbal ingenuity of the various authors. Few medical writers of the thirteenth to fifteenth centuries were willing to abandon either *scientia* or *ars*, so their solutions often involved some form of compromise or division of medicine between the two kinds of knowledge. Although some treatments of the subject stand out, such as the assertion of a fourteenth-century author, possibly Bartolomeo da Varignana, that medicine is in no way subalternated to natural philosophy,[17] and Pietro d'Abano's philosophically well-informed approach to the issue of whether any certain knowledge of nature is possible,[18] others early took on the character of routine pedagogical reviews of ancient and Arab opinion and show little sign of real involvement on the part of the author.

[15] And as was claimed in J. H. Randall, *The School of Padua and the Emergence of Modern Science* (Padua, 1961). For a general critique of Randall's position, see Schmitt, "Aristotelianism in the Veneto." Other studies of Renaissance discussions of method are referred to in Chapter 6, n. 66, above.

[16] Echoes of the debate aroused by William of Ockham's attack on sensible species and ideas about intuitive cognition are, for example, to be found in the *Summa medicinalis* of Tommaso del Garbo and are discussed in Edward G. Smith, "A Disagreement on the Need of a Sensible Species in the Writings of Some Medical Doctors in the Late Middle Ages" (Ph.D. diss., Saint Louis University, 1974). Katherine Tachau plans further study of the response to Ockham in medical circles.

[17] Biblioteca Apostolica Vaticana, MS Vat. lat. 4452, 14c, fol. 83[r]; for discussion, see Siraisi, *Alderotti*, pp. 125–27. The passage occurs in the proem of an anonymous commentary on Galen's *De interioribus*, the same commentary, without proem, being attributed to Bartolomeo in MS Vat. lat. 4454, fol. 75[v]. However, the likelihood that this proem is not by Bartolomeo (d. after 1321), but by a later fourteenth-century author, is suggested by Vivian Nutton, reviewing Siraisi, *Alderotti*, in *Medical History* (1982), 100–101.

[18] *Conciliator* (Venice, 1548), *Diff.* 3, fols. 5[v]–8[r].

For the most part, the introductory expositions of the nature of medical knowledge in the sixteenth-century commentaries on the preface and *Doctrina* 1 of *Canon* 1.1 still fall well within the tradition that has just been sketched. With the partial exception of that by Da Monte, these portions of the five commentaries show little sign of any fresh thought about such topics as evidence, proof, or proper ways of proceeding in the investigation of nature, either in general or in the specific context of medicine, anatomy, and physiology. Only with the commentary of Santorio, written in the 1620s, are distinctly new concepts introduced. However, the manipulations of conventional formulae by the sixteenth-century commentators do not simply repeat those of earlier authors, and are presumably to be related to the contemporary situation.

One change that can be detected in certain of these sixteenth-century expositions is departure from the practice of compromise, hedging, and reconciliation in definitions of medicine as science and/or art. Da Monte, Paterno, and Costeo all seem to have been readier than some of their Latin predecessors to choose one of the two definitions and entirely exclude the other, although the grounds for the choice are not always clear.

For example, much in Da Monte's professional life—his wide experience as a practitioner, his insistence on training students at the bedside of patients, his advocacy of the direct study of medicinal plants by physicians—suggests an emphasis on the practical, the empirical, and the individual. This impression is strengthened when we note that in the opening sections of his commentaries on both *Canon* 1.1 and 1.2 Da Monte stressed the need for close integration of *theoria* and *practica* and numbered himself among those who held that even the initial consideration of first principles in medicine was always ultimately aimed at actual operation. Practical, empirical, and individual aspects were of course also strongly present in the medicine of the previous three centuries and were, as we have seen, especially well developed in fifteenth-century Padua; but these were precisely the aspects that were usually associated in one way or another with the concept of medicine as *ars*. Yet Da Monte insisted that the whole of medicine (not just *theoria*, as some would have it) is properly defined as *scientia*, proceeds by demonstration, and arrives at general and eternal truths. He went on to maintain that any art was scientific to the extent that it involved consideration of general truths and the reasons for the specific activities that it entailed.[19] When these statements are taken in conjunction with

---

[19] Da Monte, comm. *Canon* 1.1 (Venice, 1554), fols. 8ʳ–9ʳ. At fol. 8ᵛ: "Dico ad hoc

the distinction between investigative and pedagogic method also incorporated into the beginning of Da Monte's commentary on *Canon* 1.1, they certainly suggest at least a desire to reexamine the relationship between medical principles and medical practice.[20] Unfortunately, however, in this passage Da Monte provided no examples of what he considered valid demonstration or universal truths in medicine.

The equally firm commitment to *scientia* as the model for medicine manifested by Giovanni Costeo, writing some forty-five years after Da Monte, was of a very different kind. According to Costeo, the question of whether medicine was or was not a science had been the subject of bitter dispute not only among the ancients but also among the *recentiores*. He proposed to resolve the issue with the assertion that art and science are two closely connected products of the human intellect that mutually assist one another. He went on to say that although the origins of medicine lay in experience, "the bosom of the whole of natural philosophy is investigated" when the physician considers pathology and disease etiology, physiology, and pharmacology on the basis of observational evidence and research into the unknown (*cum evidentibus observandis, tum abditis perquirendis*). Furthermore, "medicine frequently takes over from natural philosophy the principles of its proofs, its divisions, its definitions, and its ways of arguing."[21]

But was natural philosophy itself a science? Costeo, following "the consensus of philosophers," held that it was, but he was aware that he needed to refute "those in our age who deny natural philosophy and metaphysics to be sciences and think only geometry to be worthy of the name," because of its certainty of demonstration.[22] Although he

---

quod medicina est scientia, et proprium genus medicinae est scientia." At 9^r: "Advertatis igitur, ars consideratur dupliciter vel ut versatur circa materiam, et subiectum extrinsecum, circa quod operatur, vel ut versatur circa universalia et rationem faciendi. Primo modo considerando artem, ars vere est . . . secundo autem modo est scientia."

[20] Ibid., fols. 4^r–6^r. Da Monte naturally did not confine his discussion of method and principles relating to practice to his commentaries on the *Canon*; more extensive treatment of the subject is to be found in his lectures on Galen's treatise on therapeutic method. The dissemination and influence of these lectures in northern Europe are discussed in Nutton, "John Caius," pp. 381–83.

[21] Costeo, *Disq. phys.*, pp. 7–15. At p. 10: "Dum igitur medicina, quam ab experientia duxisse ortum constat, in spectanda morborum et symptomatum natura ac varietate, et in eorum causis, cum evidentibus observandis, tum abditis perquirendis, atque in expendenda corporum quae afficiuntur natura, ac remediorum quae iuvasse contigit, potestate, pertinacius persistit, naturalisque philosophiae universae sinus rimatur." At p. 13: "Imo ex naturali, suarum probationum principia, divisiones, definitiones, et ratiocinationes frequenter sumit."

[22] "Naturalem autem in genere scientiarum esse consensus est philosophorum, quanquam non defuere qui aetate nostra et naturalem et metaphysicam scientias esse negant,

was prepared to allow a definition of medicine that placed it in an intermediary position between *scientia* and *ars*, partaking of the attributes of both, Costeo did not really think there could be a mean between contemplative and noncontemplative, or between demonstrative and nondemonstrative, modes of knowledge. His own ultimate preference was for a definition of medicine as mostly contemplative and hence indisputably among the sciences. In defending this position, he asserted that the fact that physicians concerned themselves with individual cases did not detract from the philosophical nature of their discipline, any more than imparting ethical advice to individuals detracted from the status of moral philosophers. To the objection that the physician did not simply observe the curative powers of nature, but intervened physically by reducing dislocations, treating wounds, incising tumors, and administering medication, Costeo retorted that it was not the physician who did these things but his assistants. To the incontrovertible fact that physicians themselves did feel the patient's pulse, he replied that their objective in so doing was to observe the state of the invalid and the appearance of the body, and that such an action was comparable to an astrologer's observation of the stars.[23]

Thus, whereas for Da Monte the definition of medicine as *scientia*, whatever its ambiguities, seems to have been connected to his wish to strengthen the links between the theoretical basis and medical practice, for Costeo the same definition provided justification for the separation of medical learning and healing activity. It may be added that Costeo's discomfort (in this instance at least) with the techniques of reconciliation practiced by his thirteenth- to fifteenth-century predecessors resulted in an attempted assimilation of medical learning to natural philosophy far more thoroughgoing than most of them would have countenanced.

---

et unam geometriam scientiae nomine dignam esse ob id censent, quod ea una semper demonstret." Ibid.

[23] "At nihil hoc tamen de contemplationis prioris dignitate, nihil de scientiae natura detrahit, ut non etiam detrahit de moralis philosophiae dignitate, neque illam a scientiis excludit consultatio, quae illi frequens est etiam de privatis rebus." Ibid., p. 11. And: "At medicum (inquies) reponere luxata membra, vulnera consuere, tumores aut venam secare, ac propinare medicamenta. Haec enim natura non agit sed medicus, atque his sanitas inducitur. Imo vero nec naturae, nec medici munera haec sunt, sed ministrorum medici. Huius autem id tantum interest, quid opus sit facto ut intelligat, atque instar architecti aut imperatoris cuiusdam, ipse ab omni opera alienus, ministris quid agendum sit, committat. Quid? Nonne et admota aegris manu arteriarum motus explorare medici est? Est sane. Sed hoc, ut etiam observare aegri statum omnem, ac quicquid in eius corpore apparet, vel etiam quae ex corpore excernuntur, contemplationis, non operis, habet rationem. Ad noscendas enim aegri vires universas, accedere sine sensuum ope medico non licet, ut neque astrologo ad siderum motus observandos." Ibid., pp. 14–15.

Although in much more cautious terms, Cardano too, at least in this work, gave a qualified endorsement to the description of medicine as a kind of *scientia* and eschewed any lengthy exercises in scholastic reconciliation of the various positions on this issue. He stressed, following Avicenna, that medicine was divided not into *scientia* and *ars*, but into *scientia theorica* and *scientia practica*. Against the contemporary philosopher M. A. Zimara, he held that *scientia practica* was quite different from *ars*, because *scientia practica*, unlike *ars*, drew its first principles from contemplative science (in the case of medicine, from natural philosophy), made use of demonstration, and dealt with natural phenomena (in the case of medicine, health and sickness), rather than producing something new, as did *ars*. Cardano therefore concluded that Avicenna had meant that, although medicine did not offer perfect knowledge, something not possessed by mortals, it was a *habitus* involving reasoned demonstration from principles. Cardano's own position, however, was that medical knowledge could not be said to be true *scientia* deduced from principles but was, rather, arrived at by reasoning about sense evidence that served as its principles.[24]

By contrast, both Oddo Oddi and Paterno emphasized medicine as an art, and played down the concept of medical *scientia* and links with natural philosophy. Oddi noted that Avicenna's definition encompassed only medicine as an intellectual *habitus* and was therefore incomplete. According to Oddi, the name medicine is properly applied only to the curative part of the discipline, its most essential component and that invented first. Subsequently, the Greeks began to pay attention to bodily regimen and gymnastics for the maintenance of health, and for lack of any other term subsumed this, too, under medicine. Moreover, Oddi gave prominent place to the conventional formulation that the practical end of attaining or preserving health distinguished medicine from natural philosophy, even though the latter also encompassed the study of the human body. Furthermore, he showed preference for a def-

---

[24] Cardano, *Opera* (1663), 9:471–73. At p. 473: "[Avicenna] diceret: 'vel tu vis scientiam perfectam, et illa non habetur apud mortales, vel tu vis habitum quendam ratione ex principiis deducta demonstratum, et hic habetur in medicina.' Et circa hoc sciendum quod sunt sex habitus valde similes. Primus est intellectus principiorum, qui non est scientia sed est nobilior illa, sed non est scientia quia non est cum ratione seu discursu. Secundus est habitus qui deducitur ex principiis, et hic vocatur scientia. Tertius est habitus qui deducitur ratione ex sensibilibus tanquam principiis, et hic est habitus scientiae, non tamen scientia vera, in quo genere est medicina. Quartus est habitus deductus ex scientia per rationem, et hic vocatur scientia practica quia tendit in opus. Quintus est habitus ratione acquisitus, docente sed non demonstrante causam, et hic est ars. Sextus est habitus operandi, secundum illam rationem sine ratione, et hic est habitus operandi, quo etiam in mechanicis operarii utuntur."

inition of medicine that stressed its practical, indeed its technological, aspect. Claiming to follow Galen in *De placitis Hippocratis et Platonis*,[25] he set forth a scheme classifying *artes* according to their end products: some resulted only in speculation (*physica*), others only in action (dancing); some had as an end the acquisition of something (hunting), and others produced a result. To the last category belonged both building and medicine. In Oddi's view, therefore, Avicenna had omitted essential elements in his definition of medicine and had deviated culpably from Galen's view, and deserved to be condemned on both counts.[26] Oddi, however, certainly did not wholly repudiate the idea of medicine as *scientia* (on this subject, he seems to have been more attuned to the idea of reconciliation than Da Monte or Costeo), and elsewhere made it clear that he accepted that logic and philosophy were essential foundations of medicine.[27] While it is doubtless in a general sense true that Oddi's particular shuffling of the formulae of medical definition was a product of his Galenism, it is also evident that his was only one possible reading of Galen's opinions.[28] Whether this reading was the product of personal experience or response to the contemporary scene, or of more or less routine and unreflecting handling of texts and conventions remains unclear.

Paterno was a good deal more emphatic than Oddi in his effort to separate medicine completely from natural philosophy or general science. He began his commentary by warning the "most excellent young men" who were his audience that when Galen said the best *medicus* is also a philosopher he certainly did not mean that the *medicus* should consider such topics as time, place, plurality of worlds, the eternity of the world, the existence of a void, the nature of matter, the movement or stability of the earth, the laws of motion, "and all the other things philosophers dispute about." Paterno claimed the authority of both Galen and Socrates for the view that these subjects were "useless for the

---

[25] Oddi, comm. *Canon* 1.1 (Venice, 1575), p. 35.

[26] Ibid., pp. 34–42. At p. 34: "Expositores dicunt medicinam tripliciter capi, primo quidem pro instrumento, quod in diaetam, potionem, et chyrurgiam dividitur . . . secundo autem ab eodem sumitur, prout cibo et veneno contradistinguitur . . . ; tertio vero pro habitu intellectus, qua quidem significatione hoc in loco capitur ab Avicenna." At p. 40: "At cum Avicenna a principio essentialem constitutat diffinitione reiecta ea notionis quae ex Galeno, ut omnibus eiusdem linguae sit testata, opus est, et ad rei essentiam non aspiret, sed propria rei diffinitae accidentia una complectatur, non parum a Galeni decretis discessit; et ob id mirum in modum est reprehendendus."

[27] Ibid., pp. 70–71, and, for discussion, Schmitt, "Aristotle and the Physicians," p. 12.

[28] For example, Galen's assertion that the best physician was also a philosopher had acquired almost the force of a proverb; see Paterno, comm. *Canon* 1.1 (Venice, 1596), fol. 1ʳ, quoted in the following note.

human race," discussion of them being irrelevant not only to medicine, but also to morals and civil virtue.[29] This sweeping dismissal of the fundamental subject matter of ancient and contemporary scientific inquiry was accompanied by the assertion that all medical study, including the study of *theoria*, is and ought to be directed toward therapeutic action, and that medicine can be termed *scientia* only in the broadest and loosest sense, since contemplation is present in medicine only to the extent that it is in any of the other *artes factivae*. Furthermore, in Paterno's view *medici* who drew on philosophical authors and arguments simply for the sake of ornamenting medical discourse were gravely at fault, since nothing should be included that did not directly contribute to the overriding purpose of finding the best way to proceed in medical treatment.[30]

Probably few among the learned physicians who were Paterno's contemporaries would have gone as far as he did in his repudiation of philosophy. As already noted, it was widely accepted that logic and *physica*, including the kind of subject matter dismissed by Paterno were desirable preliminary studies for those intending subsequently to proceed to medicine, and that the content of Aristotelian teaching regarding such subjects as, for example, the elementary qualities, psychology, and mammalian biology was of some real concern to the physician. The pragmatic desire of some students and professors of

---

[29] "Optimum medicum eundem et philosophum esse oportere, multis opere ad hoc dicato Galeni demonstrare perrexit. Verum non omnia quae a philosophis tractantur a medico inquirenda esse voluit, cum ex his quaedam inutilia esse non solum morali et civili virtuti, verum et arti medicae censuerit, atque etiam toti humano generi, veluti quae de tempore, loco, et de mundo, an unus sit vel plures, genitus vel aeternus, an extra ipsum vacuum, et alia, quae a philosophis disputari solent, ut scilicet, an omnia sint unum vel multa, an omnia moveantur, vel quiescant, an omnia generentur, et corrumpantur, et id genus alia. Quae Socrates apud Xenophontem tanquam humano generi omnino inutilia despexit." Ibid., fol. 1^r. Paterno's statement does in fact echo an opinion expressed by Galen; see Galen, *On the Doctrines of Hippocrates and Plato*, ed. and tr. Philip De Lacy, Corpus medicorum graecorum 5, 4, 1, 2 (Berlin, 1980), Book 9, chap. 7, p. 589. The passage of Xenophon purporting to give the opinions of Socrates is *Memorabilia*, 4.7; Xenophon, *Memorabilia and Oeconomicus*, ed. and tr. E. C. Marchant, Loeb Classical Library (London and New York, 1923) pp. 346–51.

[30] Paterno, comm. *Canon* 1.1 (Venice, 1596), fols. 1^r–9^v. At fol. 1^v: "Quibus satis aperte indicavit, exemplo eorum quae de elementis tractantur ab Hippocrate, omnia quae philosophica traduntur in arte medica, in actionem medicam tendere, et nihil eorum in contemplationem. Atque sic nullam medicinae partem scientiam proprie dici posse, sed ut Galenus ait, communiter seu late nomen scientiae extendendo, ad artes quoque factivas." At fol. 9^v: "Nisi forte putavit Averroes, cum Aristotelis philosophica, quaedam surripi a medicis elegantibus, ad ornatum quae vere medicinae non sint, quod tamen neque Galeno neque bonis medicis placet, cum a scientia naturali nihil a medico surreptum sit ad ornatum, sed omnia ad rectam operandi rationem inveniendam sumpserint."

practica to limit the amount of time spent in medical courses on the study of material of indirect or peripheral relevance to medical practice does not seem as a rule to have given rise to denunciations of physics and cosmology as such. Nonetheless, Paterno's remarks demonstrate clearly enough that in the second half of the sixteenth century a lifelong commitment to teaching medical *theoria* did not necessarily entail any concomitant attachment either to intellectual traditions linking medicine and natural philosophy, or to a belief that at least some aspects of medicine were properly defined as *scientia*.

Yet Paterno's own commentary on *Canon* 1.1 reveals the difficulty of detaching *theoria* from these traditional concerns and concepts. In the first place, he proved unable to live up to his own recommendation, "omnia ad rectam operandi rationem," with any consistency. Although he paid much less attention than, say, Da Monte or Costeo to philosophical and scientific issues of slight or no relevance to medicine, Paterno nevertheless devoted a number of pages to such topics as the forms of the elements and the difference between Platonic and Aristotelian concepts of soul.[31] More commonly, however, he produced a thin, vague, and unspecific discourse that revealed *theoria* without philosophy as barren indeed. And he signally failed to compensate for the loss by strengthening the ties between *theoria* and *practica*. The lesson to be drawn from Paterno's opening remarks may therefore be merely that one should be cautious in accepting sixteenth-century declarations of pragmatic intent at face value. But his statements are also a reminder that the viability of *theoria* as a separate branch of the medical curriculum was vulnerable not only to the decay of the Galenic synthesis, the decline of teaching by commentary, and the growth of other kinds of medical instruction, but also to changes in the perception of the relationship between medicine and philosophy.

Despite his use of a number of by now familiar concepts, Santorio's treatment of the subject of the nature of medical knowledge and its relation to other branches of learning represents a new departure. He asserted in his preface that his objectives included not only the explication of how *theoria* served, or underlay, practice (a goal also espoused by Da Monte and Paterno), but also the corroboration of theoretical principles of physiology by physical demonstrations. In the same place he also announced that he was proceeding on the assumption that his readers, and presumably hearers, would have studied logic and philosophy before they came to medicine, and that he would expand on those sub-

---

[31] Ibid., fols. 61^r–66^v; 145^r–47^v.

jects only to the extent that they related to medical goals.[32] Although he can scarcely be said to have kept the latter promise, these two objectives informed his discussions of such questions as why medicine is conjectural, whether medicine is a science, and whether medicine is subalternated to natural philosophy.[33]

In responding to the last two standard queries, Santorio was clear and unequivocal. He held that medicine was not a science but an art, and hence that it was in no way subordinated to natural philosophy. His arguments may be summarized as follows. Medicine is not a science because science considers the works of nature, not of man. The work of the *medicus* consists in preserving health and removing illness, both of which are human activities. The subject matter of natural philosophy is considered by the *medicus* only to the extent that it can contribute to the goal of health. Furthermore, one cannot say that everything done by the *medicus* can be done by nature, because *medici* do many things that nature cannot do, such as cutting for the stone, cauterizing dog bites, and excising polyps. Nor is the converse true, because the task of medicine is essentially a repair job and the physician cannot, alas, make new body parts. Nor is it correct to say that medicine is divided into theory and practice and that the theoretical part is a science. In the first place, the division between theory and practice is itself improper; but allowing such a division for the sake of argument, it cannot be maintained that medical theory is a science. If this proposition were accepted, since every art has its theory, all the arts would be sciences and one could speak of a science of purse snatching. Nor is it valid to say medicine must be a science because an art always involves the habit of exercising it, and some learned physicians have not practiced. On the contrary, the *habitus* of an art can be acquired either from experience or from a master; hence it is possible to speak of "excellent *medici theorici* and *practici* who never exercised the art,"[34] a group in

---

[32] "Nos quidem supponemus lectores huiusque medicinae studiosos antea aliquid de philosophia intellexisse; ideo, licet saepissime et de rebus logicis et philosophicis aliquid dixerimus, illa tantum amplectemur quae nos facili manu ducent ad ultimum scopum, qui est ut habita sanitas conservetur et amissa recuperetur." Santorio, comm. *Canon* 1.1 (Venice, 1646), cols. 2–3.

[33] *Quaestio* 6: "Qua ratione ars medica sit coniecturalis." Ibid., cols. 28–35. *Quaestio* 7: "An medicina sit scientia." Ibid., cols. 39–43. *Quaestio* 13: "An medicina sit subalternata philosophiae." Ibid., cols. 140–41. Santorio's views on *Quaestio* 6 are discussed in Grmek, *Santorio*, pp. 79–82.

[34] "Respondemus dari duplicem habitus, vel acquisitum ex iteratis actibus vel a magistro; hac enim ratione possunt dari optimi medici theorici et practici qui nunquam in artem exercuerint, sicuti fuit [*sic*] Averroes, Plusquam Commentator, et alii plures." Santorio, comm. *Canon* 1.1 (Venice, 1646), col. 40.

which Santorio placed Averroes and Torrigiano. Equally invalid is Pietro d'Abano's suggestion that medicine was an art when first invented but subsequently turned into a science. If this were true, it would follow that all the sciences were at one time arts. Santorio's arguments amount, of course, to a wholesale rejection of the teaching of Avicenna, of the fourteenth- and fifteenth-century academic medical convention of maintaining that medicine was simultaneously *scientia* and *ars*, and of the opinions of those sixteenth-century commentators on *Canon* 1.1—namely Da Monte and Costeo—who claimed medicine for *scientia*.

Although Santorio cited the traditional authorities in support of the position that medicine should be considered *ars*—Hippocrates, Aristotle, Galen, and Averroes[35]—he departed markedly from the other convention of Latin academic medicine, which reserved the term *ars* for aspects of the subject that did not offer any prospect of certitude arrived at by rational demonstration. In discussing the question of why the art of medicine is conjectural, Santorio made it clear that although he thought medicine conjectural to some degree, because of individual variations and failure to ascertain either the norm or the precise extent of pathological deviations from it, this element of uncertainty could, in his opinion, be greatly reduced, if not eliminated, by means that had nothing to do with syllogistic reasoning. He asserted that the task of the *medicus* was not to treat individuals but to treat diseases; hence an effective medicine should be understood as one that cured the same disease in any number of different people, an idea that gave therapy a universal aspect and reduced the effectiveness of the argument that medicine could offer no certainty because it dealt so largely with particulars and thus did not encompass general truths. Furthermore, Santorio asserted that the "quantity of diseases" could be ascertained with considerable precision by the use of the instruments he had devised to measure the rate of the pulse, body heat, bodily humidity or dryness, and perspiration loss. Repeated use of these instruments in sickness and in health, and careful recording of even minor variations, would allow the norm for individuals to be established and deviations from the norm measured.

From this *quaestio* it becomes clear that Santorio, who from the modern standpoint is rightly regarded as a pioneer of innovative scientific

---

[35] Citing the first aphorism of Hippocrates, the title of the *Ars medicinalis* (that is, the *Microtechne* or *Tegni*) of Galen, the opening of the first chapter of the *Colliget* of Averroes, and passages in the *Ethics* and *Metaphysics* of Aristotle regarding the definitions of *scientia* and *ars* (*episteme* and *techne*) (see n. 11, above). All these citations are part of the common currency of numerous earlier discussions of the same topic.

method in medicine,[36] still adhered to an older, Aristotelian, definition of *scientia*. He placed the instruments of measurement for which he is famous—the pulsilogium, the thermoscope, and the weighing chair—not at the service of *scientia*, but at that of *ars*. In so doing, however, he evidently hoped to bring to *ars* a new precision that would approach, if not attain, certainty in a way not previously deemed possible. Thus, Santorio brings us to the threshold of an understanding of the nature and possibilities of medical and physiological knowledge very different from that expressed in the earlier commentaries discussed in this chapter.

The Elements

We now turn to the contents of the expositions of Avicenna's chapter on the elements provided by the commentators for their students in medical *theoria*. As already noted, Avicenna's brief chapter provides an essentially Aristotelian picture. The elements are the primary parts of the human body and of other bodies. They cannot be reduced to more basic components. From their admixture the diverse species of mixed bodies are made. The elements are four in number. Two of them, earth and water, are heavy; two, air and fire, are light. In the separate accounts of each element that follow, primary emphasis is laid upon the idea of natural place, and on the role of the qualities of a particular element in question in the constitution of bodies; thus, the natural place of earth, where it remains immobile, is the center of the universe; its coldness and dryness provide for the conservation of shapes and impressions in things. Finally, it is stated that in living bodies the two heavy elements assist chiefly in the generation (*plus iuvant ad generationem*) of members, and the two lighter ones chiefly in the generation of spirit and motion, although the actual mover is the soul.

This account continued to be regarded by many as orthodox and tenable throughout the sixteenth and into the seventeenth century. For academic physicians, in particular, there was good reason for conservatism. Not only was element theory an area in which there was substantial, although not total, agreement between Aristotle and Galen, still major authorities; not only were physicians explicitly instructed by Avicenna that investigation of the elements was no business of theirs;[37] but any serious revision of teaching on the elements,

[36] Grmek, *L'introduction*, passim.

[37] Aristotle devoted much of *De caelo* and *De generatione et corruptione* to discussions of the elements; see esp. *De caelo* 3 and 4, 298a24–313b21, and *De gen. et corr.* 1.1, 314a14–315a25, and 2.3, 330a20–331a5; also *Meteorologica* 1.2, 339a11–34. Galen's views are very

considered as a theory of matter, would have very grave implications for the whole of academic medicine and physiology. On the basis of the scheme of the four elements and their associated qualities rested the vast superstructure of complexional and humoral physiology and pathology and complexional pharmacology erected primarily by Galen and elaborated by his Latin heirs in the medieval and Renaissance universities. "Rational" medical treatment depended on the concept of the elemental qualities; the alternative appeared to be treatment based on the empirical, the individual, and the particular, about which it was impossible to convey any systematic teaching at all—hence some of the opposition to claims of discovery of new, empirically tested remedies for new particular diseases unknown to the Galenic system.[38] By contrast, revision of the cosmological content of traditional element theory (such as, for example, the statements about the natural place of the earth in Avicenna's chapter), however radical in other regards, had fewer implications for medicine.

In some circles, however, interest in alternatives to or modifications of the traditional scheme of the four elements was manifested from early in the sixteenth century. To name only a few celebrated examples, Fracastoro[39] and, a generation later, Giordano Bruno were both influenced by the ideas of the ancient atomists;[40] Paracelsus, who wanted to overthrow the entire intellectual system of academic medicine, discarded fire as an element, leaving a triad of earth, water, and air, and derived three additional principles from the alchemical tradition: mercury, sulfur, and salt.[41] Various factors doubtless contributed to the reopening of fundamental questions about the elements, which as Giovanni Costeo remarked, had long been regarded as settled until

fully set out in *De elementis ex Hippocrate*, Book I (Kühn, 1:413–91). According to Avicenna: ". . . medicina tractat de elementis et complexionibus et humoribus et membris simplicibus et compositis et spiritibus et virtutibus eorum naturalibus et animalibus et vitalibus et operationibus et dispositionibus corporis, scilicet sanitate et egritudine et medio. . . . Harum vero rerum quedam sunt de quibus medico nihil aliud est agendum nisi ut quid sint tantum essentiali formatione informet, et utrum sint vel non sint doctori sapientie physicalis credat," *Canon* 1.1.1.2 (Venice, 1507), fol. 1ᵛ. For discussion of Galen's theory of the elements, see Paul Moraux, "Galien comme philosophe: la philosophie de la nature," in *Galen: Problems and Prospects*, ed. Vivian Nutton (London, 1981), pp. 87–116, at pp. 90–92.

[38] On this point, see Giancarlo Zanier, *Medicina e filosofia tra '500 e '600* (Milan, 1983), pp. 18–19.

[39] See Kurd Lasswitz, *Geschichte der Atomistik* (Hamburg and Leipzig, 1890; reprint Hildesheim, 1963), 1:306–8, and *De sympathia et antipathia rerum liber unus*, Chapter 5, in *Hieronymi Fracastorii Veronensis Opera omnia* (Venice, 1574), p. 60.

[40] See Paul-Henri Michel, *La cosmologie de Giordano Bruno* (Paris, 1962), pp. 137–64.

[41] Allen G. Debus, *The Chemical Philosophy* (New York, 1977), 1:57.

"battle has been renewed in our age."[42] Such more or less practical developments as the accumulation of firsthand experience by alchemists and others of the actual properties of salts, minerals, and chemical compounds, and the multiplication of printed treatises on alchemy, spa waters, and minerals and metallurgy doubtless played a significant part in increasing the attention given to element theory.[43] However, this attention often took the form of reconsideration of long-available sources of information about ancient theories of matter other than those of Aristotle and was unquestionably further stimulated by access to fresh material about those theories in the shape of Renaissance editions and translations of hitherto little known Greek works.[44]

Whether or not they were receptive to non-Aristotelian theories of matter, all members of the sixteenth-century academic medical community in Italy were likely to be exposed to them to some extent. Obviously, the accounts of atomist and other pre-Socratic concepts provided by Aristotle and his Greek commentators remained important sources of information on these topics. Recent scholarship has emphasized the involvement of members of Italian—and especially the Paduan—philosophical faculties in the study of the Greek commentators on Aristotle and of the Greek texts of Aristotle's own works and the influence on the development of Aristotelian philosophy in Italy in the late fifteenth and sixteenth centuries of humanistic approaches to a broader range of texts and ideas.[45] Other sources of information available to physicians with philosophical or indeed classical literary inclinations included Diogenes Laertius' accounts of Zeno and Epicurus, widely disseminated in editions of the translation by Traversari,[46] Cic-

---

[42] ". . . quamvis post sedatas iam diu his de rebus controversias, a nobis accipienda citra contentionem omnem viderentur, quia tamen de his ipsis aetate nostra renovata pugna est, non temere facturi videmur, si ad stabilienda medicinae fundamenta . . . primum, unum ne sit elementum an plura." Costeo, *Disq. phys.*, pp. 40–41.

[43] Attention is drawn to some of these factors in Debus, *The Chemical Philosophy* 1:22–25; and Zanier, *Medicina e filosofia*, pp. 9–17.

[44] The interaction of literary and humanistic factors with experiential ones in the sixteenth-century approach to theories of matter is stressed in R. Hooykaas, "The experimental origin of chemical, atomic, and molecular theory before Boyle," *Chimia: Annual Studies in the History of Chemistry* 2 (1949), 65–80.

[45] See Schmitt, *Aristotle and the Renaissance*, passim, and esp. pp. 35–85; Mahoney, "Philosophy and Science," pp. 163–73, 181–89. Bruno Nardi, *Saggi sull'Aristotelismo padovano dal secolo XIV al XVI* (Florence, n.d.).

[46] Diogenes Laertius, 7.132–60, for a general acount of Stoic thought embedded in the life of Zeno (Diogenes Laertius, *Lives of Eminent Philosophers*, Loeb Classical Library, 2:237–63); 10 (Loeb, 2:528–677) for the life of Epicurus. Traversari's translation was made before 1432 and first published in 1472; the complete Greek text of the work was first printed in 1533 (ibid., introduction, pp. xxvi, xxviii). On an earlier Latin compen-

ero's treatment of Stoic thought in *De natura deorum*,[47] Plutarch's brief treatises against the Stoics,[48] and the printed editions of Lucretius.[49] Moreover, two treatises, newly available in the middle years of the sixteenth century and likely to be read by some physicians, both contained much material pertaining to the physical theories of the Stoics. These were Galen's *De placitis Hippocratis et Platonis*, one of the last of his major works to become available in the West,[50] and Alexander of Aphrodisias' *De mixtione*,[51] which had implications for the medical theory of *complexio*. The latter, in particular, was largely devoted to a lengthy rebuttal of aspects of the Stoic theory of mixtures, that is, compounds of the elements. The importance attached by physicians to this work is indicated by the fact of the three separate translations made between about 1540 and 1553, two were by medical men (one of whom was from Padua).[52] As we shall see, Stoic ideas about the elements and mixtures attracted the attention of several of the commentators on *Canon* 1.1. The actual extent and full implications of the sixteenth-century medical interest in Stoic physics are, however, topics that await further investigation.[53]

---

dium derived from Diogenes Laertius that circulated in the Middle Ages, see Gregorio Piaia, *Vestigia philosophorum: il medioevo e la storiografia filosofica* (Rimini, 1983), pp. 117–18, and literature there cited.

[47] *De natura deorum* 1.11 (Cicero, *De natura deorum, Academica*, Loeb Classical Library, pp. 446–48). Book 2 treats extensively of Stoic theories about providence.

[48] On these treatises, see K. Ziegler, "Plutarchus von Chaironea," Pauly-Wissowa (1951), 21:753–61. The extent of Plutarch's direct knowlege of Stoic teachings is debated. The treatises against the Stoics are included in the edition of Plutarch's *Opera* published (Geneva ?) in 1572 in vol. 3 (Greek), pp. 1898–1942, 1942–44, 1945–93, and vol. 9 (Latin), pp. 382–422, 422–24, 651–95.

[49] On the Renaissance *fortuna* of Lucretius, see Wolfgang Bernard Fleischman, "Lucretius Carus, Titus," *CTC*, 2:351–55.

[50] First printed in Greek, by Aldus, in 1525; the Greek text is also included in the Basel, 1538, edition of Galen's *Opera*. A Latin translation of Books 2–9 by Guinter of Andernach was published in Paris in 1534, and was followed by several other sixteenth-century Latin translations. See Galen, *On the Doctrines of Hippocrates and Plato*, editor's introduction, 1:21, 35–36, 46.

[51] Text and translation in Robert B. Todd, *Alexander of Aphrodisias on Stoic Physics* (Leiden, 1976).

[52] Regarding the Aldine *editio princeps* of the Greek text (1527), and the sixteenth-century Latin translations, see F. Edward Cranz, "Alexander Aphrodisiensis," *CTC*, 1:81, 113–14. The translators were Jakob Schegk, professor of medicine at Tübingen; Angelus Caninius Anglariensis; and Gaspar Gabriel "patavinus medicus."

[53] The sixteenth-century revival of Stoicism is discussed in Günter Abel, *Stoizismus und Frühe Neuzeit* (Berlin and New York, 1978); Julien Eymard d'Angers, *Recherches sur le Stoicisme au XVIᵉ et XVIIᵉ siècles*, ed. L. Antoine; *Studien und Materialien zur Geschichte der Philosophie*, ed. Yvon Belaval, et al., vol. 19 (Hildesheim, 1976); Michel Spanneut, *Permanence du Stoïcisme* (Gembloux, 1973), pp. 213ff.; Leontine Zanta, *La renaissance du Stoï-*

Although the most significant contributions to scientific change of the Renaissance revival of atomism belong to the seventeenth century rather than the sixteenth, discussions of corpuscular ideas took place in medical circles from 1546, when the views of Fracastoro began their rapid dissemination in the Italian medical schools.[54] Writing in France in the same decade, Fernel, whose own views on the elements were unconventional but not atomist, drew attention to the ideas of Democritus and the corpuscularism of the ancient medical Methodists.[55] As this suggests, the Galenic medical tradition was itself a means of transmission for corpuscular ideas of various kinds.[56] Information about the corpuscular physiology of the physician Asclepiades of Bythynia (first century B.C.) and the school of medical thought known as the Methodists is scattered through various works of Galen.[57] In addition, the first book of Galen's De elementis includes discussion of the atomist philosophy of Democritus and Epicurus. Moreover, although Galen repeatedly indicated his disagreements with all these thinkers, he included the idea of minimal particles in his own definition of an element.[58] Furthermore, the same idea reappears in the Latin version of Avicenna's definition, which mentions least parts into which bodies can be divided.[59] Returning specifically to the early sixteenth-century

---

cisme au XVIᵉ siècle (Paris, 1914). However, these authors deal almost entirely with the moral, religious, and ethical aspects of Stoicism. Peter Barker and Bernard R. Goldstein, "Is Seventeenth-Century Physics Indebted to the Stoics?" Centaurus 27 (1984), 148–64, call attention to the need for investigation of the influence of Stoic physical ideas.

[54] Vivian Nutton, "The Seeds of Disease: An Explanation of Contagion and Infection from the Greeks to the Renaissance," Medical History 27 (1983), 1–34.

[55] In the preface to Book 2 of his De abditis rerum causis libri duo, in his Universa medicina (Lyon, 1581), p. 589.

[56] Lasswitz, Geschichte der Atomistik, 1:230–34.

[57] For example, De constitutione artis medicae, chap. 7, Kühn, 1:249, and De tremore, palpitatione, convulsione et rigore, chap. 6, Kühn, 7:615–16. On Asclepiades, see Pauly-Wissowa (1895), 3:1632–33.

[58] For an example of Galen's attacks on the ancient atomists, see De elementis, 1, Kühn, 1:416–17. Many other similar passages are cited in Lasswitz, Geschichte der Atomistik, 1:230–34, where Galen's views on the elements are discussed. See, especially, ibid., 1:233, for Galen's use of the concept of minimal particles. De elementis, 1, Kühn, 1:413: "Quum elementum minima sit rei particula cujuscunque fuerit elementum; minimum autem non idem sensui et appareat et re vera sit; multa siquidem prae tenuitate sensum effugiat."

[59] "Elementa sunt corpora et sunt partes prime corporis humani et aliorum que in corpora diversarum formarum dividi minime possunt ex quorum commixtione species diverse generatorum fiunt." Canon 1.1.2.1 (Venice, 1507), fol. 1ᵛ. Alpago emended this definition to read "Elementa sunt corpora simplicia"; see Canon 1.1.2.1 (Venice, 1544), fol. 4ᵛ. On the contribution of Avicenna, and of medical thought in general, to the re-

Italian university milieu, we may note that Agostino Nifo, a physician as well as a philosopher, was among those who propagated a version of Aristotelian element theory that employed the concept of *minima naturalia*. Based on Averroes' interpretation (itself derived from the Greek commentators), this concept had been the subject of some discussion and elaboration in the thirteenth and fourteenth centuries. The *minima* differed from atoms in that they were conceived as qualitatively different from one another, and as acting upon one another, when combined, to produce further qualitative differences. Nifo maintained that mixtures (chemical compounds) were formed through reactions of the *minima*.[60]

Also followed were the more particularistic and practical aspects of developing thought about the elements. The production of treatises on spa waters and their analysis was indeed an Italian medical tradition extending from Giacomo Dondi in the mid-fourteenth century (and before him Pietro d'Abano, within his commentary on the Aristotelian *Problemata*) to Gabriele Falloppia (d. 1562).[61] Furthermore, attention has recently been drawn to Falloppia's attempt, in lectures delivered at Padua in 1557, to integrate Agricola's teaching about minerals with that of Aristotle, Theophrastus, and Galen. According to his modern commentator, Falloppia was also concerned to repudiate the alchemical sulfur/mercury theory about the nature of metals and to reject all forms of panvitalism because he perceived that revision of element theory would shake the foundations of medical theory of *complexio* and degree.[62] And as will become apparent, by the 1560s Girolamo Cardano,

---

vival of atomism in the sixteenth century, see Hooykaas, "Experimental origin," pp. 73–74.

[60] For some account of the history of the theory of *minima naturalia*, see Andrew G. van Melsen, *From Atomos to Atom: The History of the Concept Atom* (New York, 1960; 1st Dutch ed., 1949), pp. 58–73, and E. J. Dijksterhuis, *The Mechanization of the World Picture*, tr. C. Dikshoorn (Oxford, 1961), pp. 24, 205–9, 277–79. Nifo's views, which were not necessarily original or peculiar to him, are set out in his commentary on Aristotle's *Physics*, which went into a number of early editions; see Lohr, in *Renaissance Quarterly* 32 (1979), 536–37.

[61] Dondi's *Tractatus de causa salsedinis aquarum et modo conficiendi salis ex eis* appears in *De balneis omnia quae extant apud Graecos, Latinos, et Arabos* (Venice, 1553), fol. 109[r–v]. Dondi's treatise was written to defend a method he had devised for extracting salt from the springs of Abano. Pietro d'Abano discussed hot springs (and mentioned those of Abano) in his exposition of the Aristotelian *Problemata* 24.11 and 24.19. Falloppia's *De medicatis aquis atque de fossilibus* first appeared at Venice in 1564. In the fifteenth century Bartolomeo da Montagnana and Michele Savonarola also wrote treatises on spa waters. For details, see Debus, *Chemical Philosophy*, 1:14–18.

[62] Zanier, *Medicina e filosofia*, pp. 10–19. George Agricola's innovative and influential *De natura fossilium* was first published in 1546. The information that Falloppia's own *De*

one of the authors of the commentaries on the *Canon* under discussion, was notorious for his unconventional ideas about the elements and about minerals, and was indeed the subject of Falloppia's attack. Toward the end of the century, moreover, controversy over Paracelsus' ideas became widespread in northern and eastern Europe; recent studies trace the penetration of some Paracelsian influences into Italy in the same period.[63] In addition to all these more or less distinct varieties of manifestation of interest in the elements, sixteenth- and early seventeenth-century authors produced general surveys of the topic in various contexts. For example, accounts of element theory found a place in commentaries on works of Aristotle, notably *De caelo*, while a number of authors, including Gianfrancesco Pico, wrote separate treatises on the subject.[64] Such works were, of course, likely to be a good deal more prolix, thorough, and sophisticated than the handful of lectures that could be devoted to the elements in a course on medical *theoria* based on *Canon* 1.1.

In addition to being confronted by problems and opportunities for speculation concerning the elements presented by reports of experience; ancient theory as transmitted in ancient, medieval, and Renaissance works; and contemporary innovations, those who expounded Avicenna's chapter were working within an established tradition of commentary that had long since identified particular topics to be discussed when expounding this or other texts upon the subject. Some of these *quaestiones* were so hallowed by time that they had probably come to seem as integral a part of the commentator's task as the text itself. Some examples are the reasons for the displacement of the sphere of water, discussed by five of our six commentators;[65] the problem of

---

metallis atque fossilibus was based on lectures on Dioscorides that he gave at Padua in 1557 comes from the work itself; see his *Omnia, quae adhuc extant, opera* (Venice, 1584), fols. 167^r and 220^v, and Zanier, *Medicina e filosofia*, p. 10.

[63] See Marco Ferrari, "Alcune vie di diffusione in Italia di idee e di testi di Paracelso," *Scienze, credenze occulte, livelli di cultura: Convegno Internazionale di Studi (Firenze, 26–30 giugno 1980)* (Florence, 1982); and Paolo Galluzzi, "Motivi paracelsiani nella Toscana di Cosimo II e di Don Antonio dei Medici: Alchimia, medicina 'chimica' e riforma del sapere," in the same volume.

[64] For examples of discussions of the elements in commentaries on *De caelo*, see Grant, *In Defense of the Earth's Centrality and Immobility*, pp. 11–12, 18. Regarding Gianfrancesco Pico, see Lohr, in *Renaissance Quarterly* 33 (1980), 641, s.v. Picus Mirandulanus; and Charles B. Schmitt, *Gianfrancesco Pico della Mirandola (1469–1533) and His Critique of Aristotle* (The Hague, 1967). Other treatments of the elements included the *De elementis libri V* of Cardinal Contarini, pp. 1–91 in his *Opera* (Paris, 1571; the treatise on the elements was first published in 1548); and the commentary *In Sphaeram Joannis de Sacrobosco* of Christophorus Clavius, S.J. (Rome, 1570, 1581, and other editions).

[65] Da Monte, comm. *Canon* 1.1 (Venice, 1554), fols. 39^r–40^r; Oddi, comm. *Canon* 1.1,

whether earth, supposedly the heaviest element, is really heavier than lead (Oddi and Santorio);[66] and the questions of whether earth or water is the coldest element (Da Monte, Costeo, Santorio),[67] and whether air is hot or cold (Paterno, Costeo, Santorio)[68]—all problems that had also been discussed by Pietro d'Abano and/or Gentile da Foligno.[69] These and other similar, questions in many cases ultimately refer to difficulties relating Aristotle's statements about the elements to physical experience, or to Aristotle's differences with other ancient authors; hence the tendency of commentators on the *Canon*, whether in the fourteenth century or the sixteenth, was to refer directly to the Aristotelian texts, more or less bypassing Avicenna. The discussion of such standard *quaestiones* could not only be used to fill out commentary as much or as little as an individual author desired, it also provided a model for the way in which fresh subject matter might be introduced. Thus, for example, the explanations of modern cosmological theory embarked on by Costeo and Santorio could be introduced as part of *quaestiones* without disturbing the basic structure of commentary on the chapter in the *Canon* and without affecting the commentators' general acceptance of a largely traditional element theory.

The commentators made free use of the flexibility of the format and of the range of options as to content. All adopted the common core of subject matter dictated by the chapter itself: the proper definition of an element; the number, qualities, and places of the several elements; elements in a mixture; and the role of the elements in the structure, continuity, and organization of the human body. All introduced supplementary *quaestiones*, some of which had been discussed by their scholastic predecessors. None explicitly rejected the fourfold scheme of the elements in this passage, although Cardano made his objections to it very clear by means of references to his other works. But they differed widely in the thrust of those of their supplementary topics that

(Venice, 1575), pp. 87–88; Cardano, *Opera* (Lyon, 1663), 9:497; Paterno, comm. *Canon* 1.1 (Venice, 1596), fols. 23^v–24^r; Santorio, comm. *Canon* 1.1 (Venice, 1646), cols. 181–82. For discussions of this topic by natural philosophers from the fourteenth to the seventeenth centuries, see Grant, *In Defense of the Earth's Centrality and Immobility*, pp. 22–32.

[66] Oddi, comm. *Canon* 1.1 (Venice, 1575), p. 86; Santorio, comm. *Canon* 1.1 (Venice, 1646), col. 176.

[67] Da Monte, comm. *Canon* 1.1 (Venice, 1554), fols. 26^v–27^r; Costeo, *Disq. phys.*, pp. 71–72; Santorio, comm. *Canon* 1.1 (Venice, 1646), cols. 176–78.

[68] Paterno, comm. *Canon* 1.1 (Venice, 1596), fols. 24^v–25^r; Costeo, *Disq. phys.*, pp. 68–69; Santorio, comm. *Canon* 1.1 (Venice, 1646), cols. 200–203.

[69] See *Conciliator* (Venice, 1548), *Diff.* 12, fol. 20^{r-v}; *Diff.* 13, fol. 21^v; Diff. 14, fols. 22^r–23^r. See also Gentile, comm. *Canon* 1 and 2 (Pavia, 1510–11), 1.1.2.1, fols. 9^v–10^r.

were not conventional; in the use they made of their scholastic predecessors; in the extent to which they drew upon classical works or aspects of classical thought little known in western Europe during the Middle Ages, on recent events or discoveries, or on contemporary writers; and in the degree to which they were prepared to explain or in rare instances endorse unconventional scientific views.

To weigh the traditional against the newer ingredients in these treatments of element theory simply by distinguishing older from more recently available sources and ideas is to oversimplify. Equally important are shifting emphases and priorities in the use of older sources and the discussion of long-standard *topoi*. It is often far from easy to disentangle innovation and tradition. For example, one might suppose that the descriptions of pre-Socratic theories about matter or the fundamental constituents of the universe provided by all the authors except Cardano[70] were the products of their contemporary milieu in which knowledge of the scope of the history of Greek philosophy had been enlarged by Renaissance editions and translations, and in which there was a growing interest in non-Aristotelian philosophical systems. Such, indeed, seems likely to be the case. Yet the provision of such information within medical books was not, in fact, a novelty. In the early fourteenth century, Pietro d'Abano had incorporated a very similar series of thumbnail sketches of concepts attributed to a fairly long list of pre-Socratic thinkers into the section on the elements in the *Conciliator*.[71] Pietro, whose source and model appears likely to have been Aristotle himself, was, moreover, only one of a number of writers between the twelfth and the fourteenth centuries who drew on a variety of sources for information about ancient philosophers and their ideas and incorporated the results into historical, encyclopedic, or philosophical works.[72]

But Pietro's interest in the historical development of philosophy does not seem to have been passed on to some of his leading successors in the Italian schools. For example, in their expositions of Avicenna's chapter on the elements, as elsewhere in their commentaries on the *Canon*, Gentile da Foligno and Giacomo da Forlì both drew extensively upon the *Conciliator*;[73] furthermore, Giacomo's commentary on this

---

[70] Da Monte, comm. *Canon* 1.1 (Venice, 1554), fol. 24ᵛ; Oddi, comm. *Canon* 1.1 (Venice, 1575), pp. 83–84; Costeo, *Disq. phys.*, p. 41; Paterno, comm. *Canon* 1.1 (Venice, 1596), fol. 21ᵛ; Santorio, comm. *Canon* 1.1 (Venice, 1646), cols. 147–48.

[71] See *Conciliator* (Venice, 1548), *Diff.* 11, fols. 18ᵛ–19ʳ.

[72] Piaia, *Vestigia philosophorum*, pp. 37–147.

[73] Compare Gentile, comm. *Canon* 1 and 2 (Pavia, 1510–11), 1.1.2.1, fols. 9ʳ–10ᵛ, and

chapter appears to lean heavily on that of Gentile, who is credited by early tradition with a perhaps excessive reverence for Pietro's erudition.[74] Nonetheless, neither Gentile nor Giacomo included any survey of ancient opinions corresponding to that provided by Pietro into his exposition of the chapter on the elements. Hence, the reintroduction by sixteenth-century commentators of explanations of atomism or of surveys of the ideas about the elements of Greek philosophers other than Aristotle probably does represent a response to the contemporary intellectual climate, a supposition confirmed by Costeo's remark that the number of the elements had long been taken as established, but that the moderns had recently reopened the question.[75] Yet for this particular topic, obviously, the Aristotelian passages already exploited by Pietro d'Abano remained major sources of information; and ready access to Diogenes Laertius did not necessarily preclude renewed attention to the equally accessible *Conciliator*.[76]

The example just cited is one of a number of instances in which a shift in emphasis in the approach to ancient authors, a renewed attention to scholastic authors of the thirteenth or very early fourteenth century, and access to some material made available by humanist editors or translators seem to have combined to produce a break in established patterns of interpretation; the difficulty is always to weigh the relative importance of the various factors. The objective of the following brief summaries of the six expositions of the elements[77] is less to discriminate innovative from traditional ingredients than to illustrate a variety

---

Giacomo, comm. *Canon* 1.1 (Venice, 1508), 1.1.2.1, fols. 7ʳ–9ʳ, with *Conciliator* (Venice, 1548), *Diff.* 11–16, fols. 18ᵛ–27ʳ.

[74] According to Michele Savonarola, writing in 1446, "Hancque rem divinus ille Gentilis Fulgineus, nostre et sue etatis medicorum princeps, facile intellexit, nam, cum Paduam profectus esset, non mediocri cum desiderio gymnasium Conciliatoris nostri visitare curavit. Qui, cum ad ostium perventus esset, flexis genibus sublatoque bireto, manus extollens, ait: Ave templum sanctum! et pre dulcedine lacrimatus id ingrediebatur, multasque cedulas parietibus affixas, manu sua scriptas, velut sanctuarium quoddam, in sinu collocavit." Savonarola, *Libellus de magnificis ornamentis regie Civitatis Padue*, p. 27.

[75] See n. 42, above. Also, Costeo *Disq. phys.*, p. 29: "Medicus quatuor vulgo cognita elementa hominis, ut reliquarum quoque harum omnium rerum, principia esse credit, ex naturali philosophia: ex eaque illorum definitionem, numerum, et singulorum naturam sumit. De quibus tamen omnibus, quando et alias, et aetate nostra, varii varia sensere."

[76] As already noted, the *Conciliator* was printed at least fourteen times between 1504 and 1595; see Sante Ferrari, *Pietro d'Abano*, pp. 136–38.

[77] Da Monte, comm. *Canon* 1.1 (Venice, 1554), fols. 23ᵛ–54ʳ; Oddi, comm. *Canon* 1.1 (Venice, 1575), pp. 81–99; Cardano, *Opera* (Lyon, 1663), 9:490–507; Costeo, *Disq. phys.*, pp. 29–100; Paterno, comm. *Canon* 1.1 (Venice, 1596), fols. 20ʳ–27ʳ; Santorio, comm. *Canon* 1.1 (Venice, 1646), cols. 141–43, 145–228.

of different strategies of approach to the task and problems of teaching element theory to medical students by means of commentary in the sixteenth and early seventeenth centuries.

The Elements and Scholastic Aristotelianism: Da Monte. Although it is possible that Oddi's commentary on *Canon* 1.1 may have been written before that by Da Monte, the latter merits consideration first, since much in Da Monte's exposition links him to the philosophical ambience of the early sixteenth century. A salient feature of Da Monte's commentary is his insistence that the correct position in natural philosophy is an Aristotelianism uncontaminated by theological considerations, coupled with the endorsement of Averroes as Aristotle's interpreter and the adoption of some of the latter's opinions. Da Monte repeatedly proclaimed his allegiance to Aristotle, "whom I admire as a god in things having to do with nature" (*quem ut Deum admiror in natura*). The efficient cause of the generation of mixed bodies was, he remarked, a topic on which

. . . theologians, philosophers, and physicians respond in different ways. I will very briefly say something about this question, but whatever I say I shall say in the capacity of a peripatetic and a physician. For when I want to speak about the subject from the standpoint of theology, I shall say completely the opposite. For I think nothing worse can happen in philosophy than to mix it with theology. It is for this reason that I have never seen anyone philosophize correctly who wanted to mix theology with philosophy. Through doing this Avicenna fell into almost infinite errors. Indeed, this is why all the Scotists and Thomists, mixing everything together, throw everything into confusion and very often stray from the true peripatetic path.[78]

---

[78] "In qua quidem generatione aliter respondent theologi, aliter philosophi, aliter medici. Ego brevissime de hac quaestione aliqua dicam, sed quaecunque dicam, dicam ut peripateticus, et ut medicus. Nam quando theologice de ea loqui voluero, totum forte oppositum dicam. Nihil autem existimo deterius in philosophia posse contingere quam cum ea theologiam commiscere. Hinc est quod nullum unquam vidi recte philosophatum, qui theologiam cum philosophia voluerit permiscere. Hinc est, quod Avicenna in infinitos pene errores incidit. Hinc est etiam quod omnes Scotistae et Thomistae, dum omnia permiscent, perturbant omnia, saepissime a vera peripateticorum via aberrant." Da Monte, comm. *Canon* 1.1 (Venice, 1554), fol. 31ʳ. As is well known, from the late fifteenth century there were at Padua two chairs for teaching theology and metaphysics, one *in via Thomae* and the other *in via Scoti* (associated with the Dominican and Franciscan convents, respectively). Both traditions were actively developed during the sixteenth century.

Da Monte followed these observations with the assertion that Averroes was superior to all the other Arabs and the only one who thought with the Greeks.[79] These and other similar remarks place Da Monte, who had been a pupil of Pomponazzi, securely within the tradition of Italian secular or scientific Aristotelianism of which Padua was a well-known, although by no means the only, center.[80] They also link him to the late fifteenth- and early sixteenth-century revival of interest in Averroes as an accurate interpreter of Aristotle's thought[81] and, more generally, to the contemporary endeavor, inspired by access to Aristotle's works in Greek, to attain a full and exact understanding of the Philosopher's own teaching, stripped of accretions from other sources. But unlike other writers on natural philosophy at Padua from the 1480s on, Da Monte seems to have paid little attention to the Greek commentators on Aristotle; for example, in his exposition of Avicenna's *doctrina* on the elements, Alexander of Aphrodisias is the only such commentator mentioned, and he is only alluded to once, briefly.[82]

In fact, Da Monte's Aristotelianism was far from being as thoroughgoing as his programmatic statements about it. Propositions that appear to contradict Aristotle can be found even in the exposition of the chapter on the elements, although Da Monte did not acknowledge, or did not recognize, them as such. Thus, he developed a rather strained argument to support the claim that his own belief that the element earth was the coldest element, and colder than the element water, represented the correct interpretation of Aristotle's views.[83] By contrast, Costeo and Santorio, like Pietro d'Abano before them, both identified

---

[79] "In hac igitur quaestione duae fuerunt opiniones apud philosophos. Prima fuit omnium Arabum, praeter Averroem, qui solus cum Graecis sensit et qui unus semper in veritate praeponderat omnibus aliis Arabibus simul collectis." Ibid., fols. 31^{r-v}.

[80] Da Monte's radical naturalism and his adhesion to Pomponazzi's ideas (including denial of the existence and powers of angels or demons) are discussed in Giancarlo Zanier, *Ricerche sulla diffusione e fortuna del "De incantationibus" di Pomponazzi* (Florence, 1975), where the passage quoted in n. 78, above, is also cited.

[81] On the widespread diffusion of and serious and favorable attention to works of Averroes in sixteenth-century Italian academic circles, see Schmitt, "Renaissance Averroism"; and on the Paduan context, Francesca Lucchetta, "Recenti studi sull'Averroismo padovano," in *Convegno internazionale, L'Averroismo in Italia (Roma, 18–20 Aprile 1977), Atti dei Convegni Lincei* 40 (Rome, 1979), pp. 91–120. Apparently Da Monte did not absorb from Pomponazzi the latter's critical attitude toward aspects of Averroism (noted ibid., pp. 118–20).

[82] Schmitt, "Aristotelian Textual Studies," passim, and Mahoney, "Philosophy and Science," pp. 163–202, for interest in the Greek commentators on Aristotle in Paduan philosophical circles in the late fifteenth century. Other sixteenth-century commentators on *Canon* 1.1 expressed considerable interest in the work of Alexander of Aphrodisias.

[83] Da Monte, comm. *Canon* 1.1 (Venice, 1554), fols. 26^{v}–27^{r}.

the position that earth was the coldest element as un-Aristotelian, and Santorio faulted Da Monte for deviating from peripatetic views on this point.[84]

More important, Da Monte was, of course, simultaneously at least as much committed to Galen as a medical scientist, and to the translating and publishing enterprise of Renaissance Galenism, as he was to Aristotle as a philosopher. On many issues, his position on the relation of the two authorities was little different from that of Avicenna himself and his earlier Latin scholastic interpreters. Like his Latin predecessors, Da Monte often explained away differences between Aristotle and Galen on specific points by scholastic distinction and reconciliation.

Although Da Monte justified the study of element theory by physicians by pointing out that it underlay the theory of temperament, which was of immediate concern to the practicing physician,[85] the aspects of the subject that aroused his own interest pertained much more to purely speculative natural philosophy than to any parts of either physical science or physiology conceivably capable of empirical verification. Thus, he devoted about one-third of his sixty-two pages on the elements to a highly scholastic and astrologically oriented discussion of the causes of the generation of the elements and of the bodies in the sublunary world produced by their mixture.[86] The elements themselves he held to be generated by the action of the motion, heat, and light of the heavenly spheres upon eternal prime matter (which Da Monte thought must have at least one definable quality, namely humidity, since he held humidity to be essential to generation). Da Monte maintained that the correct belief of "all the Greeks together with Averroes" was that mixed bodies were generated from the elements by celestial Intelligences, not through any intention on their part, but rather as a result of the influence of the heavenly bodies, the different aspects and positions of the latter being responsible for the diversification of species and the different characters of human beings.[87]

---

[84] *Conciliator* (Venice, 1548), *Diff.* 12, fols. 20ʳ–21ʳ; Costeo, *Disq. phys.*, pp. 71–90; Santorio, comm. *Canon* 1.1 (Venice, 1646), *Quaestio* 18, cols. 176–178. At col. 178: "Demum si frigiditas primo convenit terrae, ut dicit Montanus, cui conveniet caliditas? Ergo vel aeri, vel aquae, vel terrae; non aeri vel aquae conveniet siccitas, ergo terrae. Quare discedere ab Aristotele in his quae pertinent ad philosphiam naturalem est mera fatuitas."

[85] ". . . scire quomodo ex mixtione elementorum fiant generationes rerum, et hoc est utile ad artem nostram, quia ex mixtione elementorum fiunt temperaturae diversae, quae sunt causae sanitatis et aegritudinis." Da Monte, comm. *Canon* 1.1 (Venice, 1554), fol. 25ʳ.

[86] Ibid., fols. 25ʳ–35ʳ.

[87] "Opinio igitur Arabum fuit, quod causa efficiens omnium mixtorum sit idea istorum omnium mixtorum insidens in intelligentia, qua quidem idea movetur intelligentia

The thrust of these arguments is to maximize the role of the heavenly bodies in the original generation and subsequent reproduction of terrestrial species and to minimize any concepts of willed intervention in terrestrial affairs on the part of conscious spiritual beings. The general topic of the role of the heavenly bodies in terrestrial generation had of course been treated by a long line of Latin authors before Da Monte, among them Albertus Magnus and Pietro d'Abano.[88] Da Monte's own continued attachment to concepts, traditional topics, and vocabulary of scholastic natural science, his sharp divorce of philosophy from theology, and his willingness to assert strongly naturalistic explanations were not confined to his teaching on Avicenna's chapter on the elements. Similar traits, as we shall see, characterized part of his handling of the somewhat more medical topic of temperament or complexion, in which he dwelled at length on topics relating to substantial form and the human soul, and once again carefully distinguished his views speaking as a philosopher and a physician from those he would express if speaking *theologice*.

Da Monte's treatment of the individual elements contains only a few points worth noting here. Accepting without question the centrality and stability of the earth, he declared that the purpose of its location was to enable it to be the recipient of all possible celestial influences, just as its coldness and dryness was designed to retain their impressions.[89] The well-worn topic of the displacement of the sphere of water

---

ad generationem specierum mixtorum, et consequenter singulorum individuorum, non aliter quam artifex movetur ad operandum propter ideam rei efficiendae in mente habitam, et ita volunt intelligentias intendere generationem mixtorum non secus quam artifex intendit super re artificiata efficienda. Hinc ideae in universali acceptae voluit Avicenna." Ibid., fol. 31ᵛ. Compare ibid., fol. 24ʳ: "Nam Plato accipiebat quoddam universale existens extra mentem, quam appellavit ideam, at Aristoteles huius modi ideas semper monstra existimavit, aliter intellexit secundam formam, id est secundam speciem." But: "Graeci autem omnes, una cum Averroes inter Arabes, quorum melior est sententia, et vere peripatetica, voluerunt quidem et ipsi mixta ab intelligentiis generari, sed non ita sicut artificiata fiunt ab artifice" (fol. 31ᵛ).

[88] For examples of Pietro d'Abano's treatment of the subject, drawn from his commentary on the Aristotelian *Problemata*, see Nancy G. Siraisi, "The *Expositio Problematum Aristotelis* of Pietro d'Abano," *Isis* 61 (1970), 326; for similar views of other early fourteenth-century Italian medical authors, idem, *Alderotti*, pp. 173–75. Albertus Magnus' paraphrase of the *Liber de causis* associates the Intelligences with the heavenly bodies, and ascribes to celestial virtues a role in generating forms; see his *Opera*, ed. Borgnet (Paris, 1891), 10:428–30. Further evidence of widespread interest in thirteenth-century mendicant circles in topics of this kind is gathered in James A. Weisheipl, O.P., "The Problemata Determinata XLIII Ascribed to Albertus Magnus (1271)," *Mediaeval Studies* 22 (1960), 3–54.

[89] "Quoniam enim natura volebat terram esse subiectum omnium impressionum coelestium, et formarum, ideo voluit terram locum esse et centrum orbis, ut omnes influx-

led him to note that the Spanish voyages of exploration had proved that land rose above the water in both northern and southern hemispheres; the final cause of this phenomenon was to provide a habitation for animals, while the efficient cause of the distribution of landmasses was the disposition of the celestial rays, which fell differently on different parts of the globe. His disquisition on the presence of air outside its proper sphere and the effects of air in mixed bodies brought together such phenomena as earthquakes, subterranean gases, and spongy fungi and alluded, although not very explicitly, to Stoic ideas about the all-pervasiveness of pneuma.[90] Da Monte evidently felt some sympathy with the latter. Since he also held that all matter necessarily had some property of humidity and, in addition, that humidity was essential for the continued existence of elementary as well as mixed bodies, he endeavored to prove, against Albertus Magnus, that some humidity was present even in elemental fire.[91] Da Monte's belief in the all-pervasiveness of humidity was presumably extrapolated from consideration of plant and animal life and clearly owes a debt to various older discussions of radical moisture.[92]

In this as in other instances, however, although the general relationship of his exposition to the early tradition of Latin scholastic natural philosophy and medical theory is plain enough, it is difficult to identify borrowings from particular authors. The only medieval author referred to by name in Da Monte's exposition of the elements is Albertus Magnus.[93] Thus, Da Monte seems to have passed on to another generation of students a pattern noted among some of the leading philosophers who taught at Padua in the previous two generations, namely Vernia, Nifo, and Zimara, all of whom combined an interest in Averroes and in Albertus.[94] Da Monte's restriction in this chapter of the me-

---

iones coelestes, undecumque veniant, aequaliter in terram imprimerentur," Da Monte, comm. *Canon* 1.1 (Venice, 1554), fol. 37ᵛ.

[90] Ibid., fols. 39ʳ–40ʳ, 43ᵛ–48ʳ.   [91] Ibid., fols. 49ʳ–51ᵛ.

[92] See Hall, "Life, Death and the Radical Moisture," and McVaugh, "The 'humidum radicale.'"

[93] ". . . magis calescit ideo materiae istius, quae semper fuit, sicut etiam dixit Albertus in libro de quatuor causis." Da Monte, comm. *Canon* 1.1 (Venice, 1554), fol. 25ᵛ. The reference appears to be to Albertus' paraphrase of the *Liber de causis*; that is, to his *De causis et processu universitatis* (see n. 88, above), rather than to the somewhat similarly titled *De causis proprietatum elementorum*, ed. Paul Hossfeld, in Albertus' *Opera*, vol. 5, p. 2 (Cologne, 1980), pp. 47–106. Possibly the passage alluded to may be *De causis* 2.1.3 (Borgnet, 10:438), but the parallel does not seem very close.

[94] Edward P. Mahoney, "Albert the Great and the *Studio Patavino* in the Late Fifteenth and Early Sixteenth Centuries," in Weisheipl, *Albertus Magnus and the Sciences*, pp. 537–63, esp. 546ff.

dieval sources cited (other than Avicenna himself) to Averroes and Albertus, and his avoidance of any mention of fourteenth- and fifteenth-century philosophical and medical writers, was a matter of policy, since his diatribes elsewhere against Giacomo da Forlì and other similar authors reveal that he knew them well.[95] Da Monte may actually have preferred the older as distinct from the more recent scholastic tradition, at any rate as regards the subject matter of the elements. But it is also conceivable that the absence of citations of fourteenth- and fifteenth-century scholastic authors, like the presence of quotations from Homer and Virgil's *Georgics* and an allusion to the myth of Apollo and Python, is merely part of an effort to present the opening sections of the work in as classically elegant a guise as possible.[96] As one might expect, the author who is most frequently cited, together with Aristotle and Averroes, is Galen, who is here called on as an authority in philosophy as well as medicine to provide a definition of the elements, to endorse the influences of the sun and moon upon terrestrial affairs, and as a source of information about the elemental composition of *spiritus*.[97]

A brief summary of element theory written for medical students is not, of course, necessarily the best basis for an evaluation of the author's own philosophical competence, interests, or positions. Da Monte's exposition is remarkable chiefly for the apparent ease with which he managed simultaneously to accommodate radical Aristotelian naturalism, astrology, Galenism, and scholastic and humanistic approaches, a combination that calls to mind Giancarlo Zanier's suggestion that the extreme eclecticism of sixteenth-century writers in drawing upon ancient and medieval intellectual systems may in itself have ultimately contributed to their breakdown.[98] Yet of all the commentators on *Canon* 1.1 under discussion, Da Monte seems the most clearly associated with the north Italian tradition of Aristotelian philosophical teaching and the most genuinely interested in highly speculative discussions of topics such as the origin of the elements, celestial influences upon generation, substantial form, the human soul, and so on. These influences and interests were just as much part of Da Monte's in-

---

[95] See, for example, Da Monte, comm. *Canon* 1.2 (Venice, 1557), pp. 27, 70, 74.

[96] For the literary references, Da Monte, comm. *Canon* 1.1 (Venice, 1554), fols. 27ᵛ, 43ᵛ. The revival of interest in thirteenth-century scholastic writers during the sixteenth century is most noted with regard to Thomist theology, but extended to other subject areas. William A. Wallace, *Prelude to Galileo: Essays on Medieval and Sixteenth-Century Sources of Galileo's Thought* (Dordrecht, 1981), pp. 160–92, shows the use of Aquinas in Jesuit teaching of natural philosophy at the Collegio Romano during the second half of the sixteenth century. See also n. 94, above.

[97] Da Monte, comm. *Canon* 1.1 (Venice, 1554), fols. 24ᵛ–25ʳ, 33ʳ, 52ᵛ–53ʳ.

[98] Zanier, *Medicina e filosofia*, pp. 1–4, 39–43.

tellectual and scientific universe as the modernizing ideas and activities that brought him deserved renown among contemporaries and subsequent medical historians.

The Elements in Brief: Oddi and Paterno. The expositions of the *doctrina* on the elements written by Oddo Oddi between about 1540 and 1558, and Paterno, probably in the late 1570s, may appropriately be considered together, despite the generation and the commentary on *Canon* 1.1 by Cardano (1562)—and perhaps also that by Da Monte—that separates them. Both Oddi and Paterno dealt with the *doctrina de elementis* by providing routine summaries that provide a basic introduction to the subject and call attention to a few familiar problems, while eschewing the more recondite of the philosophical topics favored by Da Monte. Both emphasized the role of the elements in the living body; indeed, it seems likely that Paterno's discussion of Hippocrates' reasons for believing that the human body must be compounded of more than one element, and of whether the elements in the human body are impatible and insensible, was taken over directly from Oddi, whose commentary was published in 1575, shortly before the composition of Paterno's.[99]

Oddi gave some evidence of a modest level of interest in conventional scholastic problems of physical science. For example, he took up Aristotle's discussion of heaviness and lightness in Book 4 of *De caelo*, although examining it much less fully than Pietro d'Abano had done some two and a half centuries earlier.[100] Oddi merely isolated a problematic passage about the relative heaviness of earth and lead and used it as a basis for inquiring how, if earth is the heaviest element, a small quantity of lead can weigh more than a larger quantity of earth. After reviewing the solutions of Averroes and of Tommaso del Garbo, Oddi opted for the solution that asserted that the earth we encounter is not true elemental earth, but a mixed body that does not have the extreme heaviness of pure earth.

In addition to drawing upon works of Hippocrates, Aristotle, Galen, Averroes, and Alexander of Aphrodisias, Oddi also gave evidence of a critical reading of Italian scholastic medical authors. Besides dismissing Tommaso del Garbo's views on elements in a mixture, he also rejected the explanations of the displacement of the sphere of water given by Pietro d'Abano, who had provided a notably full discussion of the sub-

---

[99] This is suggested by a comparison of Oddi, comm. *Canon* 1.1 (Venice, 1575), pp. 83–84, with Paterno, comm. *Canon* 1.1 (Venice, 1596), fols. 21ᵛ–22ʳ.

[100] Oddi, comm. *Canon* 1.1 (Venice, 1575), pp. 85–86. One may compare this with *Conciliator* (Venice, 1548), *Diff.* 14, fol. 23ʳ⁻ᵛ.

ject in *Differentia* 13 of the *Conciliator*, and Ugo Benzi. Oddi dismissed out of hand Pietro's claim that astral influences from stars in the Northern Hemisphere caused the waters to pile up and expose the land in that region, and remarked that land had also been discovered below the equator. He found equally unsatisfactory Ugo's notion that the earth we inhabit is actually a mixed body existing on top of the true sphere of water, which encircles the true earth.[101]

Paterno's treatment of the chapter on the elements was just as unoriginal and, if possible, even more compressed and superficial than that of Oddi. Thus, when he came to the sphere of water he simply referred his readers, whom he termed *iuniores*, to *Differentia* 13 of the *Conciliator* without further comment. Moreover, Paterno honored his commitment to a retreat from natural philosophy in medical exposition in several instances in which he followed mention of one of the standard problems concerning the elements with a remark dismissing the issue as the business of philosophers.[102] However, he headed his exposition with a list of passages in works of Aristotle and Alexander of Aphrodisias, as well as Galen, which he may have intended his readers to consult. And he, or his editor, inserted into the following *doctrina* (on complexions) a *tractatus de elementis*, which takes up the subject of the forms of the elements, of Stoic views about air, and the role of the elements in mixed bodies.[103] In this tractate, discussion of the nature of mixtures leads into a consideration of whether there can ever be a perfectly balanced complexional mixture in the human body, and thus presumably justifies the inclusion of the whole tractate in the section on complexions. The actual discussion of the elements, at the beginning of the tractate, Paterno based on his reading of Ocellus Lucanus, *De universi natura*;[104] he was apparently endeavoring to construct a non-

---

[101] Oddi, comm. *Canon* 1.1 (Venice, 1575), pp. 87–88. For Pietro d'Abano's discussion, which became something of a *locus classicus* for the topic of displacement of the sphere of water, see *Conciliator* (Venice, 1548), *Diff.* 13, fols. 21ᵛ–22ʳ.

[102] For example: "De quibus motionibus magna controversia extitisse videtur inter Temistium [sic] et Averroem. Utra nempe duarum gravium et levium essentiam magis exponat. Voluit Themistius, referente Averroe, notionem [sic] per motum magis essentialem esse. Contra Averroes, datam per quietem; utra autem sententia verior sit ab eccellentissimis philosophis quaerendum est. Pro iunioribus autem sat erit notare loca in *Topicis* ubi Aristotelis de diffinitionibus agit datis per motum et per quietem." Paterno, comm. *Canon* 1.1 (Venice, 1596), fol. 23ʳ. Also: "De motu autem circulari ipsius [the sphere of fire] naturalis ne existat, vel violentus, vel supranaturalis, scio magnam esse quaestionem apud Aristotelis expositores, quam ut nobis omnino inutilem philosophis explicandam relinquemus, et ad nostra magis nos convertamus, ad ignis naturam, videlicet, quam Avicennas esse inquit calidam et siccam." Ibid., fol. 25ᵛ.

[103] Ibid., fols. 60ᵛ–70ʳ.

[104] Ibid., fol. 61ʳ.

255

Aristotelian account of the elements which modified the concept of form,[105] insisted on the tangible nature of elementary qualities, and declared that each element possessed one, not two, qualities. The little treatise attributed to the early Pythagorean Okellos, of which a Latin translation was published in 1559,[106] has been identified as in reality a Hellenistic compilation drawing on peripatetic sources.[107] Paterno's endeavor is therefore of interest only for its expression of dissatisfaction, however limited and unclear, with the concept of form, and as a manifesto of willingness to seek out supposedly non-Aristotelian ancient scientific sources.

An Anti-Aristotelian View of the Elements: Cardano. When Costeo announced that the moderns had reopened the question of the number of the elements, he had in mind principally Girolamo Cardano, who was already notorious for his iconoclastic views on that, as on many other subjects. Although the seriousness of Cardano's commitment to mathematics and the level of his achievement therein were unusual for a physician, the scope of his remaining intellectual interests was entirely consonant with the philosophical and technical culture provided by academic medicine (though his interest in the occult and supernatural seems to have been exceptionally strong even for the sixteenth century). Cardano's writings on natural science were, however, far more copious and wide-ranging than most of his medical contemporaries, so that he may properly be classified, along with Aldrovandi, among the sixteenth-century encyclopedists of nature. The best known of Cardano's books on nature, the encyclopedic *De subtilitate*, is characterized by the author's eclecticism, his empiricism, his willingness to abandon Aristotelian positions, and his endeavors to devise new solutions or systems of his own. Perhaps as a result of these characteristics the work had fairly wide dissemination among a popular readership, but was severely criticized from a conservative natural philosophical standpoint by J. C. Scaliger.[108] Among the anti-Aristotelian positions for which Scaliger attacked Cardano was his rejection of the scheme of the four elements. Cardano held that the elements were three, not four, in num-

---

[105] Ibid., fol. 62ᵛ.

[106] *Ocelli Lucani De universi natura libellus Ludovico Nogarola . . . interprete* (Venice, 1559).

[107] Pauly-Wissowa, 17:2, cols. 2377–79.

[108] For Cardano's dispute with Scaliger, and the sixteenth-century *fortuna* of *De subtilitate*, see Ian Maclean, "The Interpretation of Natural Signs: Cardano's *De subtilitate* versus Scaliger's *Exercitationes*," in *Occult and Scientific Mentalities in the Renaissance*, ed. Brian Vickers (Cambridge, 1984), pp. 231–52.

ber: earth, air, and water. He denied both that fire was an element and the existence of the supposed sphere of fire, although he retained an important role in generation for celestial heat.[109] He also expressed animistic or panvitalistic views, maintaining that stones were brought to perfection by a soul (the latter being the opinion that attracted the hostility of Falloppia).[110] The obvious similarity of Cardano's ideas about the elements to some of those held by Paracelsus raises the question of a relationship between the two theories, but the nature of this, if any, remains undetermined.[111]

In his commentary on Avicenna's chapter, Cardano's own theory of the elements is implicitly present, but it is not explicitly set forth. Although a first version of the commentary may have been composed before Cardano's theories were fully developed,[112] his ideas on the elements were certainly formulated, published, and widely known before the commentary was redacted in its present form in the early 1560s. In the commentary Cardano referred the reader to the opinions about the number of the elements expressed in his *Contradicentia medicorum*;[113] his

[109] See *Hieronymi Cardani Mediolanensis medici de subtilitate libri XXI* (Basel, 1560), Book 2, pp. 74–246, of which pp. 74–157 are devoted to the denial that fire is an element, with supporting arguments.

[110] Cardano's vitalistic views on stones are mentioned in Book 7 of *De subtilitate*; see his *Opera* (Lyon, 1663), 3:461. For Falloppia's objections, see Zanier, *Filosofia e medicina*, pp. 13–19.

[111] The resemblance was noted by Lasswitz; see Lasswitz, *Geschichte der Atomistik*, 1:310–11.

[112] The two prefaces of Cardano's commentary on *Canon* 1.1 are dated, respectively, Pavia, 1561, and Bologna, 1563; see his *Opera* (Lyon, 1663), 9:455, 458. However, in his *De libris propriis eorumque usu liber recognitus* Cardano stated that he composed a commentary on *Canon* 1.1 at Pavia in 1546; see Cardano, *Opera* (Lyon, 1663), 1:106. In his *Liber de libris propriis, eorumque ordine et usu, ac de mirabilibus operibus in arte medica factis*, Cardano noted that his commentary on the *Canon* was in two books (ibid., p. 74), a description that matches the commentary printed in vol. 9 of his *Opera*. The editor of his *Opera* seems to have been responsible for attaching to the commentary on the *Canon* the title *Floridorum libri duo*, whereas Cardano himself, in his descriptions of his own works, used the title *Liber floridorum* for a collection of medical questions in one book; see Cardano, *Opera* (Lyon, 1663), 1:65–66, 102 (dating the collection of questions 1539). To confuse the issue further, the incipit Cardano gave as that of his commentary on the *Canon* does not seem to match the commentary printed in vol. 9 of the *Opera*, but this discrepancy is presumably to be attributed to editing the work underwent at the time of the addition of the dated prefaces (certainly after the composition of the *Liber de libris propriis*, which is dated 1554 on p. 95, and possibly after *De libris propriis eorumque usu*, which includes the date 1561 on p. 118). The true *Liber floridorum* seems never to have been printed, and the commentary on Avicenna appears not to have been printed before its inclusion in the 1663 *Opera*.

[113] Cardano, *Opera*, 9:490, referring the reader "in decimo *Contradicentium*." Compare "Palam est igitur omittere ignem, et coelum intelligere, et ita nos docuimus esse tria tan-

views are also laid out in *De subtilitate*, in which the whole of Book 2 is devoted to the elements, and which was published in 1550.[114] Furthermore, Scaliger's *Exercitationes* against *De subtilitate*, which attack Cardano's teaching specifically on the subject of the elements, had appeared in 1557, the same year in which Falloppia criticized Cardano's views on minerals in lectures at Padua.[115] Cardano's exposition of Avicenna's chapter on the elements was therefore prepared for an audience who, Cardano rightly assumed, was already aware of how widely his own opinions on the subject diverged from Aristotle. He announced that he would not repeat what he had said about the number of the elements in some of his other works, not because the material was not important, but because it was available elsewhere.[116] While it is possible that Cardano's reticence was the product of an uncharacteristic attack of caution brought on by his personal difficulties,[117] it seems more likely that his remark is to be taken at face value, since his exposition of this section of the *Canon* is everywhere informed by his own opinions and interests and, in particular, is characterized by free criticism not so much of Avicenna as of Aristotle. At his most sweeping he was capable of declaring, with reference to Aristotelian concepts about forms, substance, and qualities, "All these things are false, . . . but we wish to declare the mind of the peripatetics."[118] Thus, after noting that Aristotle believed the elements to be four in number, he added that Hippocrates

---

tum" (Cardano, *Contradicentia medica*, 10.26 [*Opera*, 6:910–11]). A set of Cardano's *Contradicentium medicorum liber continens contradictiones centum octo* was published at Venice in 1545, additional *contradictiones* being added in subsequent editions. But I am not sure when 10.26 first appeared in print.

[114] For the date of the first edition, *DSB*, 3:66.

[115] I have consulted *Julii Caesaris Scaligeri Exotericarum exercitationes libri XV de subtilitate ad Hieronymum Cardanum* (Frankfurt, 1592), in which the attack on Cardano's views on the status of fire as an element occurs on pp. 45–53; the first edition was Paris, 1557. Regarding the wide attention attracted by the dispute between Cardano and Scaliger, see Maclean, "Interpretation of Natural Signs," p. 231.

[116] Cardano, *Opera* (1663), 9:490, citing "in decimo *Contradicentium*."

[117] Cardano's illegitimate birth and personal idiosyncrasies, and the scandal caused by the execution of his son for the murder of his wife (1560) were the source of much difficulty and insecurity in his professional life. His problems in this regard are described at length in his autobiography; for a modern summary, see Markus Fierz, *Girolamo Cardano, 1501–1576* (Eng. tr., Boston, 1983), pp. 5–7, 27–28.

[118] "Dubitatur cur cum aqua consistat per frigidum magis quam per humidum, calefacta manet aqua, siccata non. Respondet Alexander . . . quod frigiditas non est forma aquae simpliciter, sed cum determinato humido, igitur cum tantum frigiditatis manet, et humidum maneat debitum substantiae aquae, aqua manet, melius est dicere quod frigiditas, quae est substantia, potest manere cum caliditate, quae est qualitas. . . . Omnia haec sunt falsa, quia procedunt ex falsis principiis, voluimus tamen declarare mentem Peripateticorum." Cardano, *Opera* (Lyon, 1663), 9:497.

in *De dietis* had held them to be three, all of which were cold (earth, air, water). This assertion opened the way for an explication of Cardano's own opinions on the role of heat, of which he distinguished celestial and igneous varieties. Celestial heat he described as something divine and primary, related to light and the stars; in the image of the first good, this celestial heat seeks to generate and multiply things similar to itself. In generation it acts as the instrument of the soul, causing movement, separation, rarefaction, and other changes, and thus generally preparing matter for generation and form imprinted in the first instant by the soul. Igneous heat, on the other hand is a corrupting and destructive force, which is not linked to either the heavens or the soul. Cardano further asserted that any generation of mixtures involved life and soul, and therefore, that while the elements themselves were inanimate, "the rest are mixed and generated, for example, plants, animals, and gems, which have life."[119]

Cardano's general discussion of the element earth included a section on the formation of stones and metals in which both Aristotelian views and the notion that stones are at least quasi-animate are set forth, without any explicit choice being made between the two opinions. Perhaps more significant, Cardano led his medical students to consider assertions about the action of the elements and qualities within and upon mixed bodies in the light of the properties of a series of specific substances—among them "burnt tartar" (*tartarum adustum*), aquavit, brick, salt, oil, and honey. Cardano's model for this approach, apparently new to the *Canon* commentaries, was in part Aristotle himself in *Meteorologica* 4.6–12, 382b29–390b21.

However, parts of Cardano's treatment of matter in this commentary are both overtly anti-Aristotelian and explicitly inspired by Cardano's chemical or alchemical interests. In the course of his exposition, indeed, he claimed that it was impossible for one unskilled in the *ars chymicae* to philosophize rightly; Aristotle's errors are attributed to deficiency in this respect and paralleled with mistakes he made in the *Historia animalium* through failure to dissect. The alchemy Cardano had in mind at this point was apparently entirely exoteric, since his discussion concerns the effects on the various substances of heating, chilling, dilution, immersion in water, and so on. For example, he noted the inadequacy of Aristotle's account of the liquefaction of salt and explained that salt can be dissolved by humid vapors as well as by water, but is

---

[119] Ibid., pp. 490–91. At p. 490: "videmus quod generatio pertinet ad vitam, nam reliqua miscentur, generantur, ut plantae, animalia et gemmae quae vitam habent, non autem elementa quae vita carent."

unaffected by cold. Heat, on the other hand, resolves the aqueous part of a salt solution and greatly increases the density of the earthy part, ultimately producing concretion.[120]

The range of Cardano's mathematical accomplishments naturally could not be deployed in introductory medical teaching, but his commentary on Avicenna's subsection *de terra* nonetheless contains some echoes of his mathematical interests. This portion of Cardano's exposition in fact falls into two distinct parts, the first being in reality a commentary on *De caelo* 2.14, 296a24–98a20, in which Aristotle discussed the position, shape, and size of the earth, and the second an account of the medicinal properties of various earths drawn chiefly from Galen and Dioscorides.[121] In the first section he referred his readers to Book 4 of Euclid's *Elements*, to Archimedes, and to a treatise by the Calculator, *De motu elementi*, authors who commonly found no place in courses on medical *theoria* nor, one imagines, in the reading of many medical students.[122]

Throughout his discussion of *De caelo* 2.14, in addition to drawing his pupils' attention, however cursorily, to mathematical arguments and authorities, Cardano adopted an attitude toward Aristotle and toward scholastic natural science that varied between condescension and hostility. He asserted that Aristotle was not to be blamed for not having known of later observations, but that Aristotelian conclusions about the circumference of the earth had nonetheless been superseded both by Ptolemy and by information derived from modern voyages.[123] One can see "how much faith should be attributed to Aristotle when he speaks about obscure things, since he is blind in obvious ones."[124] As for "the philosophers," they "propound trivialities either about very obvious things or about obscure things that cannot possibly be known; about those things that really need to be investigated they either say nothing at all or nothing sensible, and when by good luck they do say something fairly explicitly and the matter comes to light,

[120] Ibid., pp. 495, 492. At p. 492: "Quis ergo dubitat quod si quis imperitus sit artis chymicae nunquam poterit recte philosophari, velut neque Aristoteles qui multos [e]videntes errores tum in hoc tamen in historia de animalibus propter dissectionis ignorantiam admisit."

[121] Ibid., pp. 494–96.

[122] Ibid., p. 495. The reference to the Calculator is perhaps to Treatise 11 of the *Liber calculationum*; see John E. Murdoch and Edith Dudley Sylla, "Swineshead (Swyneshed, Suicet, etc.), Richard (fl. ca. 1340–1355)," *DSB*, 13:198.

[123] Cardano, *Opera* (1663), 9:494.

[124] Ibid., 9:494: "Vide ergo quis sensus hoc deprehendere possit, aut quae solertia artificis, et quanta fides sit adhibenda Aristoteli de obscuris loquenti, in adeo manifestis caecutienti, veniantque isti nostri philosophi et tueantur illud."

erroneous conclusions are drawn."[125] However, although these remarks convey an impression of more penetration as regards scientific
content than some of the rhetorical expressions of disdain for "barbarous" medieval translators and scholastic question-mongering encoun-
tered earlier in the present work, it should be remembered that Cardano was himself by no means averse to topics that might reasonably be described as "obscure things that cannot possibly be known"
especially as regards celestial heat, astrology, dreams, and divina-
tion.[126]

As one might expect, when he came to the subsection on fire, Cardano returned to his favorite subject: the distinction between celestial
heat and terrestrial fire.[127] But his handling of the elements air and
water is a good deal more pragmatic and particularistic; more than any
of the other sixteenth-century commentators on this part of Avicenna's
chapter, he dealt with air in a medical context, as regards both the effect
of the environment on health (drawing upon the Hippocratic *Airs
Waters Places*) and the administration of water and other liquids to the
sick. His discussion of whether bad air or bad water is more damaging—a standard *quaestio* topic—is worth recording for its grasp of the
social and demographic factors involved in public health. Cardano began by asserting that the very worst air is more damaging than the very
worst water, since air penetrates directly to heart and brain. But he
went on to point out that, whereas it is impossible to escape the effects
of bad air, bad water can be avoided by boiling or distilling, by drawing water from a cistern or using imported water, or by drinking wine.
Owing to poverty, however, these options are not available to the
common people, even when they know perfectly well the water is bad.
Hence, in actuality, larger numbers of people are hurt by bad water
than by bad air, since corruption of water is widespread. Moreover, the
diseases induced by bad water are worse than those due to bad air, since
water is subject to more than natural corruption (presumably through
man-made pollution), whereas air is not—a reminder that Cardano
wrote in preindustrial Europe. The nobility, with their access to means
for purifying or substituting for the local water supply, are less subject
to these diseases than the common people, and so may be said to be

---

[125] ". . . nec volo imitari philosophos, qui nugantur in manifestissimis et occultis, quae
sciri non possunt, in his autem quae scire praestaret nihil dicunt aut nihil sani, et bona
fortuna quadam cum aliquid dicunt clarius et res devenerit in lucem falsi deprehendun-
tur." Ibid.

[126] His interests in the latter two areas are discussed in Thorndike, *History of Magic*
5:563–79; and Fierz, *Cardano*, pp. 117–55.

[127] Cardano, *Opera* (1663), 9:502–3.

more harmed by bad air than bad water. However, extremely bad air is more damaging for the common people than bad water is for the nobility.[128]

Finally, when he came to the subject of the role of the elements in living bodies, Cardano completely abandoned the traditional lines of commentary on this portion of the *doctrina* and substituted a discourse on plants based almost entirely on Theophrastus' *De causis plantarum*.[129] The fifteenth-century recovery of Theophrastus' botanical works and their subsequent frequent reprinting in the Latin translation by Theodore of Gaza was of central importance in the vigorous development of botany during the sixteenth century.[130] Hence, in introducing what is essentially a short account of the teaching of *De causis plantarum* into his lectures on medical theory, Cardano was demonstrating not only his versatility as a philosopher of nature and his classical learning, but also his familiarity with one of the most active areas of contemporary life science, and one highly relevant to medicine.

With a little ingenuity, the elastic format of lectures embodying commentary and *quaestiones* on Avicenna's *doctrina* on the elements could thus be stretched to accommodate the range of interests of a scholar as idiosyncratic and in some ways unscholastic as Cardano. His more conventional younger contemporary Giovanni Costeo was to use the framework of commentary to different but perhaps equally instructive ends.

Costeo on Non-Aristotelian Theories of Matter. No reputation for intellectual boldness, such as surrounds Cardano, was ever attached to Giovanni Costeo. Whereas for Cardano, the composition of a commentary on *Canon* 1.1 was a very minor project among his many other writings and interests, the *Canon* was the main focus of Costeo's scholarly activity. He devoted most of his career to editing, annotating, indexing, and commenting on the Latin text of that work. Furthermore, Costeo's stance toward Avicenna was in general protective and appreciative, while on numerous specific issues he endorsed formulations found in the *Canon*. Yet, traditionalist though he was in regard to Avicenna, Costeo had a lively interest in a variety of lines of scientific discussion that had begun to emerge or had been intensified in the generation before he published the *Disquisitiones* on *Canon* 1.1 in 1589. He took the occasion of commentary on *Doctrina* 2[131] to review a series of theories

---

[128] Ibid., pp. 501–2. [129] Ibid., pp. 505–7.

[130] On the Renaissance recovery and influence of Theophrastus' botanical works, see Charles B. Schmitt, "Theophrastus," *CTC*, 2:246–48, 265–75.

[131] Costeo, *Disq. phys.*, pp. 29–100.

about the elements that in one way or another departed from the teaching of Aristotle. Some of the concepts reviewed by Costeo were of ancient, some of recent origin; all, as he emphasized, were the subject of current debate. The main bodies of opinion thus called under review by Costeo were those of the Stoics, the atomists, Cardano, and Copernicus. Furthermore, although he described Stoic ideas about the elements only in order to dismiss them, and although he disagreed vigorously with Cardano, he was decidedly attracted by some aspects of atomism, and sufficiently informed about and interested in the views of Copernicus to discuss them for ten pages before arriving at their final rejection.

Costeo's interest in the Stoics was mainly concentrated on their opinions about the qualities of the elements, and especially the Stoic belief that air was cold (and dark), rather than hot and wet as Aristotelian theory held. In focusing on this particular Stoic teaching, Costeo was in fact following a long-standing scholastic medical practice, since *Differentia* 14 of the *Conciliator* discusses statements about the coldness and darkness of the air found in Seneca's *Natural Questions*.[132] From the standpoint of the construction of a scholastic *quaestio*, the problem of whether air is hot or cold can be paralleled with the somewhat similar inquiry as to whether earth or water is the coldest of the elements, also discussed by Pietro d'Abano, by Da Monte after him, and doubtless by many others as well (on the latter topic Pietro and Da Monte reached opposing conclusions).[133] However, Costeo, who drew on Galen and Plutarch for his information about Stoic beliefs, provided a considerably fuller and more coherent account of Stoic opinions about the coldness of the air and their reasons for them than Pietro d'Abano had. Nonetheless, Costeo repudiated Stoic arguments in order to maintain a staunchly Aristotelian position about the qualities of air.[134] He was equally disapproving of Cardano's denial of elemental status to fire, citing with approbation Scaliger's demolition of Cardano's position. Costeo thought, however, that Cardano's views were likely to sway popular opinion, a judgment shared by a recent historian of the dispute between Cardano and Scaliger.[135]

---

[132] *Conciliator* (Venice, 1548), *Diff.* 14, fol. 22ᵛ. In Pietro's account, Seneca is referred to by name, but is not called a Stoic, a term used frequently by Costeo. For Seneca's views, see *Naturales Quaestiones* 2.10, in Seneca, *Naturales Quaestiones*, tr. Thomas H. Corcoran (Loeb Classical Library, 1981), 2:114.

[133] *Conciliator* (Venice, 1548), *Diff.* 12, fols. 20ʳ–21ʳ; Da Monte, comm. *Canon* 1.1 (Venice, 1554), fols. 26ᵛ–27ʳ.

[134] Costeo, *Disq. phys.*, pp. 68–69, 75–77. The work of Plutarch is unnamed, but is presumably either *De stoicorum repugnantiis* or *De communibus notitiis adversus Stoicos*.

[135] Costeo, *Disq. phys.*, pp. 57–67. At p. 58: "Possunt ergo haec vulgarem de igne

When contrasted with his conservative Aristotelian opposition to the Stoics and Cardano, Costeo's treatment of the subject of atomism was considerably more open and eclectic. He evidently hoped to make a modified corpuscularism (which, whether he realized it or not, actually lacked some essential features of ancient atomism) acceptable to his readers by combining it with aspects of Aristotelian element theory. Although far from unique, even this degree of receptivity to corpuscular explanations of nature was probably still fairly unusual in academic circles. At any rate, it does not appear to have been shared by the four other commentators on *Doctrina* 2 reviewed in this chapter, who included in their expositions brief descriptions of the theories of Democritus and Leucippus, and who were undoubtedly as familiar with Galen's accounts of the subject as was Costeo.

Galen was without question the main source of Costeo's information about ancient corpuscular theories, since his attention was focused exclusively on the ideas attributed to Asclepiades by that author.[136] In commenting on *Doctrina* 2, Costeo made no mention of Fracastoro; of Giordano Bruno, who began to announce his atomist views in print around 1586,[137] three years before the publication of Costeo's *Disquisitiones*; or of alchemical writers or experience. However, Costeo did show awareness of Aristotelian philosophical discussions of *minima naturalia*, especially the work of Nifo.[138] Costeo informed his readers that, according to Galen, Asclepiades and the Methodists believed an infinite number of extremely small corpuscles, incapable of further division, to exist in a void. The human body, like all other mixed bodies, is made from the encounters of these corpuscles; by their disjunction it is dissolved.

Costeo acknowledged that his audience was likely to reject this theory. He thought that objections to it included the unacceptability of in-

---

opinionem perturbare." Maclean, "Interpretation of Natural Signs," pp. 233–34, notes that Cardano's views enjoyed considerable popular dissemination while remaining unacceptable to academic critics such as Scaliger.

[136] Costeo, *Disq. phys.*, pp. 51–54. Costeo did not name particular works of Galen in this passage, but cited *De elementis* 1.1 at the beginning of the chapter (p. 30). The views of Asclepiades and the Methodists were mentioned by Galen, as Costeo remarked, in many different places, in addition to the passages cited in n. 58, above.

[137] Michel, *Cosmologie*, pp. 140–41.

[138] Costeo, *Disq. phys.*, pp. 52–53. At the beginning of the chapter (p. 30) Costeo or his editor cited "6 Sue. Metaphys. tract. cap.," that is, presumably, Nifo's commentary on Aristotle's *Metaphysics*. In *Augustini Niphi . . . Expositiones in Aristotelis libros Metaphysices* (Venice, 1559; facsimile, Frankfurt, 1967) the subject matter of Book 6 does not relate to the elements and it has only two chapters. Book 5, however, devotes chap. 3 to the subject of the elements and lacks any chapter numbered 4. See pp. 270–74. The concept of *minima* is briefly alluded to on p. 273.

finity within the natural order, the presumed consequence that indivisible atoms would be incapable of qualitative change, the disturbingly antiprovidential component of chance, and the consequent absence of any explanation of the causes that led the *corpuscula* now to come together, now to separate. Nonetheless, he believed that the theory was to some extent supported by experience, and that it could be interpreted in a philosophically acceptable way. He asserted that the existence of indivisible atoms (*atomi*) in nature was real and not imaginary, citing as evidence the presence of particles in the air revealed by sunlight. (In his desire to present empirical evidence, Costeo evidently overlooked or failed to grasp that atoms were postulated at the subvisible level.) Such particles could be seen even in the middle of the ocean, where they could not possibly be dust particles brought from land by the wind. Experience also showed that some particles were always present in rain; when these fell, they entered the earth through pores or interstices and, although earthy in composition themselves, constituted somewhat lighter parts within it.

The evidence he adduced thus seemed to Costeo to indicate not only that particles existed, but also that those known to experience were all earthy in nature. He therefore went on to argue that the particles were in fact *minima* of the element earth, that is, not atoms in the sense of being distinguished only by their shape and size. Thus, since the element earth greatly predominated in bodies here below, including the body of man, such particles predominated in the constitution of bodies. Hence it was possible, according to Costeo, to interpret Asclepiades' assertion that the human body consisted of indivisible particles as meaning that it was "a mass in which the earthy element predominates, that mass indeed being reduced to *minima* for the sake of mixture," a formulation that, Costeo pointed out, was compatible with the teaching of outstanding philosophers, by whom he presumably meant Aristotle, and perhaps also Nifo.[139]

In admitting that it was equally possible that Asclepiades had not meant anything of the kind, Costeo showed his awareness of the shaky basis of his attempt to reconcile two fundamentally incompatible views.[140] That his goal in this undertaking was not merely scholastic reconciliation for its own sake, but rather some measure of defense of

---

[139] "Si quis hoc illud esse existimet, quod obscuritatis nube involutum Asclepiades proposuit, elementa hominis dicens esse corpuscula insectilia, id est: molem in qua maxime terrenum superat elementum, eam vero ad minima redactam ob mistionem, non is fortasse errabit. Sunt enim haec philosophorum praestantissimorum doctrinae non dissentanea." Costeo, *Disq. phys.*, pp. 52–53.

[140] "Haec quae Asclepiadis sententiam minori repraehensione dignam facerent, an ille senserit, non disputamus." Ibid., p. 54.

atomic theory, is revealed by his addition of arguments providing tentative and partial support for the idea of particles that are indivisible and infinite in number. He asserted that indivisible particles would not necessarily be incapable of qualitative alteration and that, while the number of the particles was doubtless known to "the wisdom of nature from which nothing whatsoever can be hidden," sense experience of the particles in the air showed them to be infinite as far as the power of the human mind to grasp their number was concerned.[141] Furthermore, in rejecting an argument frequently put forward to the effect that if the basic constituent(s) of the human body were not subject to qualitative alteration man would not be able to feel pain, Costeo claimed that there was no reason to suppose that a sentient body could not be compounded from insentient first principles. Finally, he attempted to remove the unacceptably antiprovidential aspects of atomism by asserting that it was the "immense power of nature" rather than chance that brought the particles together to form bodies.[142]

The Response to Copernicanism in Commentaries on the Canon: *Costeo and Santorio.* The first sign of awareness of Copernican theory in the commentaries on *Doctrina* 2 of *Canon* 1.1 is perhaps to be found in Cardano's rather emphatic presentation of arguments for the stability of the earth, a topic to which he devoted more attention in his exposition than earlier commentators on the *Canon* had found necessary.[143] However, Costeo was the first of the commentators under review to incorporate an account of Copernican views into his exposition of Avicenna's statement that the earth is immobile at the center of the universe.

---

[141] ". . . quae nobis infinita et innumerabilia sunt, naturae sapientiae, quam rerum nihil quidquam aut usquam latere potest, finita sunt." Ibid., p. 53.

[142] "Cuius quidem quum artifex sit natura, si quis quaerat quomodo repente tam parva, tam multaque corpuscula ad constituendum hominem cogat, ignarum ille seipsum immensae potestatis naturae facit." Ibid., p. 54.

[143] "Succedunt quaestiones de terra, quas proponit Philosophus secundo *Coeli*, cap. 14; ostendit autem terram primo quiescere, quod ad motum circularem attinet, quatuor rationibus. Prima unicuique corpori inest tantum unus motus simplex, vel ergo motus esset naturalis, atque sic inesset etiam partibus, at hoc falsum: movetur enim solum motus recto, si violentus ergo non perpetuus. Secunda ratio, quae conversione feruntur, post se relinqui videntur; at non videntur. Tertia proiecto lapide in aerem, lapis non cadet directe in eundum locum, at hoc non contingit. Quarta ratio, omnia quae moventur circulari motu praeter primam sphaeram, saltem duobus motibus moventur; quod si ita esset stellarum fixarum regressus apparet, quoniam idem apparet, si octava sphaera duobus motibus volveretur; idem autem est si terra eisdem motibus moveat ut stellae quiescant. Quinta ratio est quod non moveatur motu recto, quia partes non possunt moveri a centro, quia moventur ad centrum, ergo multo minus totum." Cardano, *Opera* (1663), 9:494.

Costeo's initial description was compressed into two and a half pages and was, as one might expect, much simplified and wholly nonmathematical.[144] Nonetheless, it provided an idea of Copernicus' main contention and indicated a series of qualitative arguments that could be used to support it, some of which had been used by Copernicus himself.

Costeo began, in what was already time-honored fashion, by noting that a few of the ancients had believed the earth to move. In addition to indicating Aristotle and Ptolemy as sources of this information, he noted the individual names of Nicetas (that is, Hicetas) of Syracuse as reported in Cicero's *Academica*, and Philolaos, via Plutarch. Opinion of this kind had been revived by the *recentiores*, Nicholas Copernicus, and others, some of whom held only that the earth rotated on its axis, others that the firmament and the sun were at rest, while the earth and the heavenly orbs moved around; yet others that the earth was moved by a motion of trepidation but not that it was in orbit. These views, Costeo noted, were really grounded in sense experience, since they were based on observation of the relative nature of perceptions of motion. In some circumstances, Costeo explained, an observer is unable to tell whether it is he or the object of his observation that is moving, or whether both of them are moving at unequal speeds. He went on to use the boat-on-the-river analogy in order to drive home the impossibility of relying on common-sense experience as evidence for the centrality and stability of the earth. And a few pages later he drew attention to Copernicus' refutation of Ptolemy's claim that objects would fly off a moving earth and that clouds would always appear to be floating westward.

Costeo also listed six additional arguments in favor of the earth's motion, namely: (1) the greater appropriateness of postulating motion for the vile earth than the noble heavens, especially since inconstancy was associated with corruption by philosophers; (2) the difficulty of seeing how the heavens could move with respect to place (conceived as containing), since there was nothing beyond the outermost heaven; (3) the likelihood that nature had placed air and water surrounding the earth to provide lubrication and thus facilitate its motion; (4) the reasonableness of supposing that the earth moves in a search for maximum exposure to the rays of the sun, by which it is warmed and which stir up the origins of things; (5) the probability that heaviness, rather than lightness, is associated with motion; (6) the inconceivable rapidity of the diurnal motion of the heavens, given a stationary earth.

---

[144] Costeo, *Disq. phys.*, pp. 90–100.

Costeo claimed firsthand knowledge of *De revolutionibus*,[145] but it seems likely that he had read only its introductory portions, since his explanation contains no signs of interest or competence in technical astronomy or mathematics. Moreover, by the time he wrote, indirect access to general information about the ancient proponents of a moving earth and about the Copernican hypothesis would probably not have been hard to come by in academic circles. Thus, the references to Hicetas, from Cicero, and Philolaos, from Plutarch, were indeed used by Copernicus; but the same citations also occur in the works of mid-sixteenth-century writers, who were less interested in astronomy than in the skeptical implications for all human knowledge of radically conflicting scientific views.[146]

Costeo began his reasonably careful explication (given the nature of his work and its intended audience) of the Copernican position in the confident conviction that Copernican arguments were easy to overthrow. In fact, he devoted about three times as much space to refuting Copernicus as he had given to the exposition of the latter's views, ending with the admonition that "students should understand how perilous it is to depart from the received opinions of the ancients."[147] Costeo's rebuttals rested for the most part on arguments of a highly speculative and teleological variety drawn from scholastic natural philosophy, with occasional reference to sense experience. Astronomical detail, whether Ptolemaic or Copernican, and theological considerations are notable only by their absence. A flavor of Costeo's line of attack will be more than sufficient, and may be gained from the following summary of just one of his counterarguments. The supposed motion of the earth must be either extrinsic or intrinsic. If extrinsic, it must be caused by some kind of force (*vis*), perhaps either the Prime

[145] "Ad quae Copernicus (si modo quae ille longa scribit verborum serie assequimur). . . ." Ibid., p. 99.

[146] For the use of these references by sixteenth-century writers who were interested in skepticism, see Charles B. Schmitt, *Cicero Scepticus: A Study of the Influence of the Academica in the Renaissance* (The Hague, 1972), pp. 90, 127–28; and Henri Busson, *Le rationalisme dans la littérature française de la Renaissance (1533–1601)* (Paris, 1957), pp. 256–58. The passages assembled by Busson show that some information about Copernicus' adoption of the heliocentric theory was available at Paris by 1550. Ugo Baldini, "L'astronomia del Cardinale Bellarmino," in *Novità celesti e crisi del sapere: Atti del Convegno Internazionale di Studi Galileiani*, ed. P. Galluzzi (Supplemento agli *Annali dell'Istituto e Museo di Storia della Scienza*, anno 1983, fascicolo 2), pp. 294–95, indicates various sources of information about Copernican theory available in sixteenth-century Italy, notably Clavius' commentary on the *Sphaera* of Sacrobosco, first published 1570, and reissued in 1581. See Clavius, *In Sphaeram* (Rome, 1570), p. 87.

[147] "Haec de terrae motu, animi gratia. Atque ut quam periculosum sit a recepta veterum sententia discedere, studiosi intelligant." Costeo, *Disq. phys.*, p. 100.

Intelligence or one of the other Intelligences. But it would be unworthy for any Intelligence to assist like a servant in moving the vile and corruptible body of the earth. Furthermore, every motion is for the sake of acquiring some perfection. But the motion of an impure body like the earth could bring no perfection to purer bodies. Nor could the earth itself gain any greater perfection through movement. An imaginable greater perfection for the earth would be the exposure of every part of the earth to every one of the stars, but this would require not just rotation from east to west, but also rotation through the poles, which is absurd, since there is absolutely nothing in the heavenly appearances that can be construed as evidence for such a rotation.[148]

Like that of Costeo, the commentary on the *doctrina* on the elements by Santorio Santorio, based on lectures given at Padua between 1611 and 1624, has as its most striking feature the introduction of material about recent cosmological theories.[149] The generation that separated the two medical authors was, however, an eventful one for the history of cosmology and astronomy; furthermore, Santorio, unlike Costeo, was personally associated with circles that were very well informed about new theories and observations in physical science and astronomy, and was himself eager to introduce innovations in scientific method, if not in underlying theory, into his own physiological area of specialization. Hence, Santorio's exposition reveals a somewhat wider (although still wholly nonmathematical) general knowledge of astron-

---

[148] "Haec et similia suadere potuerunt Nicolao Copernico atque aliis moveri terram et coelum quiescere adversus receptam veterum sententiam. Qua tamen in re eos labi non est fortasse, ut ostendamus, difficile. Quaerendum enim ab his, si movetur terra extrinsecum ne sit quod eam movet an intrinsecum. Si extrinsecum dicant, erit illud quidem aut vis sine subiecto, aut vis in subiecto. Atque si vim sine subiecto esse dicant, erit ea vel prima intelligentia vel ceterarum aliqua. Atqui indignum dictu est intelligentiam aliquam terrae veluti operarium ministrum assistere, tam vile et corruptibile corpus quale haec ipsa est, moventem. Quaerimus vero etiam, quum motus omnis perfectionis alicuius acquirendae sit gratia, quorsum ea vis terram moveat: sui ne ipsius, an terrae gratia. Non in sui ipsius certe usum. Ex impuri enim corporis conversatione accedere purioribus illis corporibus nihil perfectionis potest. Sin terrae causa, nempe ut tota eodem astrorum commodo tandem fruatur, ita necesse profecto esset nullam terrae partem esse quam aliquando singula astra directo aspectu non illustrent, quare non secundum longitudinem modo, quae, ut aiunt astrologi, ab occasu in ortum est, terram moveri oporteret, sed etiam secundum latitudinem, idest, secundum eam differentiam loci quae ad polos. Utrunque vero absurdum. Nondum enim intra tot annorum spacium quot de mundi vita, observatio est quae regiones occasum solis spectabunt nunc ortum quae arcticum polum, nunc antarcticum, aut intermedia spacia prospiciunt." Ibid., pp. 92–93.

[149] Santorio's discussion of the elements occupies cols. 141–43, 145–228 in the edition of Venice, 1646 The *quaestiones* are nos. 14 and 16–25. Most of the cosmological discussion is in cols. 162–76.

omy than Costeo's, as well as Santorio's own familiarity with other aspects of contemporary science. In preparing his commentary for publication Santorio had, moreover, to work within constraints not yet imposed upon Costeo, namely the official condemnation of Copernican theory by ecclesiastical authorities, which took place in 1616.[150]

Also like Costeo, Santorio engaged in scholastic exposition of both Copernican and anti-Copernican views, beginning with the former (in itself a prudent arrangement, since scholastic *quaestiones* normally presented the position to be refuted first). Santorio split his discussion into two separate *quaestiones*, one about the earth's position and the other about its stasis or motion.[151] On the former issue, the inequality of the seasons, the variations in brightness of the planets suggesting variations in their distance, and their stations and retrogradations all seemed to Santorio "highly effective" proofs that the earth could not be central with respect to the planetary spheres. However, Santorio proceeded, these phenomena did not invalidate Avicenna's statement that the earth was in a central position, since Avicenna had meant this not with respect to the planets but with respect to the primum mobile. That the earth was at the center with respect to the primum mobile had been shown by Aristotle, and although Aristotle's argument "is not a demonstration, it is yet not to be spurned. For in doubtful cases it is preferable to rely on Aristotle rather than on other authors."[152] Finally, Santorio gave a grudging nod to the homocentric planetary theory of Fracastoro, allowing that it might be one way to maintain the proba-

[150] The decree of the Congregation of the Index pronouncing the belief that the earth orbited a central and immobile sun to be contrary to Scripture and forbidding it to be held or defended was officially published on March 5, 1616. See Stillman Drake, *Galileo at Work* (Chicago and London, 1978), pp. 252–55, 347–48.

[151] *Quaestio* 16: "An terra sit in medio universi," cols. 162–67; *Quaestio* 17: "An terra quiescat, vel circulariter moveatur," cols. 167–76, Santorio, comm. *Canon* 1.1 (Venice, 1646).

[152] ". . . moderni astronomi putant terram non esse absolute in medio. . . . Nicolaus Copernicus in libro suarum *Revolutionum* probat solem esse in medio universi, ibique quiescere. . . . Praeterea tribus argumentis efficacissimis ab observationibus astronomicis desumptis probari potest terram non esse in medio universi. . . . Haec argumenta videntur esse efficacissima, quia revera probant terram respectu planetarum non esse in medio, id est respectu orbium deferentium quibus sydera infixa sunt, qui orbes respectu terrae sunt eccentrici simpliciter. . . . Sed revera dicta argumenta nihil probant contra Avicennam: quia Avicennas vult terram esse in medio universi non respectu planetarum, sed respectu primi mobilis. . . . Sed cum satis superque probatum sit ab Aristotele quod omne grave tendat ad centrum universi, hocque centrum non differre a centro terrae, eius ratio, licet non sit demonstratio, saltem spernenda non est. Accedit quod in rebus dubiis potius Aristoteli quam aliis auctoribus fides sit adhibenda." Santorio, comm. *Canon* 1.1 (Venice, 1646), cols. 162–164.

bility of a central position of the earth with regard to the planets as well as the primum mobile, but noting that he himself had various objections to Fracastoro's proposed solution. However, Santorio refused to indulge in any further discussion of the motions of the heavenly bodies in general, announcing that only possible movements of the earth pertained to his subject.[153]

Santorio's list of arguments used by those who believed the earth to be in motion was much the same as Costeo's, with one notable addition. On his list of the contentions put forward by some *moderni* in support of a Copernican position, Santorio included the assertion that a movement of the oceans is caused by the motion of the earth, a statement that could be, but is not necessarily, an imperfect echo of Galileo's ideas about tides.[154] Santorio himself understood the movement in question to be a motion of the whole ocean from east to west, which he alleged, on the authority of Cardinal Contarini's five books on the elements and Clavius' widely read commentary on the *Sphere* of Sacrobosco, to have been observed in the course of voyages to America and the Indies. Santorio sought both to maintain that this motion took place, although it could not be observed locally and appeared to contravene certain arguments derived from Aristotelian physics, and to attribute it to celestial rather than to terrestrial causes.[155]

Santorio also listed what he said were counterarguments produced by Copernicans against Aristotelian and Ptolemaic reasoning. To the anti-Copernican assertion that if the earth moved from east to west (*sic*) projectiles thrown toward the west would travel further than projectiles thrown with equal force toward the east ("just as if someone in a ship sailing westward were to throw a ball into the sea toward the east, the ship would leave the ball a long way behind, and on the contrary if he threw a ball toward the west, the ship would come up to it before it

<hr />

[153] Fracastoro's planetary theory is set forth in his *Homocentricorum, sive de stellis liber unus*, which was first published in 1538, but which I have consulted in his *Opera omnia* (Venice, 1574), fols. 1ʳ–48ʳ.

[154] Santorio, comm. *Canon* 1.1 (Venice, 1646), col. 168. According to Drake, *Galileo at Work*, pp. 36–37, 252, 273–74, Galileo had begun to develop his theories about a relation between tides and the movement of the earth by 1595, when the concept was known to Paolo Sarpi in Venice, and the hypothesis was fully formulated by 1616. The possibility that movements of the ocean were caused by a motion of the earth was earlier discussed by Andrea Cesalpino in his *Quaestiones peripateticae* (Venice, 1593), 3.6, fols. 70ʳ–71ᵛ. Cesalpino denied the possibility of orbital or axial rotation, but not that of some kind of trepidation of the earth (ibid., 3–4, fols. 66ʳ–67ʳ). The preface to his *Quaestiones* bears the date 1569.

[155] Santorio, comm. *Canon* 1.1 (Venice, 1646), cols. 173–74, citing "Clavius in sua *Sphaera*."

fell"), Santorio said the answer was that there was no valid comparison between an arrow shot into the air and a ball thrown into the sea; the comparison should rather be to a ball both thrown and landing within the boat.[156] And of the argument that Costeo had found so persuasive, to the effect that it would be impious to suppose that one of the celestial Intelligences would stoop to moving the vile earth, Santorio remarked curtly: "This instance is ridiculous. Because just as they concede that an Intelligence is provided to move the moon, why should not one be provided for the earth? And whoever knows whether the earth or the moon is the nobler? I incline to the opinion that the earth is much more outstanding than the moon."[157]

However, Santorio was equally scathing about some of the more trivial arguments or examples he claimed to be put forward by followers of Copernicus, including the idea that the spheres of water and air provided lubrication for a turning earth ("anile and puerile," according to Santorio), and a mysterious gem with a mark on it that rotated every twenty-four hours reported by Cardano. According to Santorio, the gem in question was discovered after Cardano's death to be a finely wrought clock![158] Santorio was, as we shall see, to use the same example again in pouring scorn on excessive reliance on occult causes. He also objected to the way in which Copernicans argued from the idea of an infinite universe, a concept he apparently considered common among them, to that of the motion of the earth.[159]

[156] "Sextum argumentum, si terra tam rapide moveretur ab ortu ad occasum, sagitta versus occasum proiecta longius iter faceret quam si in orientem: sicuti, dum quis in navi currente versus occasum proijceret in mari pilam versus orientem, navis per longum spatium pilam relinqueret, e contra si proiceret pilam versus occasum tunc etiam antequam caderet navis rederetur propinqua.

"Argumentum vanissimum: quia non est par ratio de pila proiecta extra navim, et de sagitta in terra; esset par ratio de pila proiecta in ipsa navi, sed non extra navim, et hoc modo proijciatur quocunque modo pila in navi, nulla dignoscitur differentia, sicuti de sagitta in terra." Santorio, comm. *Canon* I.I (Venice, 1646), col. 172. The first edition of Santorio's commentary, in which the sentence just quoted occurs in col. 121, was published in 1625 or 1626, so the passage is not an echo of Day 2 of Galileo's *Dialogo* (1632).

[157] "Haec instantia profecto est ridicula: quia sicuti concedunt dari intelligentiam moventem lunam, cur non poterit dari intelligentia movens ipsam terram? Quis hactenus novit, an terra, vel luna sit nobilior? Ego in hanc sententiam inclino, terram esse longe praestantiorem luna." Santorio, comm. *Canon* I.I (Venice, 1646), col. 171.

[158] Ibid., cols. 174, 175. See *Hieronymi Cardani . . . In Cl. Ptolomaei . . . Quadripartitae constructionis libros commentaria* (Lyon, 1555), Book I, textus 10, p. 22. Cardano used the story as an example of the remarkable powers of gems and the influence of the heavens upon them.

[159] "Ad primam duo committunt errata. Primum supponunt coelum esse infinitum et inde concludunt coelum non moveri, quae petitio est indigna inter viros doctos, quia prius est probandum coelum esse infinitum." Santorio, comm. *Canon* I.I (Venice,

On the issue of the motion of the earth, therefore, Santorio's own conclusion was that

. . . both those who are incited by reasons drawn from natural philosophy to maintain firmly that the earth is moved in a circular manner and those whom the same kind of reasons inspire to maintain even more firmly that it is not so moved are foolish if they believe that the arguments they propound are compelling. Because these arguments, although they seem valid, are in reality very lightweight. For the question is so difficult that there is no degree of ingenuity, in my judgment, felicitous enough to eliminate doubt and perplexity in a matter of such obscurity. We, however, incline to this opinion, that the earth does not rotate from east to west, because this motion is proper to the primum mobile; nor does it have an annual motion from west to east, because this motion is proper to the sun; nor is the earth moved by a motion of trepidation, because this motion should be attributed to the ninth sphere. Hence, we believe, along with Avicenna, that the earth is at rest in the center of the world.[160]

Other sections of Santorio's discussion of the elements reveal him to have considered some of the possible implications of recent astronomical events not only for astronomy and cosmology but also, and especially, for the theory of matter. His remarks on the subject must no doubt be placed in the context of the controversy initiated at Padua and Venice by the nova of 1604, and the similar debates that accompanied the comet of 1618, both carried on in a number of rapidly published treatises about these appearances.[161] Santorio believed the nova of 1604

1646), col. 172. The history up to the early seventeenth century of the development of the concept of an infinite universe is traced in Alexander Koyré, *From the Closed World to the Infinite Universe* (Baltimore and London, 1957), pp. 1–99, and Steven J. Dick, *Plurality of Worlds* (Cambridge, 1982), pp. 1–105. The principal sixteenth-century supporter of the idea was probably Giordano Bruno.

[160] "Quare ex his colligimus quod et illi qui firmiter putant terram circulariter moveri et illi qui certo certius tenent non moveri circulariter perciti rationibus desumptis a philosophia naturali, quae licet videantur valere sunt tamen levissimae, si credant rationes quas proponunt esse argumenta quae cogant, sunt fatui; quia quaesitum est adeo difficile ut nullum ingenium meo iudicio inveniri possit ita felix quod in re tantae obscuritatis non sit dubium atque perplexum. Nos tamen inclinamus in hanc sententiam, quod terra non moveatur circulariter ab ortu ad occasum [*sic*], quia hic motus convenit primo mobili; nec moveatur ab occasu ad ortum motu annuo, quia hic motus convenit soli, nec movetur terra motu trepidationis, quia hic motus potius nonae sphaerae est attribuendus." Santorio, comm. *Canon* 1.1 (Venice, 1646), col. 175.

[161] See Marialaura Soppelsa, *Genesi del metodo galileiano e tramonto dell'Aristotelismo nella scuola di Padova* (Padua, 1974), pp. 21–65; and Adriano Carugo, "L'insegnamento della

to have been formed from terrestrial exhalations, not celestial ether, as it had disappeared from view after three months, thus showing itself to lack the permanence demanded of celestial objects in an Aristotelian system. However, he also held that such exhalations could reach above the sphere of the moon and that this had been the case with the nova of 1604 and with a recently observed comet, presumably that of 1618. Thus, Santorio simultaneously held that comets were formed from earthy exhalations and that some, although not all, comets ascended above the moon. In his commentary on Avicenna's chapter on the elements, Santorio advised his audience of the latter fact on five separate occasions, explaining in each case the evidence afforded by the absence of parallax.[162]

Appropriately for his context, Santorio used these references to cometary theory chiefly to bolster up assertions about the spheres of earth, air, and fire. Thus, the ascent of comets above the moon showed that the exhalations of earth affected the moon, and not vice versa (a statement that relates to Santorio's views on astrology). Thus, too, the passage of comets through the sphere of fire introduced earthy exhalations into it, making it impossible to maintain that the fire in the sphere of fire was either the pure element or absolutely light, and hence indirectly supporting the concept that all the elements actually existed only as mixed bodies, not in pure form. As for comets below the moon, Santorio thought that they provided evidence for the rotation of the sphere of air, because "they are moved from east to west,"[163] and for the heat of the upper regions of the air.

Santorio also considered and rejected the opinion of "those who think the matter of the heavens and of these things here below to be of the same kind." His grounds for dismissing this opinion were that, if so, a similar chain of causes as on earth should give rise to alteration and

matematica all'Università di Padova prima e dopo Galileo," *Storia della cultura veneta* (Vicenza, 1984), vol. 4, pt. 2, pp. 188–97. For the general development of cometary theory in the sixteenth century, see C. Doris Hellman, *The Comet of 1577: Its Place in the History of Astronomy* (New York, 1944). On the relationship between cometary theory and the reception of Copernicanism, see Robert S. Westman, "The Comet and the Cosmos: Kepler, Mästlin and the Copernican Hypothesis," in *Colloquia Copernicana*, vol. 1, *Etudes sur l'audience de la théorie héliocentrique*, Studia Copernicana 5 (Wroclaw, 1972), pp. 7–30.

[162] Santorio, comm. *Canon* 1.1 (Venice, 1646), cols. 160, 171, 196, 214, 218. On early applications of the theory of parallax to comets by Western astronomers, probably beginning with Peurbach and Regiomontanus in the second half of the fifteenth century, see Hellman, *The Comet of 1577*, pp. 74–75, 80–97.

[163] "Quia aer movetur ab ortu ad occasum spatio 24 horarum, quod ostenditur per cometas qui sunt in aere et qui moventur ab ortu ad occasum." Santorio, comm. *Canon* 1.1 (Venice, 1646), col. 196.

generation and produce "rivers, seas, and living beings" in the moon. However, "not even with the newly invented spyglass" was it ever possible to see any change in the moon (a remark he repeated twice), whereas someone in the moon would be able to perceive a change in the appearance of the earth if, for example, the whole of Europe were covered with snow.[164]

The fairly elementary information about recent developments in astronomy and their implications for cosmology that Santorio chose to convey to his students or readers in the medical community was of course readily available and much discussed in intellectual circles in Padua and the Veneto by the time he lectured and wrote.[165] Moreover, on the crucial issue of the motion of the earth, he managed to combine skepticism with—at any rate in print—conservative conclusions. What is noteworthy about these portions of Santorio's exposition is therefore less their scientific content than the continued enlargement and updating of such content within basic medical education. Indeed, despite his own announced separation of medicine and natural philosophy, Santorio was at pains to provide explicit justification for the study of the elements by physicians.[166] And it could certainly be argued that the introduction of medical students to the breadth and fundamental nature of some of the issues involved in contemporary scientific controversy served a pedagogical purpose beyond that of merely enlarging their general knowledge. They could at any rate have learned lessons as valuable for medicine as for any other discipline from Santorio's convictions about the either trivial or essentially nondemonstrative character of much traditional and some contemporary natural philosophical argument, and from his occasional willingness to abandon reasoning based upon such arbitrary teleological assumptions as those about the relative nobility of various bodies.

The remainder of Santorio's discussion of Avicenna's chapter on the

---

[164] "Quare, qui putant materiam coelorum et horum inferiorum esse eiusdem generis non possunt se defendere, quin in luna sit alteratio et generatio, quoniam duplicatio radiorum in luna efficeret calores, et calores vapores, et vapores nubes, et nubes pluvias, et pluviae flumina, maria, et animantia ipsa; quod est omnino a veritate alienum. Si quis esset in luna dum magna Europae pars nive albescit, videret magnam aspectus mutationem: attamen neque specillo nuper invento ullam unquam mutationem in luna videmus." Ibid., col. 196. For the other apparent reference to the telescope, see ibid., col. 214.

[165] See Soppelsa, *Genesi del metodo galileiano*, pp. 21–65. The widespread attention attracted throughout Europe by Galileo's telescopic discoveries after the publication of the *Sidereus nuncius* in 1610 is well known.

[166] In *Quaestio* 14: "Quomodo tractatus de elementis et de temperamentis pertineat ad medicum?" Santorio, comm. *Canon* 1.1 (Venice, 1646), cols. 141–43.

elements has, if anything, even more the character of a grab bag of heterogeneous information about the subject in general than the earlier
commentaries just examined. A few of the miscellaneous topics and
questions are suggestive of genuine inquiry and/or impart straightforward information. Such for example is the *quaestio* "whether air in
mixtures makes them lighter or heavier," which takes up the issue of
whether air has weight and the objections to Avicenna's assertion that
it has only lightness, and also explains the concept of specific gravity
with reference to the story of Archimedes and the royal crown.[167] In
more instances, however, Santorio simply prolonged and rendered
more intricate the discussion of standard *quaestiones* about the hotness,
wetness, coldness, and dryness of the elements, the nature of the sphere
of fire, and so on, without changing its essentially arbitrary character.
To the examination of views attributed to ancient and medieval authors he added that of the rather wide range of sixteenth-century natural philosophical writers in whom he was well read. Thus, like Costeo
before him, he reviewed the controversy between Cardano and Scaliger at some length before arriving at his own endorsement of the reality
of the sphere of fire; but in addition he weighed the belief of Scaliger
and Zabarella that the sphere of fire was thinner over the poles.[168]
Other recent writers cited by Santorio included, in addition to those
already mentioned, William Gilbert,[169] Toletus,[170] Francisco Vallés,[171]
and Telesio, with all of whom he indicated disagreements. Santorio
waxed particularly indignant against Telesio for flying in the face of
sense evidence with the assertion that heat was a natural quality of
water. In Santorio's words:

We reply to this lunatic with Aristotle, Avicenna, and Scotus;
with Aristotle . . . , when he says that he who denies sensation

[167] *Quaestio* 24: "An aer reddat mixta leviora aut graviora?" Ibid., cols. 211–13.

[168] Ibid., cols. 214–15, 198.

[169] "Quo ad terrellam magneticam Petri Perigrini, refert Gilbertus, se de motu terrellae
intellexisse a Peregrino, sed non vidisse: mendaciorum enim conditio est, ut referantur,
sed non videantur." Ibid., col. 175. See also col. 169.

[170] "Secundo colligimus, nonnullos peripateticos, inter quos est Toletus, errasse dum
dicunt Aristotelem fuisse inventorem quatuor elementorum, cum fuerit Hippocrates qui
120 annos fuit ante Aristotelem." Ibid., col. 152. The commentaries on the *Physics* and
De generatione et corruptione of Franciscus Toletus, S.J. (1532–96) went through numerous
editions; see Lohr, s.v. Toletus, in *Renaissance Quarterly* 35 (1982), 199–200. The historical
precision of Santorio's remark is worthy of note.

[171] Ibid., col. 202. In addition to medical works, Vallés was the author of commentaries on the *Physics* and the *Meteorologica*, and of a well-known work on "Christian philosophy," *De sacra philosophia*. See Lohr, s.v. Vallesius, in *Renaissance Quarterly* 35 (1982),
209; and Zanier, *Medicina e filosofia*, pp. 20–38. Santorio disagreed with Vallés' views
about the qualities of air.

should suffer the pains of sensation; with Avicenna . . . , when he says that those who deny clear and obvious things, such as that fire is hot and water cold, should not be wearied with rational arguments but tormented with fire until they realize that it is not the same thing to be burned as not to be burned (and we add that they ought to be held in icy water until they realize that it is making them cold and not hot); and with Scotus . . . , when he says that those who deny contingency and free will, and say that everything happens by necessity, ought to be tortured, and even crucified, until they admit that it is possible either to be tortured or not to be tortured.[172]

Among medical writers, Santorio undertook to review views of Da Monte and Costeo, expressed in their commentaries on *Canon* 1.1, and Eustachio Rudio.[173] Santorio also had a tendency to fill out his commentary with examples, some of which are not without interest for the social history of medicine. Thus, in speaking of the characteristics of the element fire, he described itinerant vendors of quack burn salves who first flamed an ointment containing aquavit and camphor and then applied it to their hands, claiming to the gaping crowd that it had the power to take away burns.[174]

[172] ". . . aquam sua natura esse frigidam, ita ut omnes philosophi in hac re conveniant, praeter modernum quendam sophistam vocatur Telesium, qui lib. 3 suarum nugarum in eam devenit dementiam, ut defenderet, et admodum pueriliter, aquam esse calidam et non frigidam. Sed huic insano respondebimus cum Aristotele, cum Avicenna, et Scoto. Cum Arist. 1 *Top.*, cap. 9, ubi dicit qui negant sensum indigere poenas sensus. Cum Avicenna in sua *Metaphysica* dicente qui negant clara et evidentia, ut ignem esse calidum et aqua [*sic*] frigidam, non esse rationibus defatigandos, sed igne torrendos, donec fateantur, non esse idem uri et non uri. Nosque addimus in aqua gelida tenendos, donec fateantur quam refrigerare et non calefacere. Cum Scoto, I *Sent.*, dist. 39, ubi dicit qui negant contingentiam et liberum arbitrium, dicuntque omnia necessario evenire, esse exponendos tormentis, et eo usque cruciandos, donec concedant possibile esse eos torqueri et possible non torqueri." Santorio, comm. *Canon* 1.1 (Venice, 1646), cols. 187–88. Regarding the endeavor of Bernardino Telesio (1509–88) to substitute his own system for the Aristotelian doctrine of the elements and qualities, see Neal W. Gilbert, "Telesio, Bernardino," *DSB*, 13:277–80.
[173] Santorio, comm. *Canon* 1.1 (Venice, 1646), cols. 177–78, refuting Da Monte's view that earth is colder than water; ibid., cols. 222–23, rejecting the view of Rudio that natural and febrile heat were of two different species.
[174] "Hinc aqua vitae purissima dum ardet in summa manu, non adurit manum. Cur? Quia est purissima et tenuissima, quare tanto minus elementum ignis calefaciet, cum eius materia sit longe tenuior, aquae vitae et ipso aere qui omnino caret crassicie et opacitate. Hinc circulatores, ut bene vendant chimerica sua unguenta pro ambustis, componunt unguentum ex aquavitae et camphora, quod unguentum cum candela accendunt; quo accenso ignem tangunt, qui vix calefacit, quia unguentum est ex materia tenuissima et deinde applicant illud manibus. Dicuntque illico combustionem tolli, et sic decipiunt fatuos auditores." Ibid., col. 216.

Moreover, Santorio did not hesitate to extend the range of his conventional scholastic discussions into subject areas that had little sanction either in the earlier tradition of commentary on *Canon* 1.1 or from their relevance to medicine. For example, he was interested in the topic of tides and ocean currents. In fact, he distinguished no fewer than twelve movements of the seas and discussed them in three separate passages of his exposition of the chapter on the elements. Two of these passages were, as we have seen, part of his treatment of the subject of the possible motion of the earth; the third was inserted in his account of the element water in the form of a separate question, "De causa fluxus et refluxus maris," and introduced with the remark "The *theorici* treat this question at this point, and so we do too."[175] The pretext was scarcely valid, for while the subject of tides certainly found a place in natural philosophical treatments of the elements, both within commentaries and in independent treatises, it was not a particular focus of discussion in the sixteenth-century commentaries on *Canon* 1.1 by professors of theoretical medicine, or in the earlier expositions of the work by Giacomo da Forlì or Ugo Benzi. Santorio's main sources of information seem to have been Contarini and Clavius, although he also referred to the *Timaeus*, the *Meteorologica*, and the views of Ptolemy, Strabo, Seneca, Averroes, Thomas Aquinas, Duns Scotus, Pietro d'Abano, and Pico della Mirandola. As this list suggests, Santorio was here satisfied to present his readers with a review of ancient and scholastic opinion, with some reference to alleged experience. It is conceivable that Santorio's motivation for inserting this *quaestio* may have sprung from current cosmological and astronomical debates, but his own handling of it seems to fall wholly within the tradition of scholastic natural philosophy.

Santorio's discussion of tides, like much else in these six expositions of Avicenna's *doctrina* on the elements produced over an almost hundred-year time span, reveals very clearly the weaknesses as well as the strength of the genre of commentary-plus-*quaestiones* as a teaching tool. Whatever the merits of flexibility as to content, discursive commentary was essentially unsuited to be the vehicle of systematic instruction on a particular scientific topic. Nonetheless, most of the medical commentators evidently brought to their task an active interest in natural philosophy and a fairly good level of information about current developments as well as about classic and scholastic tradition. Hence,

---

[175] *Quaestio* 19: "De causa fluxus et refluxus maris." Ibid., cols. 184–88. The *quaestio* opens: "Theorici in hoc loco tractant hanc quaestionem, ergo et nos." References to Clavius and Contarini as sources of information about tidal theory occur in cols. 168 and 184; see *De elementis*, Book 2, pp. 30–34 in Contarini, *Opera* (Paris, 1571).

in each case their chapters both serve as compendia on the general subject of the elements and reflect something of the author's personal interests or the preoccupations of his circle. The interest in more or less metaphysical topics, so marked in Da Monte, gives way to other concerns in the later expositions. Cardano and Costeo both introduced discussion of, and to some extent endorsed, non-Aristotelian (in Cardano's case anti-Aristotelian) theories about matter. And by Costeo and Santorio medical students were introduced—albeit at an appropriately introductory level and from a safely conservative standpoint—to major and highly controversial contemporary scientific issues.

Celestial Influences and Occult Causes

In the sixteenth century, ideas about the specific relevance to medicine of celestial influences and occult causes or qualities were mostly taken up in the context of theories about drugs and diseases. Hence, extended medical discussions of such concepts, pro or contra, are more likely to be found in works on *practica* than in commentaries on *Canon* 1.1. But astrology and the occult also had a wider context, beyond medicine, in philosophical, scientific, and religious ideas.[176] It is in this context that the brief discussions of the stars and of occult qualities in the commentaries merit attention, since they help to situate these professors of medical theory in relation to a prominent feature of the culture of their age.

The thoroughness with which medieval and Renaissance medicine was permeated by belief in the existence and medical relevance of astral influences and other occult (that is, insensible or hidden) qualities and causes is well known. Not only did medical men share in the astrological and related beliefs that pervaded popular and learned culture alike throughout western Europe until the seventeenth century, but medicine was linked by especially strong ties to the entire cluster of

---

[176] I make no attempt to list here the very large modern literature that has grown up on the subject of Renaissance astrology, learned magic, occult sciences, Hermeticism, and so on, nor to review the controversy over the significance of these and related topics for the history of science. Mention must however at least be made of D. P. Walker, *Spiritual and Demonic Magic from Ficino to Campanella* (London, 1958); Frances Yates, *Giordano Bruno and the Hermetic Tradition* (London, 1964); W. Shumaker, *The Occult Sciences in the Renaissance* (Berkeley and London, 1972); *Reason, Experiment and Mysticism in the Scientific Revolution*, ed. M. L. Righini Bonelli and W. R. Shea (New York, 1975); Eugenio Garin, *Lo zodiaco della vita: La polemica sull'astrologia dal Trecento al Cinquecento* (Rome and Bari, 1976); and Vickers, *Occult and Scientific Mentalities*. In the present section the subject is only the relatively restricted one of attitudes expressed toward beliefs in astral influences, predictive astrology, and occult causes in the context of academic medical teaching.

concepts about the influences of heavenly bodies and of occult forces in nature. These ties included an emphasis, believed to ascend to Hippocrates himself, on the practical usefulness of astrology for medicine and on knowledge of astrology as the mark of a well-trained medical practitioner. Also important were those aspects of Galenic tradition (especially as developed by Avicenna and his medieval Latin followers) that, alongside the "rational" system explaining the properties of bodies in terms of Aristotle's laws of motion and of allegedly manifest combinations of the four elements and primary qualities, propounded the notion that some physical effects could be the result of quite different hidden qualities and causes. In the Italian university milieu, the connections between the conceptual underpinnings of astrology and of some medical ideas were strongly developed in the fourteenth and fifteenth centuries.[177] Moreover, despite influential critiques of astrology by Pico della Mirandola and others, it seems likely that ideas current in medieval medical thought—the role of the stars in generation, the omnipresence of knowable and medically useful astral signs and/or influences, and action by specific form as well as by complexion—were, if anything, reinforced by such Renaissance developments as the various Neoplatonic and eclectic strains in humanist thought, the astral magic of the physician-priest Marsilio Ficino, and the astral determinism of the leading Aristotelian philosopher of the early years of the sixteenth century, namely Pietro Pomponazzi.[178]

It is certainly clear that for four of the six commentators on Avicenna under consideration the real effect on terrestrial bodies of influences emanating from the heavenly bodies was among the unquestioned

---

[177] For the medieval development of some of the most important concepts, see Kibre, *Hippocrates Latinus*, pp. 94–107, on the pseudo-Hippocratic treatise on astrological medicine; and McVaugh, introduction to *Arnald of Villanova's Aphorismi de gradibus* in his *Opera medica omnia* (Granada-Barcelona, 1975), 2:1–136, on occult properties and "specific form" as explanatory devices in pharmacology. Regarding astrology and medicine in the Italian university ambience, the astrological interests of the very influential Pietro d'Abano are, of course, well known. For subsequent developments, see Graziella Federici Vescovini, "L'astrologia tra magia, religione e scienza," in her *"Arti" e filosofia*, pp. 169–93, and Giancarlo Zanier, "Ricerche sull'occultismo a Padova nel sec. XV," in *Scienza e filosofia*, pp. 345–72.

[178] The links between aspects of Ficino's thought and theories about specific form and occult properties developed by medical writers are noted in Brian P. Copenhaver, "Scholastic Philosophy and Renaissance Magic in the *De vita* of Marsilio Ficino," *Renaissance Quarterly* 37 (1984), 523–54. In turn, Ficino's ideas influenced the physician Symphorien Champier, and doubtless other medical men as well; see Copenhaver, *Champier*. Regarding Pomponazzi's astral determinism, the views of Pico della Mirandola, and the development of the fifteenth- and sixteenth-century debate over astrology, see Garin, *Lo zodiaco della vita*.

principles of natural philosophy and medicine, and likely that this was also the case for a fifth, namely Paterno. Only Santorio aligned himself with the critics of astrology and occult celestial influences. Much the most detailed and explicit support of these concepts was, however, incorporated in the two earliest commentaries, those by Pomponazzi's pupil Da Monte and Oddi.

In a metaphysical vein, Da Monte expatiated at some length upon the role of the stars and planets in causing all earthly mixtures, including the temperament of the human body. Not only did the primum mobile and the planets, especially the sun and the moon, generally affect the air in ways uniformly influencing everything on earth, but the aspects, sites, and influences of all the various stars and planets were responsible for the diversification of species and forms—hence their multiplicity—although here the celestial influences could only act in conjunction with suitable, and apparently already diversified, seeds. Da Monte wound up with the assertion that the role of the stars in generation was attested not only by astrologers and philosophers, but also by physicians.[179]

Oddi used Avicenna's remark that the air, and whatever it was associated with, was among the efficient causes of health and sickness as the peg on which to hang a discourse on the practical usefulness of astrology for the physician. Citing Galen and Ptolemy as his authorities, he reiterated with much supporting detail the medical truisms that the position of the moon in regard to the planets had predictive value for both health and sickness, and that it was essential for a *medicus* to know the nativity (that is, the celestial positions at the time of birth) of his patient before beginning treatment. Oddi also apparently accepted, with reservations, the idea that every individual in a species had a twofold complexion, one of the species and one of the individual alone, and that the latter was the result of "occult dispositions and preparations of matter, occult qualities, celestial influences, and things of this kind."[180]

[179] Da Monte, comm. *Canon* 1.1 (Venice, 1554), fols. 33^r–35^r.

[180] Oddi, comm. *Canon* 1.1 (Venice, 1575), pp. 60–61, on medical astrology; and ". . . duplex est complexio, una quidem insequens formam resultans ex actione et passione primarum qualitatum, sine qua neque forma in materia produci, neque operari possit; et haec in omnibus individuis eiusdam speciei similis secundum speciem existit, in quolibet enim homine est humana complexio; altera vero est complexio materiam insequens, quae non necessaria est pro esse, et operari formae, neque ex qualitatibus manifestis resultat, sed individuum ad determinatas actiones passionesve disponit, ut quod stomachus sanus alleum abhorreat, gignitur autem complexio haec ab occultis dispositionibus, materiaeve praeparationibus, a qualitatibus occultis, ab influentiis coelestibus, et huiusmodi, quae omnia praeter manifestas qualitates ad individui generationem concurrunt, et haec complexio occulta proprietas appellari solet, quam etiam bifariam dividunt; altera qui-

By contrast, Cardano, Paterno, and Costeo, writing between the 1560s and 1580s, gave minimal attention to the subject of celestial influences in their commentaries on the *Canon*. Cardano, who was most certainly a believer—and unlike the other commentators, a notorious practicing astrologer—contented himself with briefly advising his readers of the importance of astrology for medicine and referring them to his own other works.[181] Costeo accepted the general principle of celestial influences and a role for the stars in generation,[182] but rejected specific applications of the idea put forward by medical astrologers; thus, he denied that periods or supposed properties of the planets were directly reflected in the movements and properties of the humors. Costeo pointed out that the celestial bodies acted upon terrestrial beings only by heat (therefore not by coldness, wetness, or dryness), and that the movements of the humors did not have determined periods matching those of the planets supposedly governing them.[183] As for Paterno, he seems to have ignored the whole topic.

On the subject of occult forces in general, Costeo discussed one issue pertaining to the question of whether hidden causes were in operation, working by natural but non-Aristotelian means. This was the question whether the imagination of one person can affect another body; the possibility of such power was used to provide a naturalistic explanation of *fascinatio*, or the evil eye, as well as various other supposed natural phenomena. Costeo showed himself to be evidently uncomfortable

---

dem est in omni eiusdem speciei individuo, ut quod magnes ferrum trahat: altera vero in individuo solo reperitur, de qua superius dictum est. De prima autem egit Averroes existimans quod calor proprius sit habens trahendi proprietatem, ut in medicinis, et Avicenna ait quod ipsius rei propria natura est, et Albertus Alemanus vult quod fit a forma mixti substantiali. Verum complexio materiam insequens forte sequitur ex determinata elementorum commixtione, sicuti de proprietate dicitur, quae omnibus eiusdem speciei individuis convenit." Oddi, comm. *Canon* 1.1 (Venice, 1575), pp. 144–45. The magnet was a standard and frequently repeated example of an occult property acting by specific form; for an example of early fourteenth-century medical discussion, see Siraisi, *Alderotti*, p. 182. Pietro d'Abano, cited by Oddi later in the same passage, had attributed dislike of (or possibly allergies to) particular foods on the part of individual human beings to the stars; see his commentary on the *Problemata* 21.12.

[181] "Inter causas efficientes ponuntur solum res non naturales sumptae a Galeno libro *Artis medicae*. Et de quibus actum est alias. Inter quas causas etiam possunt connumerari coelestes influxus, de quibus hic non agam; sed dicam quod obiici solet, 10 *Contradicentium* 37, scilicet quod medicina non erit scientia perfecta cum indigeat astrologia." Cardano *Opera* (Lyon, 1663), 9:476. Cardano not only commented on Ptolemy's astrological *Quadripartitum* (see n. 158, above), inserting a paean of praise of astrology into the preface, but also prepared and published a collection of horoscopes of eminent people.

[182] Costeo, *Disq. phys.*, pp. 93, 200, 312.

[183] Ibid., pp. 318–19.

with such explanations; he even found it unlikely that a mother's imagination can affect the physical condition of her fetus, despite much folklore and medical tradition to the contrary. And in discussing the hoary supposed example of the victim's corpse that bleeds in the presence of its murderer, the only choice of explanations Costeo was prepared to offer his readers was between miracle, fraud, and accidental emissions of no significance.[184] Paterno and Costeo wrote at a time when astrology still had numerous adherents within the scientific and learned community, and when hidden or insensible causes were often invoked in efforts to supplement and in a few instances go beyond the system of the four elements and their four primary qualities.[185] Nonetheless, there were reasons ortho-

[184] Ibid., pp. 313–16. At pp. 315–16: "Quotidiano experimento constat si in interfecti alicuius hominis praesentiam veniat qui interfecit, moveri ex vulnere aut ex naribus quoque interfecti sanguinem. Id etiam num frequens est in cadaveribus vel e naribus sanguinem, vel excrementa alia, atque etiam crepitus aliunde erumpere. An igitur in his quoque propultricis facultatis ac propterea animae aliquid adhuc superest? Profecto si ex natura quaerenda huius effectus ratio est, quod ex interfecto, praesente interfectore, erumpat sanguis, cogitare licet huius motus causam esse vel in occiso, vel in occisore. An ergo impetus ille est ex cadavere? Quando enim observatio quam proponimus, in iis tantum est qui recenter interfecti sunt non alienum videtur a ratione in ipsis cum calore qui nondum prorsus extinctus sit aliquid et spirituum et irascibilis animae superesse, unde sit ob vindictam spirituum et cum iis sanguinis impetus in adversarium. An contra, haec potius opera est illius qui interfecit, e quo in interfectum irrumpant malefici spiritus, qui tanquam exposcentes si quid relinquum sit vitae quod in eo sanguinis remanet, attractrice vi quandam evocet? At vere, si hic effectus naturae vim sequitur, cur eadem observatio non est in brutis animalibus, quae in iis praesertim, quae iracundia praestant, qualis canis, lupus, leo? Quomodo vero a cadaveris corde cuius omnis vis cum vita extincta est possit in exteriores partes aut spiritus aut sanguis excitari? Aut quo argumento probare aliquis possit inesse spiritibus attractricem vim, quae ab occisore emanans, ex alieno corpore sanguinem alliciat? An hic igitur sanguinis motus supra naturam magis est quam secundum naturam, neque alia huius rei causa est quam divina vis malefici hominis indicatrix et facinorum revelatrix? Nam de quo constat a quo sit interfectus et in iis qui singulari certamine periere, nihil tale aiunt observari. Iam vero quod dehinc sequebatur, nihil habet miri. Corpore enim omnibus animae viribus destituto, et retentrice facultate abolita, coincidentibusque in se ipsos sponte sua meatibus, aut facta eorum a vicinis partibus compressione, levi quavis cadaveris agitatione, nihil difficile est liquidam cuiusque generis substantiam foras exprimi per patentes meatus." A list of other discussions of this supposed phenomenon, extending from the twelfth to the early eighteenth century, is provided in Bert Hansen, "Science and Magic," in *Science in the Middle Ages*, ed. David C. Lindberg (Chicago and London, 1978), pp. 494–95.

[185] Don Cameron Allen, *The Star-Crossed Renaissance* (New York, 1966), pp. 47–100, surveys the continuing debate over astrology in the mid- and later sixteenth and the early seventeenth centuries, and lists a number of learned treatises in its favor. On Renaissance medicine and astrology, with special reference to the views of Da Monte and Santorio, see Wear, "Galen in the Renaissance," pp. 245–56. The strength of the astrological tradition is indicated specifically for the medical milieu in the Veneto in P. Ulvioni,

dox Galenic teachers of medicine—a group that includes, in one way or another, all the commentators under review— should wish, by the latter part of the sixteenth century, to play down the idea of astral and/or occult causes. One factor was probably the endeavor of some neoterics in medicine to overcome the limitations of physiological and therapeutic explanations based on complexional combination by enlarging and developing the role in medicine and physiology of occult qualities, celestial influences, and insensible characteristics peculiar to individual diseases, remedies, or patients. Orthodox Galenists frowned upon precisely the occult and particularistic aspects of neoteric medicine and of the practice of empirics as destructive of reason, system, and *scientia*, and may perhaps as a result have become somewhat less sympathetic to the presence of celestial influences and occult forces within the mainstream medical tradition.[186] Another factor was doubtless the development of those aspects of sixteenth-century science (for example, anatomy) that emphasized the collection and precise recording of data derived from recent and verifiable sense experience. And for Catholic physicians the attack mounted by the Counter-Reformation church on most astrology and all magic certainly also played a part.[187]

All these factors doubtless contributed to the open and explicit attack included by Santorio in his lectures on the *Canon* on celestial influences, prognosticative astrology, occult causes, and belief in magic, although his onslaught must, of course, be related primarily to his other scientific interests, and above all to his demand for measurable physical evi-

"Astrologia, astronomia e medicina nella Repubblica Veneta tra Cinque- e Seicento," *Studi Trentini di scienze storiche* 61 (1982), 1–69.

[186] In the late sixteenth century, the aspects of neoteric medicine referred to were often associated with the influence of Paracelsus. However, they were also characteristic of the ideas of Fernel, whose work, as already noted, aroused a lively and often hostile response in the Italian medical milieu from the 1540s. See Linda Deer Richardson, "The Generation of Disease: Occult Causes and Diseases of the Total Substance," in Wear et al., *Medical Renaissance*, pp. 175–94. On the dislike of sixteenth-century Galenists for explanations of this kind, see Andrew Wear, "Explorations in Renaissance Writings on the Practice of Medicine," in the same book, pp. 140–44, and Zanier, "Ricerche sull'occultismo," p. 18. The issue was social and professional, as well as intellectual, in that academic practitioners feared, with some reason, the rivalry of empirics and neoterics. Ulvioni has drawn attention to a proposal submitted to the Doge, after the disastrous and highly public failure of the Paduan professors Mercuriale and Capodivacca in the plague of 1575–76, for a new medical academy for the study of plague, which would draw upon astrological and spagyric contributions; see Ulvioni, "Astrologia, astronomia," pp. 42–44.

[187] On the impact of the condemnations of judicial astrology by the Council of Trent, and by Sixtus V in 1586, in medical circles in the Veneto, see Ulvioni, "Astrologia, astronomia," esp. pp. 10–15.

dence. Thus some of his most explicit statements about the limitations of reliance on the concept of occult causes in medical explanation occur in a discussion of Fernel's theory that certain diseases should be classified as "of the whole substance" and attributed to occult (and celestial) causes rather than to complexional imbalance. Santorio was prepared to allow that some kinds of disease had qualities that were indeed occult in the sense of being unknowable to sense or intellect simply because they were the result of a complex series of imperceptible changes. However, he followed a long line of predecessors—including Galen himself—in asserting that frequent recourse to occult causes as an explanation was a sign of mental incompetence, since most so-called occult causes were hidden only because of human sloth and superstition.[188]

On the subject of *fascinatio*, Santorio had no reservations or qualifications. He flatly denied that one person's incorporeal *imaginatio* could have any effect at a distance on the bodies of others, and he illustrated this denial with examples drawn from current beliefs about witchcraft and about the accessibility of celestial influences to human manipulation, two concepts he scornfully lumped together. He divided these phenomena into two categories: those that were real, but the result of

---

[188] *Quaestio* 12: "An praeter tres formas morborum propositas ab Avicenna in hoc texto et a Galeni libro De differentiis morborum dentur alia cum Fernelio." Santorio, comm. *Canon* 1.1 (Venice, 1646), cols. 119–28. At cols. 127–28: "Ad primum quando dicebant morbos occultos non reduci ad primas sed ad secundas qualitates. Respondemus reduci ad primas, et ad secundas; sed istas occultas consurgere post infinitas fere alterationes primarum et secundarum qualitatum: hinc fit quod remedia sunt sunt quodam velamine circumsepta et obtenebrata.

"Ad secundum, dum dicebant substantiam nec intellectu cognosci posse, sed sic est quod tales sunt morborum formae pertinentes ad practicam substantiam. Respondemus non solum substandiam, sed etiam qualitates ortas post infinitas alterationes nec sensu nec intellectu cognosci posse.

"Sciendum tamen plurima ab auctoribus referri in qualitates occultas quae tamen sunt apertae. . . . Qui igitur haberet oculos lyn[c]eos videret omnes has qualitates quas vocant substantiales prodire a manifestis. Hinc Galenus iuste damnat illos qui dum nesciunt rerum causas confugiunt ad occultas; tertio enim De praesagiis ex pulsibus contra Erasistratum habet hanc sententiam: 'Qui nihil docent ad alterum de duobus confugiunt, ad qualitates occultas vel ad nomina ignota.'"

Keith Hutchinson, "What Happened to Occult Qualities in the Scientific Revolution?" *Isis* 73 (1982), 233–53, suggests that the repudiation of occult qualities by various seventeenth-century scientists involved just the distinction that Santorio seems to adumbrate here, namely between qualities that were arbitrary and unintelligible and qualities that were merely insensible. The assertion that excessive readiness to resort to the occult as an explanation was a sign of ignorance was, however, also made by some medieval authors. See, for example, Nicole Oresme, *De causis mirabilium*, prologue, lines 1–8, in Bert Hansen, *Nicole Oresme and the Marvels of Nature* (Toronto, 1985), p. 136.

causes both physical and knowable; and those for which the only possible explanation was fraud or credulity. Into the former category Santorio placed damage he thought might be done to children by exposure to the exhalations of old women with infected breath or by contact with cat fur, as well as supposedly mysterious and malign marks on mattresses that were actually harmless stains caused by the accumulation of sweat and children's urine. In the latter category Santorio put spells cast by the evil eye, the supposed harm caused by sticking pins into wax images and burying them under thresholds, the imposture of a monk who pretended to cure a melancholic by feeding him pills containing nails and hair, which were subsequently vomited by the patient and presented by the monk as evidence that his victim had been bewitched (Santorio had caught the monk in the act and denounced him to the Venetian authorities), and the supposed benefits derived from incising astral symbols or images on rings. For Santorio, the only effect that these things could possibly have was through the fear they caused; no one could believe in them who did not want to be deceived, and those who professed belief must be either ignorant or imposters.[189]

[189] *Quaestio* 104: "An imaginatio non solum in proprio corpore, sed etiam extra aliquid efficere valeat." Santorio, comm. *Canon* 1.1 (Venice, 1646), cols. 831–36. At cols. 833–34: "Quo ad fascinationem, nos admittimus mulierem maleficam propter habitum perciniosum [sic], morbo gallico, vel aliquo alio morbo saeviori infectam, inspiciendo tenera puerorum corpora propter pravos halitus qui ex oculis et ex aliis corporis partibus exhalant posse inficere, alterare, et interdum pueros interimere . . . intelligendo fascinari ad halitibus exeuntibus ab aliqua re infecta, et non ab imaginatione. . . .

"Quo ad vomitiones capillorum et clavorum, dicimus haec fieri per imposturam, quam nos semel vidimus et illam sic detegimus. Venetiis quidam monachus profitebatur hominem melancholicum sanare quem dicebat esse fascinatum, deditque septem bolos ad movendum vomitum. Ego unicum surripui, mox aeger evomuit capillos, clavosque perexiguos. Ego interim in bolo quem surripui inveni similes clavos perexiguos et capillos cum antimonio cassia obvolutos. Hanc imposturam aegro et toti familiae ostendi, quod cum monachus intelligeret statim effugit, et a judice istis imposturis destinato vocatus non comparuit; unde ob huius sceleris poenam in perpetuam exilium est delegatus. Quare quod malefici inspectione, verbis, et figuris cereis aculeis transfixis sub limine domus positis, vel alijs figmentis maleficia inserant, est a ratione et experientia ab illis observata qui nolunt decipi omnino alienum; quare inter anilia figmenta haec omnia reponenda.

"Valeant igitur illi, qui in anulos alicui planetae dicatos sub certis zodiaci signis imprimunt figuras, quoniam haec sunt mere figmenta vana et ridicula. Admittendi tamen sunt effectus prodeuntes a causa timorem, vel aliam animi passionem excitante; sicuti quod inspectio maleficae vetulae quae strabos et tortuos oculos habet [sic] incutere possit in infantes aliquem magnum timorem, ob quem in comitialem morbum incidere possint. Eadem ratione ex felium oculis lucentibus credimus infantes perterefieri [sic] et fascinati, et inde praenimio timore alios effectus ita succrescere, ut tandem sequi possit interitus; credimus ex felis respiratione super os infantis infantes saepe interire posse. Tria enim venena in fele observantur, nimirum pili, cerebrum, et aer felis expiratus. Hinc orta est

Santorio's diatribe was overtly directed against naturalistic explanations, based on various kinds of occult cause, of the supposed effects of
witchcraft and astral magic. Religious orthodoxy precluded him from
actually denying that the practices he mentioned could produce real effects through diabolical assistance. But neither did he assert the possibility of such intervention.

Santorio's remarks show considerable independence of spirit, since
they were written at a time when the Venetian Inquisition was much
preoccupied with witchcraft, sorcery, and magic.[190] His views about
these subjects were certainly not necessarily representative of those of
the medical profession as a whole.[191] But his statements probably also
reflect a shared professional concern about the addition of a new category to the various kinds of empirics long feared and scorned by academically trained physicians: exorcists who used physical remedies, as
in the case reported by Santorio. In 1603 or 1604 these characters were
the subject of a complaint by the Venetian College of Physicians, who
bewailed that "there are many men and women, priests as well as religious and laity, who claim to diagnose witchcraft, and on that account

fabula quod lamiae in feles convertantur. . . .

"Reprehendimus illos, qui in culpam morborum perniciosorum trahunt illa quae inve-
niuntur in lectis, quae varia sunt, partim quia a venditorum plumarum in lectos immit-
tuntur ut pondus augeatur, partim quia sudoribus et puerorum mictu plurima conglo-
bantur et inde accipiunt varias figurae quae nihil mali efficere possunt."

[190] The activities of the Inquisition of Venice in the period 1550–1670 are summarized
in Brian Pullan, *The Jews of Europe and the Inquisition of Venice, 1550–1670* (Totowa, N.J.,
1983), pp. 8–11. Preoccupation with witchcraft began in about the 1580s, and accounts
for roughly half of the surviving records of seventeenth-century prosecutions.

[191] For example, Andrea Cesalpino in his *Daemonum investigatio peripatetica*, written in
response to a request from the bishop of Pisa for expert opinions from the university
medical faculty, expressed the conviction that the obsessions and convulsions experienced by some nuns at Pisa were undoubtedly caused by diabolical possession; this work
is printed with Cesalpino's *Quaestionum peripateticarum libri V* (Venice, 1593), at fols.
145r–168v, and is discussed in Paola Zambelli, "Scienza, filosofia, religione nella Toscana
di Cosimo I," in *Florence and Venice: Comparisons and Relations. II. Cinquecento* (Florence,
1980), pp. 3–52. Similarly, Zanier, *Medicina e filosofia*, pp. 34–36, draws attention to the
enthusiastic demonology, in Counter-Reformation Spain, of the physician Francisco
Vallés. The suggestion that the beginnings of the breakup of the old medical synthesis
may actually have stimulated beliefs, among medical men as among others, in witch-
caused illnesses is put forward in Leland L. Estes, "The Medical Origins of the European
Witch Craze: A Hypothesis," *Journal of Social History* 17 (1983), 271–84. In addition, hostility of medical men to folk healers, especially women, to whom magical practices were
attributed, has been suggested by various recent authors as at least a contributory factor
in the spread of witchcraft persecution. Possibly Santorio's attitude may reflect a continuing influence of Pietro Pomponazzi's demonstration that Aristotelian naturalism and ra-
tionalism could not be used to support belief in demons (see Zambelli, "Scienza, filosofia, religione," pp. 8–9).

they draw blood and give medicines by mouth that are so effective and strong that usually instead of driving out devils they drive out the soul."[192]

Santorio's assault on astrology was appended to the same passage of the *Canon* that Oddi had used as the locus for its defense.[193] The onslaught was thoroughgoing; its virulence was at least partially inspired by an astrologizing physician who had been unwise enough to attack the theory of *medicina statica*. Santorio devoted several pages to an ad hominem diatribe detailing his opponent's moral failings, family troubles, and professional and financial failures and errors of judgment, always repeating the theme that a successful astrologer would have predicted and hence avoided these things, so that either the claims of astrology were futile or this practitioner incompetent.

Santorio's more general arguments against astrology incorporated little that was new. As he himself remarked, the issue had frequently been debated since the time of Pico della Mirandola, and most of the arguments on either side had long since been marshaled. Essentially, he maintained that the only way any of the heavenly bodies affect things on earth is by light, heat, and motion. Hence astrology was predicated on false principles as well as being condemned by the church. The various classical and Christian authors usually cited as having endorsed astrology were either really writing about astronomy or meteorology or, in the case of the fathers, were perhaps mistaken about areas in which they had no professional expertise: thus Lactantius had wrongly denied the earth to be a sphere. It was true that Saint Thomas had said that when someone is born his whole life can be prognosticated, but he was speaking of the effect of the light of the heavens on infancy, which can affect the whole life; in any case, however, "who can know the quantity of virtue of the temperament, I will not say of the heavens, but of the stomach, liver, and other viscera."[194] The claim of astrologers that experience offers proof of the validity of their art is specious, since they are quick to claim credit for any chance successes in prediction and equally quick to explain away failures as the result of the power of free

[192] "Sono molti huomini et donne, cosi preti come frati e seculari, che danno a creder di segnar strigarie, et per ciò cavano sangue et danno per bocca medicamenti cosi efficaci et gagliardi che per il più invece di cacciar diavoli cacciano l'anima." Document of 1603 or 1604, quoted in Ulvioni, "Astrologia, astronomia," pp. 36–37.

[193] *Quaestio* 11: "Quid intelligat Avicenna per illud quod advectitur aeri: in qua ostenditur non dari influentias et falsam esse astrologiam divinatricem." Santorio, comm. *Canon* 1.1 (Venice, 1646), cols. 102–18.

[194] Ibid., cols. 103–7. At col. 106: "sed quis est ille qui quantitatem virtutis temperamenti, non dicam coeli, sed stomachi, hepatis, et aliorum viscerum possit dignoscere?"

will to overcome the stars or an insufficiently known nativity; hence the appeal to experience is really only to chance and guesswork. Santorio particularly objected to the notion that the heavens could be malign—and pointed out that if this were so, animals as well as men would be affected. (Meat animals, said Santorio, must be under a favorable sign in Lent!)

In addition to reiterating these mostly standard arguments against occult celestial influences (arguments to which, he admitted, true believers in astrology were absolutely impervious), Santorio also attempted to devise a physical demonstration that would show his students that even the physical effects on the earth of any heavenly body other than the sun were extremely small. On numerous occasions Santorio invited his students to compare first the effect of the supposed heat of moonlight on one of his thermoscopes and then, at noon on the following day, that of the sun on the same instrument.[195] (Presumably this demonstration experiment, which required two trips outside the classroom, one of them at night, was actually incorporated into the course on the *Canon*.) Santorio's lectures on *Canon* I.1 must surely have made some contribution to the marginalization of astrology within the world of academic medicine.

The Human Soul

Like earlier products of university medicine in the same genre, the set of commentaries with which we are here concerned is overwhelmingly secular in content. However, commentary on the parts of *Canon* I.1 that were concerned with complexion, or temperaments, and with the

[195] "Quando vero dixit Plato aliquas stellas frigus et aliquas calorem inducere, per frigus intelligit calorem infra moderatum, quia lumen stellarum semper repercutiendo ipsam terram calefacit. Quod vero lumen lunae calefaciat fortasse multi sciunt; sed quantum, et qua proportione ad solem lumen lunae calefaciat, ante me (quod sciam) non fuit cognitum, quia instrumentis a nobis inventis id adinvenimus: ostendimusque magna scholarium frequentia, existente plenilunio, horo secunda noctis circiter, quantum et qua proportione ad solem lumen lunae calefaciat, sicque facimus. Accipimus speculum concavum amplum ex vitro, quod est apud nos, et in plenilunio e diametro colligimus lunae radios; deinde curamus ut cuspis illius luminis sp[l]endidissima tangat verticem vitri quo dimetimur temperamenta; tunc spatio decem pulsationum nostri pulsilogii aqua descendit per duos gradus; causa descensus est quia illud lumen rarefacit aerem qui rarefactus occupat maiorem locum, quod fit aquam deorsum impellendo. Deinde die sequenti eodem modo accipimus cuspidem solis existentis in meridie, quae cuspis adurens percutiens cuspidatim eiusdem vitri verticem per duas pulsationes eiusdem pulsilogii, statim velocissimo cursu aqua descendit per centum et decem gradus; tuncque statim intelligimus quantum et qua proportione respectu solis, luna calefaciat." Ibid., cols. 107–8. The description is accompanied by a diagram at cols. 109–10.

faculties or virtues involved concepts widely assumed to have impli-cations for the understanding of the human soul, and hence brought the commentator near issues that were theologically as well as philosoph-ically sensitive. A review of the successive treatments of one such issue suggests a process whereby such topics were more and more excluded from lectures on medical theory, serious philosophical interest being replaced over the course of the sixteenth century by brief statements consonant with religious orthodoxy but expressed in philosophical terms. The single example is provided by one aspect of Avicenna's def-inition "Complexio est qualitas." This definition, in addition to sug-gesting a range of problems about the physical nature of mixtures and compounds (exhaustively treated by the commentators) also provoked inquiry as to whether complexion, or temperament, was a substance or an accident. If the former, complexion was presumably to be identified with substantial form; but religious orthodoxy maintained that the soul constituted the single substantial form of each human being. Hence, the identification of complexion and substantial form was theologically unacceptable, since it suggested a material origin (and temporal end) for the human soul, a view sometimes ascribed to Galen.[196]

Da Monte tackled the relationship between substantial form and complexion with evident interest, at considerable length, and in a man-ner that once again revealed his ties with the Italian Aristotelianism of the early part of the century, and perhaps especially with the notorious ideas about the mortality of the soul put forward by Pomponazzi. Ac-cording to Da Monte, the subject was of the first importance, although so difficult that "great men get stuck in it." He attributed the view that temperament and substantial form are distinct to "the Arabs and more recent Latin writers," while maintaining that Hippocrates, Galen, "and perhaps Aristotle himself" had held temperament and substantial form to be identical—a somewhat hypothetical judgment as regards Hip-

---

[196] *Canon* 1.1.3.1 (Venice, 1507), fol. 2ʳ. A materialist view of the soul was ascribed to Galen largely on the basis of his treatise *Quod animi mores corporis temperamenta sequuntur* (in his *Scripta minora*, ed. J. Marquardt, I. Müller, G. Helmreich, 3 vols. [Leipzig, 1884–93], 2:32–79). On Galen's actual views and the broader ramifications of the sixteenth-century debate about them, see Moraux, "Galien comme philosophe," and Temkin, *Galenism*, pp. 85, 144–46; also Luis Garcia Ballester, "Lo médico y lo filosófico-moral en las relaciones entre alma y enfermedad: el pensamiento de Galeno," *Asclepio* 20 (1968), 99–134. Galen's views on the soul still interested William Harvey; see Vivian Nutton, "Harvey, Goulston and Galen," *Koroth* 8 (1985), 112–22. The position that the soul is the one and only substantial form of man was that of Thomas Aquinas. For an example of medieval medical discussion of the relation between substantial form and *complexio* in human beings, see Siraisi, *Alderotti*, pp. 160–62.

pocrates as well as Aristotle.[197] After reviewing various arguments pro
and con, Da Monte concluded: "If I want to be a philosopher, and to
adhere to the principles of philosophy, but not of faith, I cannot not
assent to Hippocrates or Galen. But if I want to put on a theological
form (as we certainly ought to do) it should be said that the opinion of
the Arabs is true." At this point the reader may recall Da Monte's expressed opinion, just a few pages earlier, of the relative merits of most
of the Arabs and of the Greeks. Da Monte went on:

But this, as it is true in itself [that is, that soul and *temperatura* are
separate] should be believed in the same way, without any demonstration. Because there is nothing worse than to seek to prove
by demonstrations what ought to be held by faith. Because we
should rather give thanks to God because He has illuminated our
intelligence so that it knows those things which cannot be perceived by any natural means; and the Lord ought to be asked to
increase credulity in us. And certainly in this Scotus behaved out-
standingly. For when he grasped that the soul, according to natural science and the Peripatetics, is mortal (in his commentary on
the *Sentences* IV, question 41 or 43), he turned as a poet to the Lord
and gave Him thanks because he knew by divine illumination that
to be most true which naturally seemed to be false. But because we
are now in the schools, let us acknowledge ourselves to be philosophers and *medici*; therefore we defend the opinion of Galen and
Hippocrates on the basis of the principles of philosophy.[198]

[197] Da Monte, comm. *Canon* I.I (Venice, 1554), fols. 57ᵛ–61ᵛ; at fol. 58ʳ⁻ᵛ: "Est alia
difficultas longe maior, utrum temperatura sit tantum accidens, an sit forma substan-
tialis, et in hac questione haerent maximi viri. . . . Duae sunt opiniones summorum virorum, prima est Arabum et Latinorum recentiorum, qui credunt nullo modo formam
substantialem esse temperaturam, sed temperaturam primam solum dispositionem ad
formam substantialem, in qua sententia fuit Avicenna in libro *De anima*, parte prima,
cap. primo, et Albertus secundo *De generatione*, tract. secundo, cap. 15. In parte opposita
est Hippocrates et Galenus et fortassis etiam Aristoteles."

[198] "Hic modo quid sit determinandum, si me rogetis, possum respondere dupliciter
secundum duplicem formam quam possum induere. Si velim esse philosophus et stare in
principiis philosophiae, non in fide, non possum non Hippocrate et Galeno assentire; at
si formam theologicam volumus induere, quod certe debemus facere, dicendum est
opinonem Arabum esse veram. Sed hoc ut est re ipsa verum, ita credi debet sine ulla demonstratione. Nam nihil peius est quam quaerere demonstrationibus probare quod fide
tenendum est, quia potius sunt agendae gratiae Deo qui intellectum nostrum illuminavit
ut ea sciret quae nullo medio naturali percipi possunt, et rogemus Dominum augeat cre-
dulitatem in nobis. Et certe in hoc Scotus valde egregie se gessit, qui cum tenuisset animam in via naturali et peripatetica mortalem esse in quarto libro *Sententiarum*, quaest. 41
vel 43, postea conversus ad Dominum ait illi gratias quia id cognovisset illuminatione

Among the other commentators, it appears that only the otherwise intellectually unenterprising Paterno was interested in exploring the range of philosophical views about the soul. In a brief and self-acknowledged digression inserted into his discussion of nutritive and generative faculties, Paterno explained to his readers that Aristotle, as interpreted by Alexander of Aphrodisias, had taught the existence of a separate agent intellect that alone was incorruptible and immortal, and was distinct from the rational soul that makes man what he is, and a corruptible passive intellect, which, in Paterno's view, these authors had intended to identify with the rational soul.[199] Santorio believed that Paterno had actually adopted these views as his own.[200] Elsewhere, however, Paterno gave an at least partially sympathetic account of Plato's concept of soul, in which he stressed the immortality of man's rational soul.[201] Paterno's own expressed position was that it was the task of a commentator to expound the actual opinions of ancient authors, and not to doctor them into line with theological orthodoxy: "Unless we want to torture Aristotle's words so that we can make him into a theologian and a Christian, it is necessary not to depart by a nail's breadth from the things that were handed down by Alexander."[202]

---

divina esse verissimum, quod naturalem falsum videbatur.

"Sed quia nunc in scholis profitemur nos philosophos et medicos, ex principiis philosophiae defendimus opinio Galeni et Hippocratis, quia nihil est deterius arbitror quam miscere philosophiam theologiae." Ibid., fols. 59ᵛ–60ʳ. The view that the soul is mortal according to philosophy was condemned in a bull of Pope Leo X in 1513 in the context of the controversy over Pomponazzi's views on the soul. See Lohr, in *Renaissance Quarterly* 33 (1980), 646, s.v. Pomponatius.

[199] "Ex quibus manifeste apparet Galenum existimasse mentem quandam a coelo prodire, a qua cuncta reguntur et gubernantur. . . . Quam mentem cum quae ab Alexandro Aphrodiseo de intellectu agente tradita sunt, cum iis quae a Galeno dicuntur confero, mihi videor videre eandem cum intellectu agente Alexandro esse. Quinimo eam, quam Aristoteles solum extrinsecus accedere dixit, separata ab eodem ab anima rationali, qua hominem, hominem esse dixit. . . . Et paulo post, separatum hoc solum esse, tanquam perpetuum a corruptibili, et hoc solum immortale, et perpetuum esse. Idque impassibile esse. Passivum vero intellectum corrumpi. At quem passivum intellectum intelligit? Quem alium, per Deum immortalem, intelligere potest, nisi eum quem paulo superius agenti opposuit. Ut nisi verba Aristotelis extorquere velimus, ut ipsum theologum et Christianum faciamus, oportet ne latum unguem ab iis recedere quae ab Alexandro tradita sunt." Paterno, comm. *Canon* 1.1 (Venice, 1596), fols. 130ᵛ–131ʳ.

[200] "Bernardinus Paternus praeceptor noster putabat formatricem membrorum esse mentem a Caelo pendentem, esseque intellectum agentum secundum Alexandrum Aphrodiseum, se sic est, quod Alexander putabat intellectum agentum esse Deum ipsum." Santorio, comm. *Canon* 1.1 (Venice, 1646), col. 993.

[201] Paterno, comm. *Canon* 1.1 (Venice, 1596), fols. 145ʳ–47ᵛ (the first of a set of *quaestiones* appended to his commentary).

[202] See the final sentence of n. 199, above.

From Da Monte and Paterno one certainly gets the impression of some penetration of the medical faculty by ideas and attitudes associated with the Aristotelian naturalism of the Paduan philosophical school.

Despite his interest in the subject of the soul, Paterno dealt briefly and evasively with the issue of complexion and the soul when he came to expound Avicenna's definition of the former. He suggested that Avicenna's formulation was deliberately ambiguous in order to avoid open controversy with Galen, and proposed semantic reconciliation.[203] The remaining commentators simply inserted brief denials that complexion, or temperament, was identical with substantial form or with the soul, and (except in the case of Cardano) brief defenses of Galen against the accusation of having taught such a doctrine, at any rate in the form in which it was usually understood. The most prolix on the issue was Costeo, who waxed rhetorically indignant against the *recentiores* who espoused the "false, not to say impious" doctrine of the identity of temperament and substantial form and ascribed it, incorrectly in his view, to Galen and Aristotle. Costeo invited his readers to consider the undesirable consequences of this doctrine as regards the nature of humanity, namely that noble souls were formed from vile elements and subject to corruption. But he also rejected the doctrine as absurd because it seemed to him to entail a form of panvitalism; if everything that had temperament must be considered as having a soul, then this would include stones and corpses, an objection echoed by Santorio.[204]

In the early seventeenth century, as a hundred years earlier, the teaching of medical *theoria* from the *Canon* of Avicenna in the Italian universities is properly described as scholastic and as incorporating a good deal of natural philosophical content that did not directly pertain to medicine. Nevertheless, the various treatments of the relation of the concepts soul and complexion, no less than the other topics surveyed above, suggest that changes in the focus and goals of the natural philosophy taught as part of medical *theoria* had taken place between the time of Da Monte and the time of Santorio. These changes affected only small parts of rambling commentaries, but they are sufficient to suggest that in this period academic instruction in medical *theoria* was likely to reflect considerable awareness of the contemporary philosophical and scientific milieu. Can the same be said as regards contemporary medicine, physiology, and anatomy?

---

[203] Ibid., fol. 27^{r-v}.

[204] Oddo, comm. *Canon* 1.1 (Venice, 1575), p. 110; Cardano, *Opera* (Lyon, 1663), 9:507–8; Costeo, *Disq. phys.*, pp. 110–14; Santorio, comm. *Canon* 1.1 (Venice, 1646), cols. 240–41.

8

Canon 1.1 and Renaissance Physiology

Commentators on the *Canon*, like other sixteenth- and early seventeenth-century physicians, confronted not only eclecticism and innovation in areas of natural philosophy of little immediate relevance to medicine, but also major currents of change within their own discipline. Despite the weight of authority of the Galenic medical system throughout the sixteenth and into the seventeenth century, substantial critiques of the content of traditional medicine began to emerge within the academic medical community well before 1550. No new information or approach was as yet powerful enough in itself to lead to any widespread abandonment in academic medical circles of the Galenic physiological synthesis, but the process that was ultimately to revolutionize the content of medicine and allied sciences was unquestionably initiated.

The sixteenth century produced three types of implicit or explicit critique of Galenic doctrine that became particularly significant for the teaching of theoretical physiology in the northern Italian universities. The first of these was the continuation and intensification of the long-standing debates over the differences between Aristotelian and Galenic physiology. As Bylebyl has pointed out, the discussion of standard *differentiae* between the two authorities, long a school exercise in techniques of textual harmonization and dialectical disputation or reconciliation, began to take on new and sometimes more genuinely controversial dimensions, influenced by readings of ancient texts and a nascent experimentalism. Such discussions were perpetuated and expanded by the vigorous partisans in the sixteenth-century Italian schools (notably Padua) of Aristotelian natural philosophy and Galenic medicine.[1] A second development was the endeavor of Jean Fernel to revise large areas of physiological and pathological theory. Fernel retained a great deal that was traditional, and his departures from tradition often took the form of speculative reworkings, based more on eclectic use of ancient sources than on new data or methodology.

[1] Jerome J. Bylebyl, "Disputation and Description in the Renaissance Pulse Controversy," in Wear et al., *Medical Renaissance*, pp. 223–24.

Nevertheless, his *Physiologia*, which as already noted was early disseminated in Italy, was widely regarded as both radically innovative and a serious threat to traditional *theoria*. Apart from anything else, Fernel's work clearly constituted a potential alternative to *Canon* I.I as a textbook. And third, the original and widely celebrated achievements of anatomists working in the Italian schools involved the accumulation of data and the introduction of techniques unknown or in opposition to Galen.[2] The resultant controversies drew in teachers of physiological *theoria* as well as working anatomists and teachers of *practica*, for the areas of knowledge embraced by anatomy and physiology often overlapped.

Given this environment, it comes as no surprise to find that the same group of commentators analyzed in the last chapter also displayed an ability to recognize, discuss, and occasionally accommodate innovation with a generally Galenic medical system. However, while certain crucial passages allow one to trace interactions between "old" and "new" medicine, it must be emphasized that medical innovation and controversy were never the main thrust of the commentary per se. Whether critical or appreciative of Avicenna, Renaissance interpreters took as their main task the explanation of physiology according to his organization and in the light of Galen. Moreover, their attention to Avicenna's own views was in every case greater in the exposition of the specifically physiological *doctrinae* than in the more philosophical sections, where the emphasis was often on Aristotle rather than Avicenna.

[2] On Fernel's thought and influence, see Charles Sherrington, *The Endeavor of Jean Fernel* (Cambridge, 1946); Jacques Roger, *Jean Fernel et les problèmes de la médecine de la Renaissance*, Les Conférences du Palais de la Découverte, ser. D, no. 70 (Paris, 1960); Linda Deer Richardson, "The Generation of Disease," pp. 175–94, 326–30, and also, as Linda A. Deer, "Academic Theories of Generation in the Renaissance: The Contemporaries and Successors of Jean Fernel (1497–1558)" (Ph.D. diss., Warburg Institute, University of London, 1980); D. P. Walker, "The Astral Body in Renaissance Medicine," *Journal of the Warburg and Courtauld Institutes* 21 (1958), 119–33; James J. Bono, "The Languages of Life: Jean Fernel (1497–1558) and Spiritus in Pre-Harveian Bio-Medical Thought" (Ph.D. diss., Harvard University, 1981). On the response at Padua to Fernel from the standpoint of curricular reform, see Chapter 4, above. Fernel's works competed very successfully in the academic marketplace; according to Roger, *Fernel*, p. 6, ninety-seven editions or translations of his *Medicina*, or *Universa medicina*, were published between 1554 and 1680. I do not attempt to assemble here the scattered bibliography on sixteenth-century Italian anatomy. Ongaro, "La medicina nello Studio di Padova," summarizes developments at Padua in the first half of the century, and a revisionist view of late sixteenth-century Paduan anatomy is presented in Andrew Cunningham, "Fabricius and the 'Aristotle Project' in Anatomical Teaching and Research at Padua," in Wear et al., *Medical Renaissance*, pp. 195–222.

Hence the views of the moderns were only one among many considerations to be taken into account.

Once again four themes recurring in the commentaries will be surveyed, these four chosen for the clues they yield to the essential nature of Renaissance physiological instruction based on the *Canon*. These are, first, the commentators' handling of the central and interlocking Galenic doctrines of temperament and the humors; second, the relation of Aristotelian and Galenic elements in their work, exemplified in their treatment of the issue of the primacy of the heart; third, their response to the central focus of modernism in Renaissance medicine, namely innovative anatomy; and fourth, the way in which they presented ancient and contemporary theories of disease (although in the commentaries under discussion this last subject is accorded extended consideration only in Da Monte's exposition of *Canon* 1.2).

Temperatura and the Humors

The theory of complexio or temperament treated in *Canon* 1.1.3 fulfilled useful functions for medieval and Renaissance physicians. It provided a broad and flexible concept with which to organize medical theory and interpret medical experience; it served as a bridge between theory and practice; and it bolstered the claim of medicine to be based on rational and universal principles. In addition, of course, it was supported by a long tradition of authoritative exposition, extending from Galen himself to Avicenna's notable reinforcement of the theory in the *Canon*, and its subsequent elaboration by Latin scholastic physicians. As a result, the entire system of ideas relating to temperament retained its grip on medical thought until well after the end of the sixteenth century. For example, Santorio was no more willing than Da Monte to abandon temperament as an explanatory principle, or to abbreviate discussion of the topic in any significant way. The new nomenclature that replaced the term *complexio* with *temperatura* or *temperamentum* marked no break in continuity of content. Yet Da Monte's claim that *temperatura* expressed much better than *complexio* the idea of the emergence of a new form from the mixture of qualities makes it seem likely that the change was intended and perceived as a manifesto of detachment from the earlier Arabo-Latin tradition.[3] And despite the weight

---

[3] Da Monte, comm. *Canon* 1.1 (Venice, 1554), fol. 55ᵛ: "dicitur aliquid temperari quando ex duobus vel pluribus commixtis et temperatis resultat tertium habens diversam formam temperatis extremis, ideo longe melius utemini hoc nomine temperatura, quia indicat vobis essentiam ipsius rei." *Temperatura* or *temperamentum* was the preferred usage of all the Renaissance commentators on the *Canon* discussed in this volume, except for

of tradition, the substance of teaching about temperament also shows some signs of penetration by nontraditional ideas, data, and sources.

Sets of lectures on temperament based on the *Canon* fell naturally into two different parts, basic principles and specifics. The latter included temperament and disease; how temperament should be estimated; the separate temperaments ascribed to various parts of the body; and the effects on temperament of age, sex, climate, and so on. In all the commentaries, explanations of the fundamentals of temperament continued to engender highly speculative philosophical discourse. For example, Da Monte noted with enthusiasm that the definition of temperament contained "very beautiful difficulties badly handled by the moderns"—by whom he meant Latin scholastics.[4] Da Monte's interest in the role of the heavenly bodies in determining temperament and the relationship of temperament, substantial form, and the soul has already been noted. Although others did not always share his consuming interest in this range of topics, they used the introductory lectures on temperament to expand upon other equally speculative problems about it: whether temperament was an accidental or an essential quality, how the mixture of qualities making it up should be interpreted, whether it should be regarded as a fifth quality distinct from the primary four, and whether and how the primary qualities continue to exist once it has been formed.[5] The antecedents of these disquisitions reach back to thirteenth-century scholastic debates on the subject of mixtures, as Santorio was aware when he appended to his exposition of Avicenna's definition of *complexio* a *quaestio*, "Whether the forms and qualities of the elements remain in a mixture," in which he announced his own adherence to the views of Thomas Aquinas and Scotus.[6]

Oddo Oddi, who seems to have hesitated between *complexio* and *temperatura*. *Complexio* was the universal terminology of late medieval Latin medical writers. On the history of the term, see Danielle Jacquart, "De *crasis* à *complexio*: Note sur le vocabulaire du tempérament en Latin médiéval," Centre Jean Palerme, Memoires 5, *Textes médicaux latins antiques*, ed. G. Sabbah (Saint-Etienne, 1984), pp. 71–75.

[4] ". . . in hac definitione sunt pulcherrimae difficultates male a modernis tractatae." Da Monte, comm. *Canon* 1.1 (Venice, 1554), fol. 55r.

[5] See Oddi, comm. *Canon* 1.1 (Venice, 1575), pp. 99–115; Cardano, *Opera* (Lyon, 1663), 9:507–14; Paterno, comm. *Canon* 1.1 (Venice, 1596), fols. 27–29r; Costeo, *Disq. phys.*, pp. 101–17; Santorio, comm. *Canon* 1.1 (Venice, 1646), cols. 228–70.

[6] "An formae elementorum et eorum qualitates maneant in mixto." Santorio, comm. *Canon* 1.1 (Venice, 1646), *Quaestio* 30, cols. 255–60. On the medieval discussions of elements in a mixture, see Annaliese Maier, *An der Grenze von Scholastik und Naturwissenschaft: Die Struktur der materiellen Substanz, das Problem der Gravitation, die Mathematik der Formlatituden* (Rome, 1952), pp. 1–88.

In the middle years of the sixteenth century, however, two fresh developments provided a further stimulus for attention to these and similar topics. The first was the reception of the *De mixtione* of Alexander of Aphrodisias, which provided a comparison and analysis of atomist, Stoic, and Aristotelian views on juxtaposition, mixtures, and blending. The review of Avicenna's definition in the light of *De mixtione* seems to have begun with Oddo Oddi. His source was presumably the Aldine edition of the Greek text published in 1527, although it seems likely that he also knew one or both of the Latin translations made in the Veneto in the 1540s.[7] Oddi's pupil, Andrea Graziolo, in the scholia to his translation of *Canon* 1 (1580), Costeo, and Santorio all drew on *De mixtione* for their discussion of the fundamentals of complexion theory.[8]

The second event to inject a new stimulus into discussions of complexion theory was the publication of Fernel's *De naturali parte medicinae* (1542), subsequently reissued as the *Physiologia* section of his *Universa medicina* (1554). Fernel's tendency to restrict the role of complexion theory in physiology and pathology and to emphasize the importance of *spiritus*, innate heat, and idiosyncratic or individual factors was rightly perceived by orthodox Galenists as undermining the claims of their medicine to be a rational science based on the analysis of qualitative or complexional balance. Furthermore, Fernel had sharply and explicitly attacked Avicenna's definition of *complexio*, terming it "absurd" and referring to the "feeble minds" of those who accepted it. Fernel objected to calling temperament a quality, since this implied that a separate, fifth quality emerged from the primary four; and he also objected to the associated idea that the four qualities ceased to exist in their original mode once complexion had come into being.[9] (Like many of Fernel's other positions, this one was not without antecedents in scholastic medicine; for example, Giacomo da Forlì had noted around 1400 that "it can probably be held that *complexio* is not any quality distinct

---

[7] On this work and its reception see the previous chapter. Oddi's discussion is found in Oddi, comm. *Canon* 1.1 (Venice, 1575), pp. 99–100.

[8] *Canon* 1, ed. Graziolo (Venice, 1580), fols. 13ᵛ–14ʳ; Costeo, *Disq. phys.*, p. 102; Santorio, comm. *Canon* 1.1 (Venice, 1646), cols. 229–30.

[9] "Hanc temperamenti rationem cum minime perspiceret, nec satis animo complecteretur Avicennas, subabsurdam commentus est definitionem: qua primarum qualitatum effectione mutua, quintam qualitatem eamque simplicem emergere confirmat. . . . Itaque novam illam qualitatem pro temperamento invehere, cum vanitas quaedam sit opinionis, quae multorum animos imbecilles diu multumque vexavit, nos clarissimorum philosophorum imitatione ut elementorum substantias, sic omnino et qualitates in composito teneri fatemur ex harumque perfusione et concentu temperamentum consistere." Fernel, *Physiologiae libri VII*, 3.1, in his *Medicina* (Lyon, 1581), p. 56.

from the whole aggregate of the primary qualities," although Giacomo himself thought it more probable and more consonant with reason to hold that *complexio* did constitute such a distinct quality.)[10] Accordingly, Graziolo, Costeo, and Santorio all undertook the dissection and repudiation of these opinions of Fernel in their scholia and commentaries on *Canon* 1.1.3.[11]

Although the treatments in the commentaries of the fundamental definition of *temperatura* thus do reflect current concerns and are in part based on sources that are in some sense new, in essentials these analyses clearly belong to the same genre as their medieval predecessors. In both, a physiological concept is discussed not in terms of any generalizations, however arbitrary, from clinical or other physical experience, but on the basis of philosophical reasoning about processes of mixture, which were by definition supposed to be imperceptible to sense. It is thus hard to imagine any conceivable physical evidence that would be held to invalidate any of the arguments presented.

When it came to more specific areas of complexion theory, even the scholastic discussions to be found in fourteenth- and fifteenth-century commentaries on *Canon* 1.1 were always to some extent oriented toward physical experience. It would therefore be wrong to suggest that evidence of attention to such experience in the corresponding sections of the Renaissance works necessarily implies the penetration of changing scientific ideas into lectures on medical *theoria*. Nonetheless, in different ways, three of the six commentaries under review—those of Cardano, Costeo, and Santorio—reveal the development of approaches to teaching this part of complexion theory, which shifted the emphasis somewhat toward the questioning of medical truisms, toward a demand for concrete evidence, and toward the test of personal or recent experience.

Cardano indeed cast doubt on the very basis of the claim that a knowledge of complexion theory was necessary to medical practice, and hence an essential part of medical education, since he was highly skeptical of Galen's own contention that temperament could be de-

---

[10] ". . . probabiliter teneri potest complexionem non esse qualitatem aliquam distinctam a toto aggregato ex primis qualitatibus taliter refractis. Patet quia quascunque operationes attribuimus complexioni si esset simplex qualitas attribuere possumus huic toto aggregato . . . probabilius et rationi magis consonum est complexionem mixti saltem perfecti esse qualitatem secundam simplicem specifice distinctam a quacunque qualitatum primarum que tamen qualitates primas in virtute sua activa continet." Giacomo da Forlì (Jacobus Forliviensis), comm. and *quaestiones* on *Canon* 1.1 (and 1.2) (Venice, 1508), fol. 173ᵛ.

[11] *Canon* 1, ed. Graziolo (Venice, 1580), fols. 13ᵛ–14ʳ; Costeo, *Disq. phys.*, pp. 194–98; Santorio, comm. *Canon* 1.1 (Venice, 1646), cols. 224–50.

tected by touch. In the first place, Cardano pointed out that touch was not in fact the only way in which physicians reached their judgments about a patient's temperament.[12] He scarcely deserves credit for a new insight here, for he drew attention to a passage of Gentile da Foligno's commentary on the *Canon* in which Gentile had noted that although physicians were wont to claim that complexion was known by touch, in reality the differences in complexion ascribed to different parts of the body could not be felt, since *complexio influens* was not found in dead bodies, and in living bodies nominally cold parts felt warm. Gentile went on to remark that physicians actually also determined complexion by three other means, namely the *via syllogistica*, citations of authorities, and what Gentile called the *via experimentalis*. As an example of the last, he offered the assertion that the brain must be cold because it is watery and earthy; it must be watery and earthy because when watery parts have evaporated—presumably in a dead body—solid (hence earthy) residue remains.[13]

Cardano's solution to the problem of the imperceptibility of the variations in temperament between the different parts of the body was no advance on Gentile: Cardano suggested that, for example, among supposedly cold parts, the teeth although not on their surface cold to the touch in a living body were nonetheless colder than other parts and internally cold.[14] However, in another passage Cardano manifested a general skepticism, truly radical in its implications for traditional therapy, about the possibility of using touch to detect the complexional norm of any individual patient. He pointed out that the most celebrated physicians after frequent visits over a long period of time were often unable to agree about a patient's temperament; that the sick often—indeed more frequently—recovered when treated by unskilled people who paid no attention to temperament; and that it was in any case sufficient for a physician to know the cause and severity of the disease, which could be determined from the nature of the patient's incapacity without any attention to temperament. And in an early example of the practice of criticizing Galen on the basis of a supposed truly Hippocratic medicine, he added as a clinching argument that Hippocrates had laid little emphasis on the entire concept of temperament.[15]

---

[12] Cardano, *Opera* (Lyon, 1663), 9:537.

[13] Gentile da Foligno, comm. *Canon* 1 and 2 (Pavia, 1510–11), 1.1.3.1, *dubium* 4, fol. 22ʳ.

[14] Cardano, *Opera* (Lyon, 1663), 9:537.

[15] "In universum magna incidit dubitatio circa temperaturae cognitionem, quam adeo extulit Galenus *Primo ad Glauconem*, ut velit medium non esse medium, nisi propriam temperaturae mensuram non solum qualitatem cognoverit, et licet tacta sit supra et in *Tertio contradicentium*, dico tamen quod multa huic opponantur; nam nunquam primum,

Unlike Cardano, Costeo strongly defended the traditional role ascribed in medical practice to temperament. In an attack on Fernel's notion that it was not modified by changes in the humors, but was more like a kind of permanent constitution peculiar to each individual, Costeo protested, in words that express very well the centrality of the concept of temperament to the entire traditional medical system: "But if it is true, Oh most learned Fernel, that the temperament of the parts is not changed by variations in the humors, to what end was such diligent study instituted by physicians for the regulation of diet? Who will hope to use cold things to bring back bodies that are too hot, hot things to bring bodies that are too cold, dry things to bring bodies that are too moist, moist things to bring bodies that are too dry back to a state of moderation?"[16]

Yet in at least one instance, Costeo showed that he was just as capable as Cardano of skepticism about the evidential basis for venerable truisms. Although medical and Renaissance physicians devoted interminable debate to *quaestiones* relating to the supposed complexional differences between the sexes, very few of them failed in the end to endorse the proposition that in general the temperament of women was colder and more humid than that of men. Even when a few sixteenth-century authors, among them Paterno in his commentary on *Canon* 1.1.3, pointed out that certain passages of Hippocrates supported the opposite opinion, such passages were usually explained away. And rare indeed was any serious questioning of the fundamental notion that not

---

quod non vidi hominem aliquem qui ad hoc cognitionis pervenerit, imo quod maius est, clarissimi medici etiam post longam visitationem invicem saepe litigant. Secundo quod repente advocamur vel ad curandos morbos acutos, vel ad consulendum in morbis diuturnis. Tertio quod videamus plures sanari infirmos et ab imperitis, tales ac longe plures quam quorum temperies nota sit. Quarto quod sufficit medico scire causam morbi et quanta sit; sed haec deprehenditur a magnitudine laesae operationis, qualiscunque sit temperatura, ergo absque conditione [*sic*; ? cognitione] temperaturae dignoscemus et morbum, et quantitatem morbi, et causam, et omnia necessaria. In oppositum est istud quod videmus saepe homines eodem vitio laborantes, et unus moritur, alter sanatur, et unus iuvatur vehementer ab uno auxilio, et alter nihil prorsus, et unum cogimur regere uno modo, alium alio modo, et non potest causa neque in morbo, neque in causa morbi, cum supponantur paria, neque in compositione; igitur restat ut temperatura sit causa horum. . . . Et vult huiusmodi ut statum adventitium et abundantiam humorum consideret Hippocrates, tum etiam morbos diuturnos et excessus temperaturae. Sed temperaturam membrorum non principaliter considerat, neque ut indicem affectus, sed potius permittit, ut siquis velit, temperaturam ex affectu dignoscat, non ex temperatura affectum." Cardano, *Opera* (Lyon, 1663), 9:558–59. Regarding Cardano's own *Contradicentia medica*, see Chapter 7, n. 113.

[16] "At vero si verum est, doctissime Ferneli, pro humorum varietate partium temperamentum non immutari, quorsum tam diligens medicorum studium in instituenda victus ratione? Quis corpora calidiora frigidis, frigidiora calidis, humidiora siccis, sicciora humidis, in mediocrem referre statum speret?" Costeo, *Disq. phys.*, p. 195.

only physical sexual characteristics, but also a wide range of stereo-
typed and conventional psychological characteristics ascribed to either
sex were the result of sexual temperament and thus of nature.[17]

Costeo, however, took the position that various supposedly female
characteristics usually attributed to sexual temperament could just as
well be the result of social conditions. He pointed out that timidity,
considered in women a cold trait, was also common in boys, who were
held to be complexionally hot; perhaps in both it was simply the fruit
of inexperience of the world rather than of temperament. Similarly, the
supposed propensity of women to humid diseases was, where it existed, in Costeo's view likely to be the result of inactivity rather than of
temperament, since active women did not suffer from diseases of this
type. As for the more rapid aging and shorter life span of women than
of men, this was probably due less to natural frigidity than to overwork
and excessive childbearing, for "we observe daily that those of them
who are more fecund grow older more quickly and die sooner." Costeo added that it had not been observed whether the greater heat of men
was due to natural male temperament or to the activities expected of
them, and he ended by comparing the effect of sex roles on temperament to the practice of "some nations in which the natural shape of the
head is changed in tender infants by art, and with long use becomes
natural and proper to them, and they are observed to retain a different
shape of the head."[18]

---

[17] Paterno, comm. *Canon* 1.1 (Venice, 1592), fols. 57ᵛ–58ʳ. On Renaissance discussions of sexual *temperatura*, see Ian Maclean, *The Renaissance Notion of Woman: A Study in
the Fortunes of Scholasticism and Medical Science in European Intellectual Life* (Cambridge,
1980), pp. 33–35; for examples of medieval *quaestiones* on the same subject, see Siraisi,
Alderotti, pp. 320, 323, 325.

[18] "Ab his non valde diversa argumenta sunt quae ex foeminarum constitutione universa desumuntur. . . . Et quanquam timiditatem ad cordis frigiditatem sequi medicis
plane constitutum est, cur tamen deiectum mulierum animum in parvum rerum usum
non referamus? Nam et pueri alioqui calore affluentes, ipsi quoque foeminarum instar
omnia timent. Propensio autem in lachrymas vere non frigiditati sed humiditati succedit;
neque is vere affectus est, ut proponitur, cordis, sed cerebri. Et inutilium quoque suc-
corum abundantiae illius quae in mulieribus est authorem esse non tam naturam quam
ocium, earum exemplo docemur quae exercentur, quas etiam morbi ex bile frequentius
quam ex pituita corripiunt. Demum vero, senectam atque interitum foeminarum celeri-
orem non tam insitam frigiditatem quam labores ac veluti diuturnos in filiorum gesta-
tione et procreatione morbos efficere, illud persuadet quod quae ex iis foecundiores sunt
celerius senescere atque interire quotidie observamus. Itaque quum ex propositis
utrinque rationibus nihil sit firmi, an forte mulieres quae pueris mollitie et natura quo-
dammodo consentiunt, eodem, ut illi modo, miti quidem calore superiores, acri autem
inferiores; et contra, mares non miti, sed acri caliditate superare dicamus? Non est hoc
quidem rationi dissentaneum. At neque hoc fortasse ut mares plerunque calidiores esse
dicamus, observata ea natura quae illis est vel ab ortu vel per se, vel post ortum et per

Costeo's remarks should not be read as a denial of the existence of sexual temperament, nor as necessarily indicating disapproval of conventional sex roles and their effects on temperament—although he certainly sounds more sympathetic to women than Santorio, who countered the argument that the lustfulness of women indicated a hot temperament with the assertion that female concupiscence was not directed toward sexual pleasure, but was merely a means of gaining tyrannical control over men.[19] What is noteworthy about Costeo's comments is his clear appreciation of the arbitrariness with which the traditional scheme ascribed differences associated with gender roles to nature and of the need to question the evidential basis for such assertions.

Costeo and Cardano may well have been to some degree responsive to intellectual currents connected with the revival of philosophical skepticism, of which, as has recently been pointed out, Galen's works were one source.[20] Perhaps, although he drew on an ancient source to illustrate the point, Costeo was also influenced by dawning contemporary awareness of the variety of human behavior and social organization around the globe and the consequent variability of human nature, an awareness that doubtless also contributed to the development of a skeptical turn of thought.

---

accidens comparata. Si enim qui frigido natura temperamento sunt exercitatione calescere, et contra qui calido, perfrigerari ocio solent, rursumque si nationes quasdam quibus naturalis capitis figura alias in teneris adhuc infantulis arte mutabatur, longo tandem usu tanquam naturalem propriamque et ab aliis diversam capitis figuram retinere observantur, cur non etiam virilem naturam ob continuatam longa iam annorum serie exercitationem calidiorem, foeminam vero contra, frigidiorem ob contrarium victum evasisse concedamus?" Costeo, *Disq. phys.*, pp. 216–17. Costeo's remarks may be compared with the entirely dialectical and scholastic treatment of the problem that some women appear to have signs of a hotter temperament than some men in Oddi, comm. *Canon* 1.1 (Venice, 1575), pp. 247–49. An influence of life style on the physiological characteristics of the sexes was, however, acknowledged by Galen: "Nec hic consistamus, sed incolat ille Pontum, haec Aegyptum, praeterea vir in umbra vivat et otio ac multis in delitiis molliterque, mulier ruri agat ac multa in exercitationibus sit et victu utatur modico, hujus mulieris pulsus quam viri major erit." *De causis pulsuum* 3.2 (Kühn, 9:109). The source of Costeo's information about head binding is Hippocrates, *Airs Waters Places*, chap. 14 (*Hippocrates*, ed. and tr. W.H.S. Jones, Loeb Classical Library [London and New York 1923], 1:110–11). Hippocrates believed the shape of the head thus acquired would become hereditary.

[19] "Nec dicant foeminas maxime concupiscere mares, ideo calidiores; quia respondemus concupiscentiam illarum ut plurimum non ess gratia voluptatis, sed ut viros reddant amore perditos hoc solo fine, ut in ipsis tyrannidem exerceant." Santorio, comm. *Canon* 1.1 (Venice, 1646), col. 538.

[20] J.-P. Pittion, "Skepticism and Medicine in the Renaissance." *Skepticism from the Renaissance to the Enlightenment*, ed. R. H. Popkin and C. B. Schmitt (Wolfenbüttel, 1986).

Santorio, who was, on the contrary, clearly concerned primarily to confirm complexion theory, possibly as a counter to skeptical criticisms, adopted an approach that in the long run was likely to prove more destructive to the entire concept than any isolated expressions of skepticism about particular aspects of it. His lectures on this subject, as on many others in his commentary on *Canon* 1.1, are marked by an effort to engage his pupils with the use in physiological science of instrumentation, quantification, and the recording of observed data, and with the findings of sixteenth-century anatomists. To this end, eight instruments of physiological measurement are illustrated and described in Santorio's discussion of the specific applications of temperament. These consist of different types of thermoscopes and pulsilogia and are clustered in the section dealing with the subject of the different *temperaturae* attributed to different parts of the body. Instructions stressing the accurate timing of the use of the thermoscope and the need for recording observations are intended to assist the physician in using these devices not to determine the heat or coldness of the body as a whole, but that of the heart. The stress is on the prognostic and practical usefulness of this information, but Santorio was evidently also concerned to solve once and for all the problem about perceptibility raised in turn by Gentile de Foligno and Cardano. Like Gentile, Santorio was espousing a *via experimentalis*, but Santorio's concept of experiment, or rather of controlled observation was very different from that of the medieval author.[21]

Anatomical considerations also come from time to time into Santorio's elucidation of highly abstract and traditional *quaestiones* about temperament. Thus in his treatment of complexional differences between the sexes, Santorio took the opportunity to rebut the theory of the parallelism of male and female genitalia, remarking that neither the cervix of the uterus nor the "clitoris Falopii" corresponded to the penis, and noting various differences in size, shape, position, and so on between the *foeminarum testes* (i.e., the ovaries) and the testicles.[22] (Costeo, who took the same position, discussed this subject as part of his commentary of the *doctrina* on the members, not temperament.) Again, in the course of responding to the *quaestio* of whether bile is hotter than blood, Santorio gave his readers an account of the functioning of the valves in the heart. On the whole, however, despite the opportunity

---

[21] Santorio, comm. *Canon* 1.1 (Venice, 1646), cols. 307–12. Other instruments designed to measure the temperature and humidity of the air are illustrated and described in cols. 425–30. The remaining instruments illustrated in the chapters on *temperatura* are either therapeutic or unrelated to the four primary qualities and their admixture.

[22] Ibid., col. 542.

afforded by Avicenna's lists of temperaments of different bodily parts, the subject of *temperatura*, unlike that of the humors, seems not to have inspired much anatomical discussion.

Like temperament, with which it was closely connected, the doctrine of the humors, treated in *Canon* I.I.4, continued to provide a central explanatory concept in sixteenth-century physiology and pathology. Chyle concocted from nutriment was further concocted into the humors, which in turn nourished the body. Imbalance among or deterioration of the humors produced complexional imbalance, that is, illness. But unlike *temperatura*, a quality or mixture of qualities that could only be physically perceived by its effects (and the extent to which even that kind of perception was possible roused disagreement), the humors were conceived of as fluids physically present in the body. Accordingly, practicing physicians paid a good deal of attention to the manifest characteristics of bodily fluids. For example, the widespread practice of phlebotomy ensured that all practitioners were familiar with the gross appearance of venous blood, which was often interpreted in accordance with the notion that all four humors, not blood alone, were contained in the veins. Cardano thought that only beginners would need to have it explained that if drawn blood was left to stand, all four humors could be seen (dark substance at the bottom being interpreted by him as melancholy, yellowish or foamy matter at the top as bile, and the middle layer as a mixture of blood and phlegm).[23] Also unlike *temperatura* or the elements, the subject of the humors did not readily lend itself to metaphysical speculation. The protracted scholastic discus-

---

[23] "Relinquuntur duo quae pro tirunculis practicae declaranda sunt. Primum ut dignoscatis partes sanguinis. Facta igitur sectione venae in duabus cyatis absque suppressione et dimisso sanguine in umbra per horam, videbitis quinque illas partes positas prima *Aphorismorum*. In suprema parte spumosam quandam ac flavam congeriem, quae est bilis procul dubio; et haec ut plurimum est crassitudinis medii digiti. Deinde proicietis serosam partem, quae non differet ab urina nisi quia non sit in renibus [!]. Hac eiecta, ponetis sanguinem ut iacet super tabulam et dividetis per mediam; et pars una est nigra, et si fuerit homo melancholicus videbitis interstinctum lividis maculis et quasi nigris; pars vero media est sanguis admixtus pituitae, et pro hoc dignoscendo debetis cum acie gladii trahere, et si facile dividitur et est valde ruber, parum est de pituita; et si tenax et subalbidis multum, debetis etiam pondere experiri, et si levis est pro quantitate abundat bilis et pituita; si gravis atrabilis et sanguis qui crassus est ac nigrior, est significans super caliditatem vehementem, quia calor resolvit partes aqueas, et hoc de sanguine crasso dicebat Galenus libro *Quod animi mores*, etc.; aquosus autem significat frigiditatem, sed haec potest provenire merito pauci caloris et ciborum." Cardano, *Opera* (Lyon, 1663), 9:561. (In this passage Cardano seems to have forgotten his own cautions about the difficulty of determining *temperatura*.) Others argued that only three humors were present in blood, however (blood itself, bile, and black bile); Costeo, who opposed this position, thought the *pituita*, though present, was not apparent to sense. See Costeo, *Disq. phys.*, p. 230.

sions about the humors indulged in by medieval and Renaissance physicians centered instead upon differences between authorities as to their number and properties (taste, color, consistency, etc.) and upon obscure aspects of real or supposed physiological processes in which the humors were involved.[24] In addition, the subject of the production of the humors and their distribution in the body inevitably touched on aspects of anatomy.

The foregoing considerations help to provide the context for two features that appear worthy of note in the treatment of the humors in the commentaries under review: the presence of a few passages of anatomical material and, perhaps more important, the efforts of Da Monte and Santorio to integrate theoretical and practical aspects of teaching about the humors.

The infrequent allusions to anatomical organs connected with the humors are for the most part quite traditional in content. However, there are occasional signs that the teaching of *theorici* on this subject was affected by the enhanced contemporary awareness of the importance of anatomical understanding. We may take as a single example in which the commentators (other than Cardano, who broke off his commentary before the point in question) treated a group of organs to which particular importance was attached in humoral physiology since they were specialized for storage and distribution of humoral fluid: the gall bladder, cystic duct, hepatic ducts, and common bile duct. It should first be noted that according to Galen in *De naturalibus facultatibus*, the gall bladder was endowed with an attractive faculty, which drew yellow bile (choler) from its site of manufacture in the liver; a retentive faculty, which enabled the fluid to be stored; and an expulsive faculty, which from time to time caused its release into the stomach. In *De temperamentis*, or *complexionibus*, Galen presented a slightly different account in which he said that in some individuals there were paired bile ducts, one discharging into the stomach, the other into the duodenum. However, in his more detailed and anatomically oriented description in *De usu partium*, although Galen referred to bile ducts in the plural he denied that yellow bile flowed into the stomach and correctly asserted that bile was released into the duodenum. In their twelfth-century translations the first two of the works named were well known to learned physicians of the thirteenth to fifteenth centuries, many of whom were in any case more interested in the physiology of faculties, *complexiones*, and humors—the main subject of these works—than in

[24] For examples of medieval *quaestiones* on the humors, see Siraisi, *Alderotti*, pp. 326–28.

anatomical detail. The account in *De usu partium*, although available from the early fourteenth century, appears to have attracted less attention prior to the sixteenth century. On the basis of Galen's brief and somewhat cryptic remarks in *De naturalibus facultatibus* and of his description in *De temperamentis*, the generally accepted belief in late medieval medicine was that bile flowed into the gall bladder from the liver, and was transported out of the gall bladder by two ducts, one leading to the stomach, the other to the duodenum.[25]

This belief was partially corrected by Vesalius, who devoted special attention to the gall bladder. In the first edition of the *Fabrica* (1543), he described the bile duct as leading into the duodenum, and asserted that an extension from the gall bladder into the stomach, which he had seen in only a single individual, must be an anomaly.[26] Subsequently, in his *Operationes anatomicae*, first published in 1561, Gabriele Falloppia presented additional information about the structure and relationship of the parts and the way in which bile was transmitted to the duodenum. Falloppia denied that the common hepatic duct, formed by the junction of the right and left hepatic ducts in the liver, led into the gall bladder, and pointed out, correctly, that this duct led into the common bile duct, which in turn emptied into the duodenum. He further explained that at certain times the meatus where the common bile duct joined the duodenum was closed, since a continuous flow of bile was not required for digestion. In order to prevent bile from being regurgitated into the liver at these times, nature had provided a passage (i.e., the cystic duct) branching off the bile duct into the gall bladder. The function of the gall bladder was to store any bile that flowed up the cystic duct and to release it when needed for digestion. Falloppia also denied that the gall bladder had either an attractive, a retentive, or an expulsive faculty as far as bile was concerned.[27] From the time of their first appearance, not

[25] *De naturalibus facultatibus* 3.5 (Loeb ed., p. 244); *De temperamentis* (*De complexionibus*) 2.6 (Kühn, 1:631–32); *De usu partium* 5.1 (tr. May, 1:244–49, and, for discussion, 1:244, n. 1). The relation between Galen's views and the development of Renaissance ideas about the physiology of the gall bladder is discussed in Owsei Temkin, "The Classical Roots of Glisson's Doctrine of Irritation," in *The Double Face of Janus and Other Essays in the History of Medicine* (Baltimore, 1977), pp. 290–316. On the currency of belief in the two bile ducts, one leading into the stomach, among medieval and Renaissance physicians, see C. D. O'Malley, *Andreas Vesalius of Brussels* (Berkeley and Los Angeles, 1964), pp. 115–116.

[26] *Fabrica* (1543), pp. 509–11. For discussion of Vesalius' contribution to understanding of the anatomy of the gall bladder and related ducts, see O'Malley, *Vesalius*, pp. 115–16, 172.

[27] *Gabrielis Falloppii medici mutinensis Observationes anatomicae* (Venice, 1561), fols. 177ʳ–179ʳ.

only Vesalius' *Fabrica*, but also Falloppia's *Observationes anatomicae* (the demand for which was sufficient to justify a second edition within a year from the same Venetian press that had produced the first)[28] were, of course, well known and widely discussed in the Italian medical milieu.

In the early 1540s, Da Monte evidently did not regard anatomical discussion of the gall bladder and related organs as forming a necessary part of commentary on Avicenna's *doctrina* on the humors. Although he subjected Avicenna's remarks on bile to the same thorough and hostile examination as the rest of the section on humors, and although this part of his commentary was sufficiently leisurely to find room for a lengthy excursus of vision and colors, he seems not to have mentioned the gall bladder and ducts at all, merely remarking that natural yellow bile was manufactured in the liver.[29]

By contrast, Oddo Oddi introduced a decidedly anatomical emphasis into his treatment of the subject. He inquired whether Aristotle's list of animals that lacked a gall bladder meant that not all animals produced choler and melancholy, and concluded that such was not the case. And he defended Avicenna against the accusation that he was the source of the "common error" that asserted that a duct carrying choler ran from the liver to the stomach. Oddi was right in pointing out that Avicenna had not said bile flowed into the stomach, but his defense seems rather disingenuous. The real source of the "common error" was most likely a simplified rendering of one of Galen's somewhat divergent accounts, but to this possibility Oddi did not draw attention. Indeed, his main purpose in discussing the bile duct or ducts at all seems to have been to defend the account in *De temperamentis* as Galen's true position. Oddi insisted that the authentic Galenic, and correct, teaching was that the bile duct was normally one and normally led into the duodenum, although in some cases the bile duct was twinned, with a larger branch leading into the duodenum and a smaller one into the stomach, and in a very few instances the duct leading into the stomach was the larger one.[30] Although the existence of criticisms of Galen's accounts of the bile duct(s) is not acknowledged in this passage, it seems fairly clear that it is in fact a response to such criticisms, and possibly to the *Fabrica* itself; as already noted, Oddo Oddi's commentary may

---

[28] Venice, 1562.

[29] Da Monte's discussion of bile occupies fols. 186ʳ–213ʳ of his comm. *Canon* 1.1 (Venice, 1554), with the digression on color occurring at fols. 197ᵛ–210ᵛ. The generation of bile in the liver is briefly mentioned on fol. 187ᵛ.

[30] Oddi, comm. *Canon* 1.1 (Venice, 1575), pp. 324–25. On the discussions by Aristotle and Galen of animals lacking a gall bladder, see May, tr. *De usu partium*, 1:221–22, n. 45.

have been begun in the late 1530s, but it was still unfinished at its author's death in 1558, and was thereafter revised by his son Marco for publication in 1575.

Paterno merely briefly mentioned the function of the gall bladder, which he described as that of attracting and storing part of the common bile and black bile, and Costeo was almost equally reticent. After devoting several pages to a consideration of how chyle reached the liver—in which he expressed doubt that the mesenteric veins (*mesariacae venae*) could be, as Galen had taught, the only route and postulated a shorter route via capillary veins leading from the intestines—Costeo turned to the site of manufacture of the humors. He noted that the *medici* had not yet reached agreement as to whether blood was manufactured in the liver, the heart, or even, as some of the moderns thought, in the spleen; or on whether, if the blood was manufactured in the liver, this process took place in the tissue of the liver itself or in its veins; or on whether the liver also manufactured the other humors. However, he did not here embark on any description of the structure or function of the gall bladder or ducts.[31]

Only with Santorio do we arrive at any explicit account of the work of sixteenth-century anatomists on these organs. Santorio provided a reasonably accurate summary of Falloppia's findings—but immediately went on systematically to reject them. Santorio taught his students that Falloppia's observations were simply erroneous; furthermore, he asserted that Falloppia's explanation contradicted Galen, Averroes, and reason, the last because if the gall bladder lacked an attractive faculty, gravity would prevent any bile from being retained in it. Finally, Santorio claimed that "most certain experiments" involving inflation of first the hepatic ducts (*rami fellei*) and subsequently the gall bladder showed that the direction of flow and relation of the parts was not as Falloppia proposed.[32] Given that Falloppia had died in 1562, at

---

[31] Paterno, comm. *Canon* 1.1 (Venice, 1596), fol. 95ᵛ; Costeo, *Disq. phys.*, pp. 327–28.

[32] *Quaestio* 77: "An vesica fellea trahat bilem. . . . Falopius tenet bilem non attrahi a vesicula, sed pelli ab hepate in vesiculam. Deceptus fuit Falopius, quia putabat meatum felleum duodeno intestino insertum non provenire a vesica fellea, sed ab hepate; addebatque vesicam tunc solum recipere bilem quando intestinum duodenum ob flatus vel ob nimios cibos distenditur et ob distentionem ita interclauditur meatus felleus ut per illum bilis in hepate genita non possit expurgari, quo casu dicebat bilem recurrere ad vesicam felleam, quae sit facta a natura tanquam diverticulum in quo conservetur bilis ne illa occasione sanguis illa inficiatur.

"Haec Falopii opinio reluctatur Galeno, Averroi, rationi, et experimentis. . . . Demum Falopius his experimentis certissimis adversatur, quia si immittatur tubulus in ramos felleos et inflentur, statim vesicula et non intestina inflantur. Pari modo si immittatur tubulus in vesiculum et infletur, statim distenditur ramus felleus qui in duodenum

least fifty years before Santorio wrote (as well as before the commentaries of Costeo and Paterno were written or that of Oddi published),
the passage illustrates well the durable hold of Galenic ideas—and also
that "experimental" techniques did not always necessarily produce superior information.

Five out of the seven commentators made little or no discernible effort to link their lectures of Avicenna's *doctrina* on the humors to any
practical applications of humoral theory. However, the strong commitment of Da Monte and Santorio to the development of integrated
medical teaching, and no doubt also their own extensive involvement
in medical practice, plainly did affect the way they explicated the humors in the course of *theoria* based on *Canon* 1.1.

Although Da Monte made a few references to the state of humors in
various diseases, he did not introduce extended discussions of diagnosis
or therapy into his exposition of *Doctrina* 4. His occasional asides on
pharmacological terminology are chiefly noteworthy for a passage in
which he described "true" *mumia*, in order to warn his hearers or readers off the false and useless substitutes available in Venetian pharmacies. In Da Monte's version, *mumia* had once been collected in Arabia
from the exudations of corpses that had been impregnated with unguents, but was no longer available; the substitute, dried bodies from
Africa, which he claimed could be purchased in Venetian pharmacies,
was of no medicinal use whatsoever.[33] Yet the underlying reason for

insertus est, quare meatus felleus implantatus duodeno intestino provenit a vesica et non
ab hepate; rami vero fellei hepatis, inflata vesica, non inflantur quia habent valvulas quae
impediunt inflationem. Haec inflatio commode fit cum tubulo vitreo, qui potest inveniri
valde exilis." Santorio, comm. *Canon* 1.1 (Venice, 1646), cols. 657–58. Santorio did not
claim actually to have performed these three experiments himself. The first result seems
unlikely, but may depend on the site where insufflation was introduced; the second result
appears possible, but does not, of course, counter Falloppia's argument; in the third case,
Santorio has provided an explanation for a result that does not correspond with his own
theory. Santorio recorded that he had personally seen two autopsies in which the gall
bladder was opened, although "many years before" (ibid., col. 656).

[33] "Cum igitur advenit caliditas et siccitas corpori quod erat concretum a frigiditate,
tunc eliquatur a vi caloris; uti patet in febribus colliquativis, in quibus materia crassa et
pinguis defluit, pariter idem fit de cadaveribus quae suspenduntur in cruce, in quibus fit
colliquatio talis per calorem solis. Idem fieri dicitur de cadaveribus illis quae in Aphrica
suffocantur sub harena, liquantur omnino corpora illa ab ingentissimo ardore solis et sic-
citate harenae, unde remanent corpora illa prorsus arida, quae sic arefacta reportantur a
mercatoribus vel a nautis ad nos, eaque vendunt pro mumia. In illis enim exaruit totum
humidum per eliquationem factam a calore igneo.

"Haec tamen non est vera mumia cum in se nullam habeat qualitatem ut ea, habet enim
nisi summam terrestreitatem, et faciunt nos devorare talia cadavera sic torrefacta et
adusta. At vera mumia est aliud diversum ab huiusmodi cadaveribus, et alias afferebatur
ad nos a mercatoribus arabibus, de qua, quia hic non est locus nihil dicam, dicam tamen

the diatribe against Avicenna's teaching on the humors, to which, Da Monte devoted almost all this portion of commentary, is clearly connected with his ideas about integrated medical education. Da Monte particularly criticized *Doctrina* 4 of *Canon* I.1 precisely because he was convinced that knowledge of the humors was "extremely useful" for the practicing physician. He announced that proper understanding of the humors was essential not only for comprehending the structure of the human body, but also its growth, nutrition and reproduction, health and sickness, human character, and medical prognostication.[34]

In commenting on *Doctrina* 4 he therefore abandoned the philosophical bent for speculation that had marked his exposition of earlier sections and instead tried to demonstrate how minor misunderstandings incident upon the process of transmission from one language and cul-

---

unum verbum. Dico quod mumia vera et antiqua ea erat quoniam mos erat arabum, virorum nobilium maxime, quando quis nobilis moriebatur ung[u]ebant corpus aloe et myrrha quemadmodum patet in evangelio de unguento Domini Iesu Christi, posteaque unxissent induebant et cooperiebant pannis linneis, et ita conservabant in suis sepulchris. Postea, tractu temporis adveniente calore illi putredini, colliquabatur pinguedo illius corporis ita ut commisceretur cum myrrha et aloe illa, ex qua unctione fiebat fermentatio quaedam et mixtura optima quam tunc portabant ad nos mercatores illi furantes e sepulchris, et haec mumia mirandum in modum iuvabat ad convulsionem tollendam, habebat enim hoc fermentum vim resolvendi et molliendi, quam dabant etiam in potu, et maxime conferebat ad contusiones, tam interiores quam exteriores, sic igitur mercatores illi furabantur tempore noctis corpora arabum nobilium mortua eaque ad nos portabant, quod arabes intelligentes providerunt, constituerunt enim corpora locanda esse in loco tuto ne praedarentur. Unde non possunt nunc huc transferri. At isti medici ignari qui occupantur tantum imposturis ignorant quae sit vera mumia, et comprobant pro vera mumia corpora illa in harena suffocata delata ad nos his temporibus a nautis. . . . Horum autem corporum aliqua videri solent Venetiis tempore ascensionis in pharmacopoliis valde nigra et horrida visu, et sunt maxime arida." Da Monte, comm. *Canon* I.1 (Venice, 1554), fols. 228ʳ–229ʳ.

[34] ". . . omnium quae tractantur in arte medica pulcherrima speculatio et utilissima est speculatio de humoribus . . . nam sine hac cognitione non potestis cognoscere fabricam humani corporis. . . . Secundo non possumus scire quo modo nutritur, augeatur, conservetur corpus in suo esse, quia ex his humoribus non tantum generatur homo, sed etiam nutritur et primo servatur in vita. Tertio sine cognitione istorum humorum non possumus cognoscere sanitatem, quia sanitas consistit in bona proportione istorum quatuor humorum, at si non cognoscetis sanitatem, non cognoscetis etiam aegritudines, quia fiunt diversae aegritudines ex diversitate humorum, et omnia genera morborum oriuntur ex his humoribus, non potestis etiam scire occultos affectus corporis, quia affectus indicantur per excrementa, excrementa autem discernuntur per humores, praeterea operationes omnes gubernantur per dominium humorum. . . . Praeterea mores ipsi tales sunt quales sunt humores. . . . Praeterea sine cognitione horum humorum non potestis scire prognosticationes . . . et ita videtis totam fere artem fundari in cognitione humorum." Ibid., fols. 141ᵛ–142ʳ. The section of Da Monte's commentary devoted to the humors extends from fol. 141ʳ to 246ʳ.

311

ture to another could have severe consequences for the content of medical education, and hence of medical practice. His goal was simply to eradicate as many such errors as possible. Da Monte's methodology involved identifying in the Latin text of the *Canon* instance after instance of intentional or accidental divergence from Galen's teachings; no difference seemed too minor to escape his censure. In a number of instances, he was by no means the first to point out a particular discrepancy or inconsistency; but where earlier commentators had reconciled, Da Monte condemned.

Da Monte's 200-page critique of Avicenna's teaching on the humors is far more detailed than some of the condemnations of Avicenna found in works expressly directed against Arab medicine. Space does not permit a full listing of his objections, but some have already been noted in discussing his attitude toward Avicenna and toward the commentator's task (Chapter 6). One good illustration of Da Monte's technique is provided by his handling of Avicenna's account of natural *pituita*, or phlegm, which in *Canon* 1.1.4.1 is described as "sweet" (*dulcis*). Two hundred years before Da Monte wrote, Gentile da Foligno had noted in commenting on this passage that both Johannitius and, elsewhere, Avicenna himself described natural phlegm as insipid; in a conciliatory spirit Gentile had opined that Galen must have used the term "sweet" simply to mean without taste, as when ordinary people speak of "sweet water," and hence that either "sweet" or "insipid" could properly be used to describe natural phlegm.[35] Taking up the same point, Da Monte explained, with appropriate textual citations, that Avicenna had probably been trying to reconcile a discrepancy within the Galenic corpus, since in *De naturalibus facultatibus, pituita* was termed sweet, in the sense Gentile had understood, whereas in *De atra bile* it was called insipid. Da Monte did not find Avicenna's effort at reconciliation culpable in itself, but he pointed out that Avicenna's failure to appreciate that "among the Greeks and Latins waters are called sweet in order to distinguish them from those that are nitreous and saline" had led him into the "venial sin" of supposing that natural *pituita* partook of some real sweetness. And this mistake had in turn been responsible for Avicenna's "mortal sin" of supposing natural *pituita* not to be extremely cold, a teaching completely opposed to that of Hippocrates and Galen, and a false foundation on which many false conclusions were based.[36]

---

[35] Gentile da Foligno, comm. *Canon* 1 and 2 (Pavia, 1510–11), 1.1.4.1, *dubium* 19, fol. 32ᵛ.

[36] "Avicenna interpretatus est dulce pro dulcedine actuali, et non intellexit quod apud Graecos et Latinos aquae dicuntur dulces ad differentiam aquarum quae sunt nitrosae et salsae . . . sed istud est peccatum veniale, veniamus ad peccata mortalia . . . dixit con-

In his critique of Avicenna's teaching on the humors, Da Monte's canon of correctness was usually in agreement with the text of Galen, although this had to be considered in conjunction with "the truth of the thing itself." Da Monte did not discuss the question of how the latter was to be arrived at, apparently assuming that it would always be self-evident. For example, Da Monte disapproved of the classification of fever caused "by putrescent blood" as *febris synocha*. After demolishing Avicenna's views on this topic, Da Monte exclaimed: "You see therefore how vain it is to consider authorities, when you might consider the thing itself; from the very nature of the thing you will find fever caused by putrescent blood to be very different from *febris synocha*. And that is enough on this subject."[37] Moreover, Da Monte did not hesitate to propose his own classification of the humors and other bodily fluids and to assert its superiority, without reference to Galen. The suggested change was organizational only and involved grouping the humors and other fluids first as useful or nonuseful, and then by site (inside or outside the veins) and function (nourishment of the body or its offspring, provision for excretion, production of disease); its announced purpose was the elimination of time-wasting debates over ambiguities in Avicenna's scheme.[38]

Subsequent commentators seem to have been unconvinced both by Da Monte's critique and by his claims to present authentic Galenic doctrine. It is likely that Paterno had Da Monte in mind when he referred disapprovingly to "very ingenious and equally learned men" who strove to destroy the teaching of both Galen and Avicenna on *pituita salsa*.[39] By the time Santorio came to review the history of criticism of Avicenna's assertion that the kind of bile known as *vitellina* was a mixture of yellow bile and thick *pituita*, he found Da Monte's methodology of textual comparison of Avicenna's statement with passages of Galen correct as far as it went, and an advance on the practices of older commentators, but nonetheless inadequate. Santorio remarked that the earlier scholastic commentators had resolved the discrepancy between Avicenna and Galen on this topic by reading into the texts factually in-

---

sequenter et necessario pituitam naturalem non esse valde frigidam. . . . Ideo iam posito uno fundamento non vero, necessarium est postea dicere multa quae sunt falsa." Da Monte, comm. *Canon* 1.1 (Venice, 1554), fol. 173ʳ.

[37] "Videtis igitur quam vanum sit considerere authoritatibus, et quod rem ipsam consideretis; ex ipsa rei natura invenietis febrem a sanguine putrescente longe aliam esse a synocha, et de hoc satis." Ibid., fol. 168ᵛ.

[38] Ibid., fols. 153ʳ–154ʳ.

[39] "Atque haec sunt quae de salsa pituita a Galeno et Avicenna hic habentur. Adversus quae insurrexerunt viri ingeniosissimi pariter et doctissimi qui omnia ab utrisque proposita explodere nixi sunt," Paterno, comm. *Canon* 1.1 (Venice, 1596), fol. 85ᵛ.

correct distinctions between various kinds of vitelline (i.e., egg yolk) color in bile, while Da Monte and other sixteenth-century authors had pointed out that it looked as if the statement in the *Canon* depended on a partial or hasty reading of Galen. In Santorio's own view, Avicenna's statement, and apparent reading of Galen, could be defended if it was considered to apply to only one subspecies of *bilis vitellina*, since it then accorded with practical medical experience of the characteristics of the sputum of patients with tertian fever.[40] Santorio here certainly gave the appeal to medical experience higher priority than it had usually enjoyed in earlier theoretical medical expositions; nonetheless it should be noted that he rejected neither the goal of reconciliation nor reliance on textual analysis.

Santorio, like Da Monte, described the *doctrina* on the humors as "most useful" for the practitioner, noting especially its utility in diagnosis.[41] But as the example just cited shows, in Santorio's commentary, unlike that of Da Monte, the effort to enhance that usefulness is no longer exclusively, or even primarily, rooted in an analysis of divergences from Galen. In this as in other instances Santorio's commentary appears more scholastic than those of his sixteenth-century predecessors largely because he sought to weigh all previous opinions, and in so doing did not necessarily give much more weight to sixteenth-century Galenists than to the *veteri interpretes*. His conception of the proper way to increase the actual usefulness of lectures on the humors

---

[40] *Quaestio* 80: "An vitellina bilis sit mixtura ex citrina et pituita crassa. . . . Antiqui interpretes Avicennae, et Hugo Senensis, qui inter antiquiores est postremus, conciliant Avicennam cum Galeno dicendo dari duplicem vitellinam, alteram magis coloratam, alteram vero minus. . . . De hoc duplici colore vitellinae bilis dant exemplum de ovis recentibus et vetustis. . . .

"Caeterum hac distinctione de duplici colore vitellino non conciliant Avicennam cum Galeno, quia ex Avicenna omnis vitellina videtur esse mixta ex bile et pituita. Praeterea in vitello ovi recentis non potest esse mixtura diversorum humorum . . . si vitellina simillima luteo ovi recentis esset mixta ex pituita et bile citrina sequeretur quod citrina esset intensioris coloris quam illa vitellina quod reluctatur experientiae. . . .

"Hinc Montanus, Valesius, et quam plurimi alii tenent Avicennam fuisse deceptum dum legeret Galenum. . . .

"Quod vero detur haec vitellina Avicennae patet ex Galeno et ex ipsa practica medicinae . . . quia in tertianis sputis haec mixtura ex bile et pituita quotidie excernitur." Santorio, comm. *Canon* 1.1 (Venice, 1646), cols. 666–69. Yet another way of tackling the problem had been chosen by Oddo Oddi, who attempted to determine Galen's actual position by comparing two modern translations (those of Leoniceno and Linacre) and the Greek text; see Oddi, comm. *Canon* 1.1 (Venice, 1575), pp. 327–28.

[41] "Tractatus iste est utilissimus, quia cognita natura et cognitis humorum differentiis dignoscuntur febrium putridarum, tumorum, et innumerabilium morborum differentiae; ignoratis vero, haec omnia ignorantur." Santorio, comm. *Canon* 1.1 (Venice, 1646), col. 545.

in a course on *theoria* appears in the interlarding of this part of commentary with accounts of symptoms; recommendations for therapy; and illustrations, descriptions, and instructions for the operation of instruments and apparatus for use in the treatment of humoral disorders. These devices included a water bed, a humidifier, a trocar for drawing off dropsical fluid, a perforated ball to be filled with liquid and used for moistening the mouths of fever patients, a device for stopping nosebleeds, and a clyster.[42] How closely Santorio was still tied to the traditional system of temperaments and humors is indicated by his humidifier, which was intended to cool as well as moisten the air: the cooling function was to be accomplished by filling the vase with a potion made from complexionally cold herbs and heating it until steam was given off.[43] Yet Santorio also incorporated into his exposition of the *doctrina* of the humors an illustration of his famous weighing chair, and an account of his own novel theories about the importance in physiology of insensible perspiration and the desirability of measuring its emission.[44]

Aristotle and Galen

All traditional physicians were simultaneously both Aristotelians and Galenists, in the sense that by and large Aristotelianism and Galenism were mutually reinforcing systems of thought. However, as already noted, discussion of differences between the two authorities in the specific area of physiology was a staple of academic discourse among both philosophers and physicians. These debates both helped to determine some of the directions of sixteenth- and early seventeenth-century anatomical and physiological investigations and were ultimately rendered obsolete by their results. Discussions of the differences between Aristotle and Galen were often described as occurring between philosophers and physicians, but in fact the situation was more complex. Aristotelian natural philosophers might normally be expected to defend Aristotle's physiological ideas against those of Galen, but it did not necessarily follow that all physicians were monolithically Galenist on all disputed issues. Aristotelian doctrine had of course been present in Western medicine since at least the thirteenth, or even the twelfth, cen-

---

[42] Ibid., cols. 567–68, 569, 615–16, 609, 700, 835, 836. Santorio appears to have been the inventor of the trocar; see Grmek, *Santorio*, p. 82.

[43] Santorio, comm. *Canon* 1.1 (Venice, 1646), col. 569.

[44] *Quaestio* 98: "Ex quibus signis dignoscatur illa humorum quantitas quae inservit pro sanitate conservanda." Ibid., cols. 778–83, with illustration at cols. 781–82. Regarding other works of Santorio describing his theory, see Chapter 6, above.

tury.[45] But physicians who might incline toward Aristotelian concepts regarding, say, the primacy of the heart or the role of the female in conception (to name only two of the major topics of debate), were nonetheless trained within a generally Galenic medical system. By the same token, even the most devoutly Galenist physicians had of course received some training in Aristotelian natural philosophy and usually espoused a generally Aristotelian world view. Hence, the interaction of Aristotelian and Galenic ideas in sixteenth- and early seventeenth-century physiology is a complex topic, the history of which is far from completely written. Hitherto, it has attracted attention chiefly in terms of the intellectual formation of major figures, notably William Harvey.[46] From the commentaries on *Canon* I.I one can gain, more modestly, a glimpse of the routine teaching offered to their students by professors of *theoria* about areas in which the authority of Aristotle and Galen appeared to be in conflict.

In *Canon* I.I, the subject of the difference between Aristotle's view that the heart was the primary or ruling organ of the entire body, including its sensory motor, growth, and reproductive faculties, and Galen's picture of brain, heart, and liver as principal members, each governing a separate bodily system and set of faculties, was twice prominently mentioned, once in the first chapter of *Doctrina* 5, on the members, and again in the opening section of *Doctrina* 6, on the virtues. This twofold account indicated not only the importance attached to the subject, but also its many-faceted nature. The problem could be regarded as an anatomical one, since Galen's position was in part based

[45] On the use made of Aristotle by thirteenth- and fourteenth-century learned physicians, see Siraisi, *Alderotti*, chaps. 5 and 6.

[46] See, most recently, Charles B. Schmitt, "William Harvey and Renaissance Aristotelianism: A Consideration of the *Praefatio* to '*De generatione animalium*' (1651)," in *Humanismus und Medizin*, ed. Rudolf Schmitz and Gundolf Keil (Weinheim, 1984), pp. 117–38; nn. 2, 3, and 4 on p. 118 contain a bibliography of earlier studies of Harvey's Aristotelianism. See also Jacques Roger, "La situation d'Aristote chez les anatomistes padouans," in *Platon et Aristote à la Renaissance. XVIe Colloque International de Tours* (Paris, 1976), pp. 217–24. An example of the participation of philosophers in physiological debates between Aristotelians and Galenists is provided by Cesare Cremonini's *De calido innato et semine pro Aristotele adversus Galenum* (Leiden, 1634). From the medical side, the Renaissance debates may have been somewhat further stimulated by the reception of *De placitis Hippocratis et Platonis*, which contains lengthy attacks on Aristotle's views on the heart. On Aristotelianism and Galenism at Padua in the early sixteenth century see Antonio Antonaci, "Aristotelismo e scienza medica a Padova nel primo Cinquecento. Il pensiero medico di Marcantonio Zimara," in *Aristotelismo veneto e scienza moderna*, ed. Luigi Olivieri, Atti del 25° anno academico del Centro per la Storia della Tradizione Aristotelica nel Veneto, 2 vols. (Padua, 1983), 1:415–34, which, however, reached me too late to be incorporated into the discussion here.

on an understanding superior to Aristotle's of the anatomical relationship of brain, spinal cord, and nervous system. But it also pertained to the faculties and spirits, since the Aristotelian arguments were linked to ideas about the heart as the source of vital spirit, vital faculty, and innate heat. Inevitably, too, the argument had philosophical or metaphysical overtones, not only because of Aristotle's status as a philosophical authority, but also because his arguments in favor of the primacy of the heart were supported by statements about the need for a unified government in a society and the priority of one over many.[47] And the argument touched on ideas about the soul, since Galen's three principal members could be associated with Plato's tripartite soul, located in the same organs. Furthermore, Avicenna's own solution was itself matter for debate, since he both urged his readers to be satisfied with the knowledge that Aristotle's solution was "truer" while Galen's was "more manifest to sense," and also suggested that although the brain and the liver were indeed the seats of faculties, these in turn somehow depended on the heart.[48]

When Renaissance commentators on *Canon* 1.1 came to expound these passages they were the heirs to a long tradition. While the earliest medieval discussions of this and other differences between the physiology of Aristotle and Galen had served the then important purpose of focusing medical attention on the nature and scope of the divergences, and while medieval physicians were often perfectly capable of making a definite choice between the two authorities on particular points, it must be admitted that later medieval *quaestiones* about the heart and principal members were often routine pedagogical exercises, directed toward teaching the opinions of the ancient authors. In these works nominal reconciliation was usually achieved, either in the way Avicenna suggested or through the construction of syllogistic arguments displaying the verbal ingenuity of the disputant. Such characteristics did not entirely disappear when the topic was taken up in the Renaissance commentaries, but the penetration of other elements is also marked.

Of the commentators on *Canon* 1.1 who wrote on the controversy over the heart and principal members (Cardano's commentary breaks off before either of the relevant passages is reached), two took an Ar-

---

[47] E.g., *De motu animalium* 10, 703a4–36, and *De partibus animalium* 3.4, 666a14–15.

[48] See the passages quoted in Chapter 2, nn. 32 and 33. And: "Aristoteli videtur quod omnium istarum operationum principium existit cor; sed primarum operationum earum manifestatio in his predictis existit principiis quemadmodum apud medicos cerebrum est sentiendi principium, et post hoc quisque sensus habet membrum in quo eius apparet operatio." *Canon* 1.1.6.1 (Venice, 1507) fol. 23ʳ.

istotelian and three a Galenic position. No doubt the connections between medical *theoria* and philosophy ensured that professors of *theoria* were somewhat more likely than their colleagues in *practica* to take an Aristotelian stand on the primacy of the heart.

Da Monte was both the most committed to traditional modes of reconciliation between authorities and the most strongly Aristotelian. He taught his pupils that the discrepancy between Aristotle and Galen was not so great as usually thought, and that it only seemed major because of our limited capacity to understand the thought of these great men.[49] On the primacy of the heart, however, Aristotle had "determined far better" than the *medici* and his reasoning "seems more efficacious."[50] But Aristotle's superiority, Da Monte made clear, lay in grasping the philosophical concept that all things in one genus must have one cause or principle; this, however, is not to deny physical connection between the brain and the nervous system asserted by the *medici*: "For Aristotle does not deny that the brain gives sense and motion and is a principle, but afterwards these nerves have their principle from the heart."[51] This was scarcely an adequate presentation of Aristotle's position, as Da Monte must surely have known; Aristotle repeatedly asserted that the heart was the source or principle of sensation and motion, and did not distinguish between nerves and ligaments.[52] Equally tendentious seems Da Monte's assertion that Galen had recognized that brain and liver were somehow subordinate to the heart. It may be added that Da Monte also took an unambiguously Aristotelian stand on another major area of difference between the two authorities, that over the female role in conception.[53]

[49] ". . . inter Aristotelem et Galenum et medicos non est discrepantia tanta quantam aliqui putant, sed pauca est. Magna videtur propter nostram ingenii debilitatem contemplantis opinionem illorum insignium virorum." Da Monte, comm. *Canon* 1.1 (Venice, 1554), fol. 252ʳ.

[50] "Aristoteles autem longe melius determinat," ibid., fol. 251ᵛ. And: ". . . ratio Aristotelis videtur efficacior." Ibid., fol. 252ᵛ.

[51] "Nam Aristoteles non negat quin cerebrum det sensum, et motum, et sit quasi principium, sed postea isti nervi habent principium a corde." Ibid.

[52] Aristotle asserted the primacy of the heart in *De juventute et senectute* 3, 469a 10–12, *De partibus animalium* 2.1, 647a 21–32, *De generatione animalium* 2.6, 743b 25–26, and elsewhere, and this was the position normally identified as Aristotelian in the Middle Ages and Renaissance. However, in *De partibus animalium* 3.11, 673b 9–12, he termed both heart and brain ruling parts, a passage that provides some justification for Da Monte's claim. On Aristotle's failure to distinguish nerves and ligaments, see May, intro. to *De usu partium*, 1:16.

[53] Da Monte, comm. *Canon* 1.1 (Venice, 1554), fols. 257ʳ–58ᵛ; similarly, and in even stronger terms, in the additional chapter edited by J. M. Durastante, in the second edition

In strong contrast to both Da Monte's approach and his opinions stand those of the two Oddi. (Marco, who wrote the portions of their commentary dealing with the problem of the so-called principal members, explained that he shared his father's views on the subject.) Writing between 1558 and 1575, Marco was sharply critical of the Avicennan formula that Aristotle's belief in the primacy of the heart was somehow philosophically truer, even though sense experience endorsed Galen's findings about the connection between the brain and nerves of sensation and motion; Marco Oddi pointed out that to divorce ratiocination from a basis in sense experience was entirely contrary to Aristotle's own method of procedure in natural science. In Oddi's view, to dismiss sense experience in favor of the text of a philosopher was the sign of a weak intellect. He noted, further, the Aristotelian position on the primacy of the heart was based on a false analogy, that of the government of a human state by a king, which did not necessarily correspond to the physical organization of a plant or an animal. Similarly, the contention that the heart stood at the center of the body was purely dialectical, since in physical reality it was the umbilicus that was at the center of the body.

As for the more genuinely physiological claim that the heart was the principal organ and the fountain of life because it was the first part to take shape in the embryo, Aristotle had never observed embryos as Hippocrates and Galen had done and was, furthermore, inexperienced in dissection (in this, Oddi was doubtless unfair to Aristotle). The observations of Hippocrates and the study of aborted fetuses and anatomy clearly showed that in reality the first stage of the formation of the fetus was the enclosure of the semen by a membrane; then the liver, heart, and other organs began to be formed from the blood and spirits attracted by the semen; next heart, brain, and liver appeared clearly formed along with the rudiments of the other parts. Nor was it true, as his supporters claimed, that Aristotle said the heart was the source of the natural and vital faculties, since Aristotle had not known of the distinction between those two faculties. On the other hand, the views of Galen and the *medici* were based on solid demonstration from things perceived by sense; for example, anatomy clearly showed the nerves to be linked to the brain and the veins to the liver. Oddi further claimed that in some animals the vena cava "does not . . . touch the heart." These anatomical considerations were, Oddi asserted, demonstrated by "sense and experience, the mistress of all things," so that the opin-

(Venice, 1557), p. 605: "videtur quam fuerit malignus Galenus et quam frivola fuerint eius argumenta contra Aristotelem, et e contra quam argumenta Aristotelis sint valida."

ions of the *medici* were clearly consonant with truth, whereas the arguments of Aristotle and his followers were merely dialectical sophistries.[54]

It would, however, be highly unwise to read Oddi's hostility, in this instance to Aristotle and to philosophy in a medical context, as evidence that contemporary medical students at Padua were likely to learn about the heart/brain controversy solely from a Galenic or anatomical standpoint. Writing probably in the 1570s or 1580s, Bernardino Paterno was of the opinion that the very success of the revival of Galenic and the development of contemporary anatomy had been responsible for what he perceived as a reactive neo-Aristotelianism on the subject of the primacy of the heart. Paterno's own Galenism on the issue of the principal members was in fact responsive to philosophical as well as anatomical considerations. Moreover, various passages of Paterno's commentary in which heart and brain are discussed are not distinguished by their clarity; in his case, the modernization of commentary often seems to have resulted merely in the loss of the scholastic ability to set out different intellectual positions clearly. However, in the question appended to the end of his commentary, "whether the principle of sensation and motion is in the heart or the brain," Paterno plainly asserted that anatomy and vivisection "if they are well demonstrated to us" really do show conclusively that sensation arises in the brain and not the heart.[55] In Paterno's opinion, the medical Aristotelians of his own day had been obliged to recognize that such demonstrations constituted a final refutation of the kind of defense of Aristotle's ideas about the heart put forward by Avicenna and Averroes; but this recognition had merely had the effect of stimulating Aristotle's followers to come up with a new defense of the primacy of the heart, based not on the claim that it was the source or ruling principle of nerves and veins, but rather on the notion that it was the fount of vital heat, the instrument of the soul. Paterno was wrong in regarding vital heat as a

---

[54] Oddi, comm. *Canon* 1.1 (Venice, 1575), pp. 402–4. At p. 404: "vena cava cor non semper contingit, siquidem in quibus dexter non adest cordis ventriculus"; and "amplius eodem sensu et experientia rerum omnium magistra monstrarunt ipsi ex substantia cerebri paulatim indurata nervos oriri. . . ."

[55] ". . . de principio facultatum sentiendi et movendi secundum electionem, an in cerebro existat, vel in corde. . . . Recurrendum autem ad anatomen et corporum viventium dissectionem, quae si bene nobis demonstrata sit, nobis apparebit cor, et cerebrum copulari arteriis, venis, et nervis. . . . At vinculo constricto nervo medio inter utrumque, si cor viderimus sensum amittere, in reliquis vero partibus servari omnibus cum cerebro nexum habentibus, nonne iure optimo iudicabimus, non cor facultatem sentiendi cerebro tribuere, sed ab hoc cor ipsum eam suscipere?" Paterno, comm. *Canon* 1.1 (Venice, 1596), fols. 150ᵛ–151ʳ. The *quaestio* continues to fol. 153ʳ.

new theory, but it certainly received fresh emphasis and new applications in the thought of Fernel, against whose followers Paterno's remarks were probably directed. Paterno himself rejected the idea that
the arteries or veins were the channels through which vital heat flowed
from the heart on the grounds that such a flow could not be shown by
anatomical demonstrations.[56]

As far as the introductory teaching of medical *theoria* is concerned,
Paterno's observations about the reinvigoration of Aristotelian ideas
about the heart seem to be confirmed by Costeo's commentary. Costeo's treatment of the subject was complex, cautious, and conciliatory,
but he nonetheless appears to have moved from an initially Galenic toward a more or less Aristotelian position. In his exposition of the *doctrina* on the members, Costeo espoused a number of fairly standard arguments on behalf of the *medici* against Aristotle: he noted that
sensation could be destroyed without the heart being affected; he remarked that the seat of the soul is the body as a whole, not the heart; he
observed that the distribution of functions among several principal
parts provided better protection against injury to the body as a whole,
and doubted whether any one part could possibly direct all the body's
complex functions. He conceded that the heart was the seat of innate
heat, which perfected all the body's actions; but he denied that this
meant that the heart was the principle of all those actions. Likewise he
denied that the claim that the heart was the first organ to live and the
last to die, if true, meant it was the principle of all the faculties. As for
the question of the ruling principle of the nerves and veins, this was still
sub judice, although sense experience appeared to favor the *medici* rather
than the peripatetics.[57]

By the time Costeo came to comment on *Doctrina* 6, on the virtues,
he was more sympathetic to the Aristotelian position. In a rare instance
in the commentaries of acknowledgment of an exact contemporary by
name, he indicated that he had been persuaded by a disputation of
Agostino Bucci, professor of philosophy at Turin, "who fights for the

---

[56] "Coeterum ex Aristotelis sectatoribus haec quae dicta intelligentes sunt, iis refutatis
quae ab Averroe et Avicenna dicta sunt, novum modum defendendi Aristotelem a Galeni
rationibus introduxerunt, dicentes in proposita difficultate explicanda, neque venas, neque arterias, neque nervos respiciendos esse, sed id tantum calorem vitalem, quod animae instrumentum est in omnibus suis operationibus, a corde tanquam principio prodire." Ibid., fol. 151ʳ. And: "Hoc si est, rationi utique consentaneum calidum hoc
ingenitum vim eandem deferre, aut per venas aut per arterias. At cur ergo ligatis venis
aut arteriis facultas ea in membra diffunditur, ligatis nervis statim deperditur . . . ?"
Ibid., fol. 151ᵛ.

[57] Costeo, *Disq. phys.*, pp. 361–64.

Peripatetics with arguments that are not vulgar."[58] Here, Costeo examined a form of conciliatory argument that stressed the role of the heart as the source of the vital spirits from which animal spirits, responsible for sense and motion, were manufactured in the brain. (Medieval authors, including Avicenna himself, had often sought to achieve reconciliation by means of essentially similar arguments, which in one way or another presented brain and liver as secondary centers of activity that were, however, ultimately dependent on the heart.) Costeo noted that the *recentiores* found this argument unacceptable, both because it bore no relation to Aristotle's actual statements about the brain, and on anatomical grounds: crushing the nerves destroyed sensation and motion, whereas in some animals sensation and motion appeared to persist for a time after evulsion of the heart. But Costeo now thought that these arguments, far from being unanswerable, were "easily solved" by the peripatetics; Aristotle had not been as inept nor his arguments as futile as his opponents held. For example, it was not true that Aristotle had always treated the brain as a relatively insignificant organ with the sole function of cooling the heat of the heart, since in De partibus animalium 3.11 (673b9–12) he had referred to heart and brain as "the main governing powers of life"; furthermore, Galen had shared his view that the brain had a cooling function. Why should we not assume that Aristotle understood that communication between heart and brain via the arteries was necessary to allow heat and spirits to travel up and down? As for the notion that sensation and motion persisted in some animals after removal of the heart, it must be recognized that the loss of the heart inevitably produced loss of life; the movements that were perceived were simply the residue of an "impetus of spirits" sent by the heart into the rest of the body.[59]

However up-to-date the sources of his defense of Aristotle, Costeo's essential goal was evidently the traditional one of reconciliation. The indifference to conciliation and the hostility to Aristotle that mark Santorio's comments on heart and brain present a sharp contrast, yet by the time Santorio wrote, these attitudes, too, represented a set of intellectual conventions that were equally well established, if of more recent origin. Thus, Santorio's remarks that anyone who thought the nerves

<hr />

[58] "De qua re prodiit nunc in lucem Augustini Buccii Taurinensis primarii in ea Academia philosophiae professoris disertissima disputatio, qua non vulgaribus argumentis pro Peripateticis pugnat." Ibid., p. 490. According to Lohr, in *Studies in the Renaissance* 21 (1974), Bucci (who held a medical as well as a philosophy degree and had studied under Da Monte) held a professorship in philosophy at Turin from 1569 to 1592. He published *Naturales disputationes VI ad De anima libros* (Turin, 1572).

[59] Costeo, *Disq. phys.*, pp. 487–90.

originated in the heart was imbecilic, and that the analogy between the human body and the state was purely dialectical, recall, and may indeed derive from, those of Marco Oddi, who wrote some eighty years earlier. And Marco, it will be recalled, claimed to share the opinions of his father. (Santorio, however, added the republican comment that a state could be just as well ruled by a group magistracy as by a king.)[60]

If Santorio's treatment of the problem of the supposed primacy of the heart is compared with those of Oddi and Paterno, the two sixteenth-century commentators on *Canon* I.I who adopted an anti-Aristotelian position on this issue, the chief difference seems to be Santorio's own more careful listing of the kinds of physical evidence supposed by Aristotle and his followers to substantiate the primacy of the heart. The assertions he noted, along with the implications drawn from them, were as follows: sensation requires heat, and the heart is the source of heat and therefore sensation; blood is found outside the veins only in the heart, therefore blood must be manufactured in the heart; if a carotid artery is compressed, an animal is deprived of sensation and motion, therefore these faculties must depend on the heart, as the arteries depend on the heart; the brain itself has no sensation, therefore cannot be the principle of sensation; the brain palpates on account of the arteries, which shows that all motion has its origin in the heart; death inevitably follows serious injury to the heart, whereas it is possible to survive some degree of injury to the brain, so the heart must be the body's king. Santorio denied all the conclusions drawn from these assertions, and in some cases also rejected the assertions themselves. In just one instance, when he noted that survival was possible despite some damage to the heart, he drew on the findings of named sixteenth-century writers on practical medicine and anatomists. Otherwise, he relied for his arguments entirely on texts of Galen, even for *experimenta* to disprove the Aristotelian contentions.[61]

Santorio's handling of the question of the primacy of the heart thus stands in striking contrast to his readiness to introduce into his commentary new material—descriptions of his own instruments or theories, accounts of non-Aristotelian cosmology and of very recent anatomical findings—on topics that were not among the major traditional

---

[60] "Secunda ratio Aristotelis est in civitate unus debet esse rex; est argumentum dialecticum, quia posset etiam triumviratus aeque bene ac rex gubernare civitatem." Santorio, comm. *Canon* I.I (Venice, 1646), col. 876. The discussion continues in *Quaestio* 108: "An cor sit membrum tribuens et non suscipiens, id est an a corde omnes corporis facultates proveniant" (cols. 877–86).

[61] Ibid., cols. 878–84; the Galenic *experimenta* (tortoise walking after evulsion of the heart, effects of injury to the heart, effects of injury to the brain) are at col. 881.

323

subjects of controversy between Aristotelians and Galenists. As the example just examined shows, Renaissance commentators on the *Canon* were capable of transforming the main Aristotelian/Galenic *quaestiones* in response to current concerns and attitudes, but only up to a point. All appear to have regarded themselves as engaged in genuine controversy, rather than a routine academic exercise; Costeo, indeed, explicitly drew on contemporary polemic. The three Galenic authors taught their pupils to reject reconciliation and attach importance to anatomical evidence. Even in some courses on *theoria*, therefore, the argument over the primacy of the heart seems to have shifted somewhat away from philosophical and toward anatomical grounds, though this does not mean that the students were invited to consider physical evidence for themselves or without the baggage of interpretation preformulated by medical tradition and the requirements of controversy. Rather, what happened was that assertions about anatomy took their place alongside other kinds of argument. The nature and traditions of teaching by commentary on the *Canon* provided a context in which it was difficult if not impossible to treat the subject of the function of the heart as anything but an instance of controversy between the ancient authors. The appeal to anatomy hence remained largely an appeal to Galen's texts. Thus, Santorio's handling of the question of the primacy of the heart in the second or third decade of the seventeenth century differed relatively little from that of the elder Oddi at the height of the Galenic revival some eighty or ninety years before, despite the fact that in other respects Santorio's commentary belonged to a different world of thought from that of the two Oddi.

Physiology and Anatomy

In sixteenth-century medical science the two areas of most active and lively innovation, and those in which the greatest actual additions to knowledge and advances in methodology occurred, were anatomy and pharmacological botany. Of these, the latter was of little relevance to physiology, to the course in medical *theoria*, or to commentary on the subject matter of *Canon* 1.1, and hence it is not surprising that the commentaries reflect little or nothing of contemporary activity. Anatomy was a different matter, since in certain respects it was highly relevant both to physiological theory in general and to the content of *Canon* 1.1 in particular. The parts of the body constituted one of the standard subdivisions of medical *theoria*, and to it Avicenna had devoted the whole of the fifth *doctrina* of *Canon* 1.1. Furthermore, and perhaps more important, to the extent that they provided a basis for or substantiated

324

theories of physiological function, anatomical considerations found an appropriate place in the exposition of the *doctrinae* on humors and virtues. Hence although professors of *theoria* and their students, in those capacities, played no part in the practical development of anatomy, they could not be indifferent to the revival of Galenic anatomy or to the findings of sixteenth-century anatomists and the controversies those findings engendered.

Thus, the already noted anatomical material in the commentators' teaching on the humors and in their presentation of traditional themes of Aristotelian/Galenic debate is part of a wider pattern in their work of responsiveness to this major area of development in sixteenth-century medical science. Unquestionably, the sixteenth- and early seventeenth-century commentaries on *Canon* 1.1, especially those of the two Oddi, Costeo, and Santorio, had a markedly more anatomical focus than their medieval predecessors. Yet a variety of factors ensured that the response of the Renaissance commentators on *Canon* 1.1 to the anatomists remained partial, frequently superficial, and always highly restricted in scope.

In the first place, the anatomical *Doctrina* 5, *de membris*, included in *Canon* 1.1 was itself partial in coverage, surveying only bones, muscles, arteries, veins, and nerves. The practice established by early commentators of excluding from commentary all but the first chapter of *Doctrina* 5 cut back the anatomical content still further, since this first chapter is largely devoted to principles of classification of bodily parts and contains almost nothing in the way of actual anatomical description. Second, by the time the significant expansion of anatomical studies began around the end of the fifteenth century, the curricular division between *theoria* and *practica* was firmly established. It was of course no part of the duties of professors of *theoria* to provide detailed anatomical instruction or to conduct anatomical demonstrations. Hence, their level of competence and interest depended on individual predilection, on their past careers, and no doubt to a large extent on whatever anatomical training they happened to have received in their own student days.

Moreover, professors of *theoria* could not assume that their audience would have received much (if any) specific anatomical instruction. Jean Fernel echoed Gentile da Foligno in deploring this state of affairs and asserting that anatomy belonged at the beginning of medical studies, but to no avail.[62] Although at Padua and elsewhere lectures on *Canon*

---

[62] See Bylebyl, "Disputation and Description," pp. 225–26, and nn. 15, 16; for Gentile's views, see Chapter 3, above.

1.1 formed part of a three-year cycle of courses in *theoria*, and thus presumably in principle need not have been attended only by beginning students, in practice, courses on *theoria* often seem to have been treated as introductory surveys. It is true that Da Monte was able to assume that the audience for his lectures on *Canon* 1.2 already knew at least something of anatomy, but these lectures were not part of the normal cycle of courses in *theoria*—they were probably given as extraordinary lectures—and may have attracted a special audience.[63] Those students who did not manage to evade the courses on *theoria* altogether would usually be exposed to specific and practical instruction and demonstration in anatomy as in other branches of medicine only after they heard lectures on *Canon* 1.1.

Finally, the interest of the commentators in anatomy was of course limited by the very nature of the task of teaching physiology by means of commentary on the last three *doctrinae* of *Canon* 1.1. The main objectives of such commentary (even in discussing the first chapter of *Doctrina* 5) were to present theories of physiological function and to explain difficulties, problems, or controversies that had arisen. The anatomical teachings of the *moderni*, whether Galenic or neoteric, were relevant to this undertaking only to the extent that they were perceived to have bearing on particular physiological controversies, usually ones that had been long-standing subjects of discussion. Within these boundaries, however, six out of seven commentators—Da Monte, the two Oddi, Cardano, Costeo, and Santorio—made appreciable efforts to direct the attention of their pupils and readers toward the significance for *theoria* of anatomical work done since 1500.

Da Monte deserves mention in this connection not because of anything in his commentary in *Canon* 1.1, in which the anatomical component is extremely slight and, as far as I have been able to determine, almost wholly traditional, but because at least one passage in his exposition of *Canon* 1.2 suggests that on occasion his teaching inculcated in students of *theoria* an attitude toward immediately contemporary anatomy that was positive as well as attentive. The commentary on *Canon* 1.2 was probably written in the mid-1540s, and is mainly devoted to the subject of the classification of diseases. In the course of discussing cataract, Da Monte criticized Giacomo da Forlì for misunderstanding Avicenna's description, attributing Giacomo's errors to his never having actually treated a case of cataract. Da Monte's own ac-

---

[63] "Credo vos scire ex anatome quo modo septem sunt tunicae oculi, et tres humores." Da Monte, comm. *Canon* 1.2 (Venice, 1557), p. 45. Regarding the teaching of *Canon* 1.2, see Chapter 4, above.

count, which followed, included several pages of explanation of ocular anatomy to support the view that the cause of cataract was not, as Giacomo had held, "repletion of the optic nerves," but rather a distinct "impediment" residing in the eye. In addition to thus making understanding of a medical condition contingent upon understanding of anatomy, Da Monte's description, while preserving the traditional terminology of the eye's seven tunics and three humors, showed awareness of Vesalius' work on the eye; in particular, Da Monte referred with approval to the "excellent" description of the ciliary body by "Vesalius, the light of the whole art of anatomy."[64]

Returning to *Canon* 1.1, we may first note that both Cardano and Santorio included explicit defenses of anatomy in the opening sections of their commentaries. Cardano was concerned only to uphold the standing of anatomy as a science. The objection to classifying anatomy among the sciences was of course that it consisted merely in knowledge of particulars gained through sense experience, did not involve reasoning or logical demonstration, and hence was, at best, an art. Cardano pointed out that anatomy did indeed involve demonstration of *posteriora ex prioribus* and that this was precisely the kind of science contained in Aristotle's works on animals. In Cardano's views, sense knowledge of parts of the body might be only an art, but it was transformed into true anatomical science when it involved knowledge of connections and causes. He concluded, abrasively as always ("whatever you may say about this, I shall say . . . "), that anatomy was not only a true and outstanding science, but more worthy of the name than some other parts of natural philosophy.[65]

Half a century or more later, Santorio took up the issue anew, this time in the form of a *quaestio*: "Should anatomy pertain to the physician?" (*An anatomia pertineat ad medicum*).[66] Like Cardano, Santorio defended the standing of anatomy as a science, and thus worthy of the physician's consideration, but he also found it necessary to rebut the idea that, given that it was a science, anatomy properly belonged only to natural philosophy and to the study of Aristotle's works on animals, and not to medicine at all. In the course of so doing, Santorio strongly asserted the fundamental importance of data derived from sense expe-

[64] Da Monte, comm. *Canon* 1.2 (Venice, 1557), pp. 44–48; at pp. 45–46, "Vesalius lumen totius artis anatomicae." For another example, see Nutton, "Montanus, Vesalius."

[65] "Concludo ergo quod anathomia est vera scientia sicut sunt reliquae quicquid enim dixeris de hoc, dicam ego de aliis etiam obiiciam partibus philosophiae naturalis, anathomia ergo scientia est et praeclara." Cardano, *Opera* (Lyon, 1663), 9:487.

[66] Santorio, comm. *Canon* 1.1 (Venice, 1646), *Quaestio* 15, cols. 143–45.

rience alone in both natural philosophy and medicine;[67] as for the role of reasoned argument in anatomy, Santorio thought the very proliferation of anatomical controversy—"so that everything is *sub judice* even up to the present day"—was sufficient to guarantee anatomy's status as a science involving reasoning as well as observation, and not just a collection of facts: "for if anatomy were known by sense alone, there would not be so many questions in anatomy which are considered by Du Laurens, and before Du Laurens by Vesalius, and by an infinite number of others; there would not be so many questions between Aristotle and Galen about the origin of the veins and the nerves . . . so that the opinion that anatomy is understood only by sense without the use of reason is manifestly false."[68]

Although Costeo introduced into his commentary no formal defense of anatomy of the kind put forward by Cardano and Santorio, he nonetheless made it plain that he not only shared their opinions about the importance of the subject for *medici* in general, but also thought it should have a place of its own within the course on *theoria* based on *Canon* 1.1. Santorio and Marco Oddi no doubt expressed the standard justification for the normal practice of omitting commentary on all except the general and introductory first chapter of *Doctrina* 5 in their remarks to the effect that despite the presence in Avicenna's text of a descriptive account of bones, muscles, nerves, veins, and arteries, detailed teaching on these subjects was best left to anatomists.[69] Costeo, however, unlike any other of the Renaissance commentators, and

[67] "Praeterea non valet, hoc sensu cognoscitur sine ratiocinio, ergo non pertinet ad philosophum vel medicum; quia innumerabilia sunt quae solum sensu cognoscuntur quae tamen pertinent ad philosophum, ut dari motum, locum, tempus, dari gravia et levia, dari coelum, alterationes, generationes, dari caliditatem, frigiditatem, humiditatem, et siccitatem, dari quinque sensus et quamplurima quae cognoscuntur sine ratiocinio, quae pertinent ad philosophiam naturalem. Idem dicimus in medicina plurima cognosci sensu tantum quae revera pertinent ad medicinam vel philosophiam." Ibid., cols. 144–45.

[68] "Sed concludimus anatomiam cognosci ratiocinio; si enim sensu solo anatomia cognosceretur, non essent tot quaestiones in anatomia, quae a Laurentio considerantur, et ante Laurentium a Vesalio, et ab infinitis aliis; non essent tot quaestiones inter Aristotelem et Galenum de origine venarum et nervorum . . . quare manifeste falsa est illa sententia quod anatomia solum sensu sine ratiocinio intelligatur." Ibid., col. 145. The *Historia anatomica* of André du Laurens (1558–1609) was published in 1600; see Bylebyl, "Disputation and Description," pp. 226–27. Sixteenth- and early seventeenth-century concepts of the kind of knowledge offered by anatomy are further discussed in Andrew Wear, "William Harvey and the 'Way of the Anatomists,' " *History of Science* 21 (1983), 223–49.

[69] See Oddi, comm. *Canon* 1.1 (Venice, 1575), p. 441; and Santorio, comm. *Canon* 1.1 (Venice, 1646), col. 962.

unlike most if not all of their medieval predecessors, extended his commentary on the *doctrina de membris* beyond its first chapter. His reasons for so doing seem to have been twofold. First, if one may judge by the amount of effort he contributed to editing the *Canon*, Costeo was probably the most strongly committed of the commentators to the value of Avicenna's work as such (see Chapter 5); part of Costeo's motivation may therefore have been simply a desire to do justice to Avicenna's text. However, he was also clearly concerned both to make his readers aware of the importance of anatomy in current medical science and to weigh the relative merits of ancient and modern anatomical descriptions of particular parts of the body.

Although Costeo's enterprise gave anatomy an exceptionally prominent place in a physiological textbook and in the teaching of traditional *theoria*, he certainly did not devote the whole of his commentary on the *doctrina de membris* to that subject. Of the 150 pages he allotted to this section, well over one-third are devoted to an exposition of the introductory chapter essentially similar in its general tenor to those of the other commentators.[70] In this, although some anatomical description is present, it is subordinated to the theme of classification—similar and dissimilar, simple and composite parts, "contributing" and "receiving" members, the question of the primacy of the heart, and so on— and to the exposition of standard topics of physiological controversy. Thus, Costeo gave a good deal of attention to apparent or real inconsistencies in Galen's, and hence some of Avicenna's, accounts of the coats, and fibers within the coats, of various organs—notably arteries, bladder, and intestines—a subject that also preoccupied Paterno and Santorio, among many other authors.[71] Discussions of this subject— and Costeo's was no exception—tended to be couched in terms of the attractive, expulsive, and retentive qualities ascribed respectively to longitudinal, horizontal, and oblique fibers, and to have as their goal the reconciliation or explaining away of Galen's inconsistencies. In this chapter, too, Avicenna provided the text for lengthy expositions, often leading to reconciliation, of the Aristotelian and Galenic theories about conception; Costeo's treatment included a fairly detailed description of the female testes (i.e., the ovaries), but is otherwise unremarkable.[72]

---

[70] Costeo's exposition of the *doctrina de membris* occupies *Disq. phys.*, pp. 334–484, with that of the introductory chapter at pp. 334–97.

[71] Ibid., pp. 395–97; compare Paterno, comm. *Canon* 1.1 (Venice, 1596), fol. 121ʳ⁻ᵛ, and Santorio, comm. *Canon* 1.1 (Venice, 1646), cols. 950–59.

[72] Costeo, *Disq. phys.*, pp. 372–90. The description of the "female testes" is on p. 377: "substantia autem dura, magnitudine longe quam in maribus inferiores; ex quibus comprimendo veluti ex vesica aliqua aqueus tenuisque humor exilit. Iis coniuncti non sunt,

Furthermore, Costeo's expositions of the later sections of *Doctrina* 5 on nerves, veins, and arteries seem little different in character and not much more anatomical in focus than the discussions of the same subjects included by other commentators in their treatment of the introductory chapter of the *doctrina de membris* or elsewhere. Aristotle's ideas about the relations of the nerves and the heart, the much vexed question of the nature and causes of pulse, whether the arteries carry *spiritus*, blood, or both, the differences between the views of Aristotle, Galen, and Averroes on the subject of the veins—all these topics could be and were taken up by the other commentators, as well as by a host of other writers on academic physiology, in contexts other than commentary on the later chapters of *Canon* 1.1.5.

The real innovation in Costeo's treatment of *Doctrina* 5 lies in his introduction of the subject of the anatomy of bones and muscles, to which he devoted a total of some fifty pages.[73] Even so, he did not expound every one of Avicenna's thirty chapters on bones and thirty chapters on muscles. On the muscles, Costeo commented only on Avicenna's introductory statement defining the relationship of nerves, muscles, tendons, and ligaments. The subject had also been taken up by Marco Oddi, who, in the course of discussing *virtus motiva* in his exposition of *Doctrina* 6, had criticized Avicenna's account of voluntary motion from the standpoint of Galenic anatomy.[74] Costeo, however, gave the subject more prominence by placing his account within a separate anatomical section, and a different emphasis by criticizing Galen's account of the role of muscles and nerves in voluntary motion from the standpoint of the *moderni*.[75] Costeo's discussion of the bones, in which he commented on Avicenna's eight chapters on the bones of the head and neck and two chapters on the ribs and thorax, seems to have little precedent in the tradition of commentary on *Canon* 1.1.

Costeo was unambiguous in his recognition of the superiority of the contribution of Vesalius and other recent anatomists to the knowledge of skeletal anatomy, declaring that "as far as the division of the structure of the bones is concerned, the *recentiores* should in my opinion be

---

ut in maribus, seminarii meatus; imo eo intervallo ab iis disiuncti, quod dimidii digiti crassitudinem aequet; neque alia ratione quam tenuissima membranula adnexi. Sunt hi etiam graciles, atque angusti, minusque quam in maribus flexuosi, longe vero breviores."

[73] Ibid., pp. 398–451.

[74] See Oddi, comm. *Canon* 1.1 (Venice, 1575), pp. 490–92.

[75] "Ceterum non contemnenda hoc in loco est alia recentiorum in Galenum pugna, qui licet voluntarii motus instrumenta musculos esse censeant, habere tamen eos id muneris non ex nervis, sed ad Averrhois exemplum ex carne, probabilius censent. Patere enim id ex dissectione." Costeo, *Disq. phys.*, pp. 444–45. The discussion continues until p. 451.

taken into account and followed."[76] Yet he was evidently also concerned to salvage as much as possible of ancient anatomy, and praised the work of Bartolomeo Eustachi for its contribution to saving Galen.[77] Costeo called the attention of his readers to numerous specific instances in which the opinions of the *recentiores* together with data from observation and dissection confirmed conclusions different from those of the Hippocratic and Galenic works on bones, or from those of Aristotle or Avicenna: varieties of joints, the number of sutures in the skull, the conformation of the sphenoid bone, the number of vertebrae, the number of pairs of ribs, the respective roles of nerves and muscles in voluntary motion, to name only a few.[78]

But in a good many of these instances he then proceeded to adopt one of several strategies that absolved the ancient authorities, and especially Hippocrates and Galen, from blame. Hence Costeo admitted the existence of numerous errors in Galen's *De ossibus*, but attributed them to copyists, thus freeing Galen from responsibility.[79] On several occasions, moreover, he suggested that apparent inconsistency or error in the views of Hippocrates or Galen was due to corruption of the Greek text, showing his awareness of some of the intensive activity devoted to editing Greek texts by mid-century medical philologists. By the time Costeo wrote, mistranslation into Arabic or Latin could no longer be used as a blanket excuse for palpable errors or inconsistencies.[80] And he also suggested once or twice that the ancient authors

[76] "Itaque, quod ad divisionem structurae ossium pertinet sunt (ut arbitror) laudandi et sequendi recentiores." Ibid., p. 402.

[77] Ibid., p. 404. Bartolomeo Eustachi's two earliest works, on bones and on the motion of the head, both published in 1561, were, according to C. D. O'Malley "directed against the anti-Galenism of Vesalius, for whom he [Eustachi] had developed a unilateral hostility" (*DSB*, 4:486). Regarding Eustachi's subsequent career and own important contributions to anatomy, see *DSB*, 4:486–88.

[78] Costeo, *Disq. Phys.*: varieties of joints, pp. 400–401; sutures, pp. 404–8; sphenoid bone, p. 413; vertebrae, pp. 425–28; ribs, pp. 429–30; regarding nerves and muscles in voluntary motion, see n. 75, above.

[79] "Qua profecto de re, quando obiectis in Galenum rationibus sensus assentitur, fatendum quidem est esse in libello *De ossibus* errores; at eos tamen descriptorum potius quam Galeni culpa incidisse ut pro certo habemus; ita confirmare posse videmur ex Avicenna, qui ossium structuram praeter libelli eius seriem hoc loco prosecutus nulla de sententia eius scriptoris, a quo tamen dissentit, facta commemoratione." Ibid., p. 402.

[80] "De Hippocrate vero, illud apertum est libellum *De ossium natura* conspersum erroribus multis ad nos pervenisse. Cuius in vulgata graeca editione principium totum ad hanc usque de qua agimus sententiam desideratur." Ibid., p. 425, and similarly p. 428. Examples of the activities, during the 1540s and 1550s, of a circle of medical philological scholars in collecting and collating manuscripts and editing or reediting Greek medical texts (including Galen's *De ossibus*) are discussed in Nutton, "John Caius and the Eton Galen."

331

must have obtained their information from the consideration of some special case or situation different from that of dissection of the adult human cadaver, on which the *recentiores* based their findings. Thus he opined that Hippocrates had been engaging in conjectures about the sutures in the living skull, not in describing a dead one; and he expressed surprise that Aristotle had said there were only eight pairs of ribs, since it was manifest there were no fewer than twelve, but added that anomalous individuals had been observed to have eleven or thirteen.[81] And from time to time he resorted to the assertion that the *recentiores* had simply misunderstood Galen's teaching and criticized him unjustly.

Despite Costeo's persistent concern to defend the reputation of the ancients, no reader of this section of his commentary could fail to come away with the impression that in numerous specific instances the anatomical teaching of the moderns was superior to that of the ancients. Furthermore, although he certainly did not abandon traditional techniques of textual harmonization and scholastic argument, Costeo on a number of occasions made it clear that the standard by which the correctness of a statement about anatomy should be judged was that of conformity with data provided by recent, perhaps even preferably personal, observation. Of course, definitive conclusions reached on the basis of data patent to sense were likely to be more easily obtainable in the case of skeletal anatomy than in such long-standing physiological controversies as, say, the debate over whether and in what sense the veins originated in the liver. Yet Costeo's repeated assumption that if the results of observation differed from an ancient text it was likely to be the text that was at fault (even though he was almost always careful to exonerate the ancient author) was surely a useful lesson for students of *theoria*. Although Costeo was the first to admit that his anatomical coverage was partial and superficial, owing to the "immense labor" involved in providing a complete account, it seems likely that he sent his students away with the beginnings of an appreciation of "this whole part of medicine [which] in our age has been illustrated and enlarged by extremely learned men."[82]

The endorsements of anatomy as a part of medical science by Car-

---

[81] "In costarum historia mirum quod eas Aristoteles scribit homini utrinque esse octo, quas non pauciores esse quam duodecim apertum est, licet in aliquibus tredecim, in nonnullis etiam undecim aliqui observarint." Costeo, *Disq. phys.*, p. 430.

[82] "Sane autem, si cui in reliqua quam hic deince[p]s prosequitur et ossium et partium reliquarum privata historia, vel expendere singula, vel veterum recentiorumque dissidit tractare componereve animus sit; immensi is laboris opus sumat et temporis iacturam faciat, quum aetate nostra universa haec medicinae pars sit a doctissimis viris et illustrata et aucta." Ibid., p. 431.

dano and Santorio, and Costeo's insistence that the subject should have some place in the course on *theoria*, did not represent mere lip service to a fashionable ideal. Various passages in the commentaries of Da Monte, the two Oddi, Costeo, and Santorio indicative of knowledge of specific recent or contemporary developments in anatomy have already been noted; to them should perhaps be added Marco Oddi's fairly detailed description of the way in which "certain neoteric anatomists" had revised Galen's assertion that the nerves of sense took their origin from the front of the brain.[83] Santorio, in particular, was extremely well read in all aspects of contemporary as well as older medicine, anatomy among them. An attentive pupil would certainly have come away from Santorio's lectures on *Canon* 1.1 familiar with the views of modern anatomical and physiological writers on a variety of topics, even if he also gathered that most of these writers were most of the time wrong. The latter portion of Santorio's commentary is a mine of information about sixteenth- and occasionally early seventeenth-century anatomo-physiological thought and is rich in references to mid- and late sixteenth-century authors who wrote on such topics; among those cited are Vesalius, Falloppia, Realdo Colombo, Laurent Joubert, and André du Laurens, along with a variety of other more theoretically or philosophically inclined authors.[84] As this list suggests, in all the commentaries, including Santorio's, appeals to anatomical experience are frequently just as textbound as any other form of argument; the statement that a phenomenon is attested by sense or can be seen in dissection is just as likely to be based on a text of Galen as on a record of sixteenth-century observation, and more likely to be based on either than on the commentator's personal experience. Yet Santorio from time to time clearly and unambiguously appealed to his own experience in dissection and perhaps to anatomical experiments that he attempted himself (as in the case of the gall bladder).[85]

Although most of the commentators were both convinced of the importance of anatomy and reasonably well informed about it, the actual function within their expositions of material drawn from anatomy or appeals to anatomical experience was limited, more often than not, to

[83] See Oddi, comm. *Canon* 1.1 (Venice, 1575), p. 476. For sixteenth-century changes in dissecting techniques, which produced an improved understanding of the anatomy of the brain, see Edwin Clarke and C. D. O'Malley, *The Human Brain and Spinal Cord* (Berkeley and Los Angeles, 1965), pp. 820–23.

[84] See, e.g., Santorio, comm. *Canon* 1.1 (Venice, 1646), cols. 542, 808, 861, 1069. Laurent Joubert's *Medicinae practicae . . . tomus primus* was published Lyon, 1582.

[85] ". . . in cadavere in quo tamen ipsa observavimus." Santorio, comm. *Canon* 1.1 (Venice, 1646), col. 1044.

furnishing additional arguments in the discussion of standard topics of physiological debate. The kind of limited and partial attention to anatomical considerations that has already been noted in the commentators' treatment of Aristotelian/Galenic controversy was entirely characteristic of their use of the subject. Anatomical evidence could also serve a similar purpose in controversies that mingled traditional topics of debate and more modern physiological theories. Two examples, both topics of some importance in sixteenth- and early seventeenth-century medical thought are the problem of whether or not heartbeat and arterial pulse are synchronous and questions relating to the generation of vital and animal spirits.

The complex nature and history of Renaissance controversy over pulse has recently been effectively analyzed by Jerome Bylebyl. The problem of the synchronous or alternating character of heartbeat and pulse is in fact only one of a cluster of related questions about the movement of the heart and arteries, no one of which can be fully considered in isolation from the rest. However, for the present purpose it may suffice to note, that, as Bylebyl has shown, the question of whether diastole and systole in the heartbeat and arterial pulse were synchronous or alternating was, like other related issues, already discussed by Galen and his Alexandrian predecessors; became a topic of scholastic physiological disputation in the Latin Middle Ages; and was subject to further debate and review in the light of experimental and other considerations in the sixteenth and early seventeenth centuries. Galen's own position was that heartbeat and pulse were synchronous—that is, that diastole in the heart coincided with diastole of the arteries—and that both were caused by an active vital faculty in the heart and arterial walls. However, Erasistratus, whose views were reported by Galen, the author of an anonymous *Compendium de pulsibus* attributed to Galen in the Middle Ages, Pietro d'Abano and other scholastics, and Jean Fernel all for one reason or another held some version of the theory that heartbeat and pulse alternated in the sense that systole in the heart coincided with diastole of the arteries, because the heart mechanically impelled *spiritus* into the arterial vessels. In the sixteenth century the debate was reopened by textual scholarship that rejected the *Compendium de pulsibus* as spurious and thus clarified Galen's authentic position, by attention to Galen's own descriptions of anatomical techniques for investigating the problem, and by the work of Realdo Colombo and other practicing anatomists. Much controversy ensued and was duly reflected in the teaching of professors of *theoria* commenting on *Canon* I.I.[86]

---

[86] See Bylebyl, "Disputation and Description," passim, and esp. pp. 228–32, on which

As a result, Marco Oddi, Costeo, and Santorio all introduced the problem of the relation of heartbeat and pulse into their discussions of Avicenna's account of the functions of heart and arteries. Oddi's main goal was to defend the Galenic position that the two movements were synchronous. He briefly mentioned the view of Erasistratus and spent a little more time repudiating the Aristotelian view, further endorsed by Torrigiano in the early fourteenth century, that the movements were a mechanical consequence of the ebullition of blood, but it is clear that his principal adversary was Fernel. According to Oddi, Fernel had put together the opinion of Erasistratus with certain misunderstood sentences of Galen and arrived at a very false result. Oddi maintained, with Galen, that the simultaneity of heartbeat and arterial pulse could be detected manually (on the assumption that the heart strikes the chest at the moment of diastole, instead of, as actually, in systole). He also followed Galen in asserting that the motion of the arteries took place in the arterial walls (not in the contents), which led him to devote some attention to explaining the appearance presented by the arteries in dissection.[87]

The commentary of Marco Oddi, written to perpetuate the views of Oddo Oddi, is a product of the Galenic revival at its height and of a period when Fernel's physiological views were still a relatively new contribution to medical debate. However, around 1620, Santorio still defended the Galenic position on the relationship of heartbeat and arterial pulse, and still cast his defense in the form of an attack on Fernel. Santorio's treatment of this subject supplies one of the many passages serving as a reminder that the teaching of *theoria* by means of commentary on the *Canon* helped to perpetuate not only aspects of the medieval tradition of scholastic physiological disputation, but also the controversies of the middle years of the sixteenth century. Santorio's only real addition to Oddi's arguments was the remark that the simultaneous diastole of heart and arteries could be observed in a vivisected animal.[88]

Up until the end of the sixteenth century, working anatomists continued to produce conflicting reports of observations of the timing and sequence of the movement of heart and arteries in vivisected animals, and conflicting interpretations of which observed movements of the

---

the foregoing summary is based. On Galen's own pulse lore, see also C.R.S. Harris, *The Heart and the Vascular System in Ancient Greek Medicine* (Oxford, 1973), pp. 397–431.

[87] See Oddo, comm. *Canon* 1.1 (Venice, 1575), pp. 383–89.

[88] "Patet quoque experientia, dum mactatur aliquod animal vivum, in quo arteriarum et cordis diastole eodem tempore fieri inspicimus." Santorio, comm. *Canon* 1.1 (Venice, 1646), col. 862. He also constructed an instrument with which he claimed it would be possible to measure whether systole was more rapid than diastole in any individual (ibid., cols. 510–11).

heart in vivisection constituted systole and which diastole,[89] so that Santorio should not perhaps be blamed overmuch for selecting an observation to suit his argument. Nonetheless, the passage is a good illustration of the highly arbitrary manner in which data attributed to anatomical observation were apt to be used in the course of physiological arguments that were still confined within a framework that was both Galenic and scholastic. In Santorio's case, a keen interest in physiological-anatomical problems connected with the structure and movements of the heart and arteries and their contents, which led him to write quite extensively on these topics within his commentary on *Canon* 1.1, was combined with a rigid Galenism on a good many anatomical points (including the existence of foramina in the septum of the heart).[90] Santorio was indeed capable of writing on occasion as if "Galen and anatomy" were almost interchangeable terms.[91] Moreover, for Santorio anatomical considerations remained only one, and not necessarily the most persuasive, form of evidence; thus he found nothing incongruous in citing views of Thomas Aquinas to bolster an argument about pulse and respiration.[92]

Yet a generation before Santorio, Costeo's brief comment on the pulse controversy suggests that a different attitude toward anatomical evidence—and by extension toward experimental or observational data in general—may occasionally have been inculcated by teachers of *theoria* even when dealing with long-standing physiological debates. Costeo mentioned the problem of pulse only as an aside in the course of an otherwise unremarkable discussion as to whether the action of the arteries depended on the heart. Unlike Oddi and Santorio, he refused to take a position on whether diastole in the heart coincided with diastole in the arteries, although he evidently inclined to the view that it did not. But on this issue he did not retreat into scholastic reconciliation. Rather, he made it plain that in his opinion the dispute could be settled only on the basis of observations of the living animal (presumably in vivisection), "the only suitable judge of this disagreement." Since Cos-

---

[89] See Bylebyl, "Disputation and Description," pp. 237–38.

[90] ". . . foramina perexigua septi, seu membranae, quae separat sinum dextrum a sinistro . . . eadem tamen foramina in vivo debent esse magis aperta quam in cadavere, in quo tamen ipsa observavimus." Santorio, comm. *Canon* 1.1 (Venice, 1646), col. 1044. Santorio, like Fabrizio (see Chapter 4, above) and Galen himself, took the pits in the septum of the heart to be the termination of passages through which a significant amount of blood could pass. The question was not easily determined by inspection, and even Vesalius remained in doubt. See Harris, *Heart and Vascular System*, and n. 98, below.

[91] ". . . reluctatur anatomiae et ipsi Galeno" (Santorio, comm. *Canon* 1.1 [Venice, 1646], col. 951); ". . . ostendimus ex Galeno et anatomia" (ibid., col. 1117).

[92] Ibid., col. 1075.

teo stated that the dispute was still unresolved, he was presumably conscious of the ambiguous character of the observations already reported. Here the use of selected anatomical evidence in conjunction with ancient texts to support a predetermined position has given way, however fleetingly, to a willingness to allow experimental evidence alone to determine the outcome of a controversy or the validity of a hypothesis. However, it seems likely that Costeo found it possible to take such a position in this particular instance only because he believed that Galen himself had been of two minds on the question, and because he thought the solution of the problem essentially irrelevant to the main issue of whether the arteries depended on the heart.[93]

Although the subject of *spiritus* is not allocated any separate section of *Canon* 1.1, it occupies a relatively prominent position in that work, notably in chapter 4 of the concluding *doctrina* on the virtues, where an account of the generation and distribution of spirits in the body is to be found. Hence ample opportunity was present for the commentators to take up any of the various controversies about the subject that preoccupied Renaissance medical writers. On the whole, however, the treatment of the subject in the commentaries was relatively restrained. Certainly these academic Galenists showed little taste for exploring at any length the kind of ideas about connections between *spiritus* in the human body and celestial *spiritus*—somewhat perilous from the standpoint of religious as well as medical orthodoxy—that are associated with the thought of Fernel.[94] The commentators tended to deny, if in

---

[93] "Quod autem deinceps proponitur contrahi arterias quum cor dilatatur, an ita vere habeat res adhuc quidem controversum est, Galeno hac ipsa de re nunc in unam, nunc in alteram partem inclinante. Quicquid tamen ex sensu, solo idoneo huius dissidii iudice, in vivente animali statuendum fuerit; pendere arteriarum motum a cordis motu, nihil proposita dubitatio impedit. Sed si quidem dilatato corde arterias quoque dilatari verum sit, insitam cordi vim arteriarum motus originem esse per se dandum est. Sin autem non nisi contrahente se corde, et spiritus in arterias exprimente, arteriarum fiat pulsus; erit quidem earum motus a corde per accidens, sed quem tamen negare non liceat habere originem a corde." Costeo, *Disq. phys.*, p. 479. Bylebyl, "Disputation and Description," p. 229, notes that in *De anatomicis administrationibus* 7.12 (Kühn, 2:626–41) Galen left open the question of the conclusions that would result from an investigation of the issue by vivisection, although he suggested procedures by which investigation could be undertaken. Hence, Costeo's belief in Galen's uncertainty on the issue may not be without foundation.

[94] See Walker, "Astral Body," pp. 119–27. For the ancient history of theories about *pneuma*, or *spiritus*, see G. Verbeke, *L'évolution de la doctrine du pneuma du Stoïcisme à S. Augustin* (Louvain and Paris, 1945); and for medieval developments, James J. Bono, "Medical Spirits and the Medieval Language of Life," *Traditio* 40 (1984), 91–130. Much information about medieval and Renaissance ideas about *spiritus* (not always in a physiological context, however) is to be found in the essays collected as *Spiritus: IV° Colloquio*

some cases rather hesitantly or regretfully, that *spiritus* should be thought of as animate or ensouled[95] and to concentrate on strictly physiological aspects of the topic.

Among the commentators, only Da Monte treated problems about *spiritus* solely in terms of speculative natural philosophy and reconciliation of texts; he inquired whether, given Galen's hesitancy on the issue, natural as well as vital and animal spirits should be postulated, and into the relationship between *spiritus* and innate heat. Moreover, Da Monte's brief discussion of the elemental nature of *spiritus* hints that he had somewhat more sympathy than the other commentators for ideas about the celestial relations of *spiritus*. There he attempted to reconcile Avicenna's assertion (characterized by Da Monte as Platonic) that the elemental components of *spiritus* are air and fire with the Galenic position that *spiritus* is compounded from air and water. Da Monte's solution was that *spiritus* should be considered as formed from air and fire when connected with innate heat and affecting mores; otherwise, it should be treated as a compound of air and water.[96] The later commentators all included some attention to anatomy in their discussions of *spiritus*.

By the time Paterno, Costeo, and Santorio took up the subject, controversy over the generation and transmission of vital and animal spirits had long rested to a significant extent on anatomical considerations. As is well known, in the traditional account of the generation of *spiritus* a small amount of blood passed through pores in the septum of the heart into the left ventricle, where it was mixed with inspired air to form vital spirits and thence discharged into the arteries; the vital spirit was carried by the arteries up to the retiform plexus, or rete mirabile, where it was either prepared for transformation into animal spirits or actually so transformed; the animal spirits resided in the brain, whence they streamed through the hollow optic nerves to the eyes. The essen-

---

Internazionale del Lessico Intellettuale Europeo, Roma, 7–9 gennaio 1983, Atti, ed. M. Fattori and M. Bianchi (Rome, 1984).

[95] See Oddo, comm. *Canon* 1.1 (Venice, 1575), pp. 56–58, denying the animation of *spiritus*; Paterno, comm. *Canon* 1.1 (Venice, 1595), fol. 55[r], asserting that the spirits of our body are of the nature of ethereal lucid body diffused from the heavens; Costeo, *Disq. phys.*, pp. 548–50, denying the animation of *spiritus*; Da Monte, comm. *Canon* 1.1 (Venice, 1554), fol. 248[r], "spiritus implantatus non erit proprie animatus."

[96] Ibid., fols. 247[r]–49[r]. In the additional chapter appended to the second edition (Venice, 1557), p. 558, Da Monte noted that some of the *moderni* "nihil scientes nisi ex commentariis" denied the existence of animal spirits. Here again, his *moderni* may be thirteenth- to fifteenth-century Latin authors. For Da Monte's discussion of the elemental components of *spiritus*, see comm. *Canon* 1.1 (Venice, 1554), fols. 53[r]–54[r], which also includes a reference to *spiritus* as the "instrument" of the soul.

tial anatomical features of this narrative—the perforate septum, the human retiform plexus, and the hollow optic nerves—were all called into question early in the sixteenth century, although all continued to find defenders into the seventeenth. Writing in 1536, Nicolò Massa called attention to moderns who questioned the existence of the rete mirabile in man (as Berengario da Carpi had done a generation earlier).[97] Subsequently, Vesalius asserted that dissection showed the optic nerves to be solid and that comparative anatomy revealed that Galen had described the rete found in the ox, but not in man; and Vesalius also expressed doubts about the pores in the septum.[98] Furthermore, in 1556, the well-known neoteric physician Giovanni Argenterio published a treatise in which he denied the existence of separate animal spirits.[99]

Paterno dealt with these issues by avoiding them. His most extended discussion of *spiritus*, in one of the *quaestiones* appended to his commentary, was designed to show how animal spirits were formed in the brain and not in the retiform plexus, which served only the purpose of preparing the vital spirits for transformation.[100] While texts of Galen could be cited on either side of this argument, it seems probable that Paterno opted for the brain as the site of manufacture of animal spirits because he was aware that the rete mirabile might finally disappear from descriptions of human anatomy; however, he made no explicit allusion to such a possibility.

By contrast, Costeo inserted a thirty-page tractate on *spiritus* into his commentary on the last chapter (on operations) of *Doctrina* 6 in which he systematically reviewed the objections of the *recentiores* to various aspects of the theory of spirits, and especially to the concept of distinct animal spirits, and equally systematically refuted them.[101] Once more, Costeo drew on immediately contemporary polemic to bolster his arguments on a theme that seemed to him especially important, acknowledging that he had drawn much of his material from a treatise,

---

[97] See his *Liber introductorius anatomiae*, translated in Lind, *Studies in Pre-Vesalian Anatomy*, p. 242, and, for the date, ibid., p. 174.

[98] *Fabrica* (1543), pp. 324[424], 310[410], 589. On the development of Vesalius' views on the pores in the septum, and the stronger expression of doubt in the second edition of the *Fabrica,* see Whitteridge, *Harvey*, pp. 45–48.

[99] *Joannis Argenterii medici De somno et vigilia*, Book 2, chaps. 7–10, in his *Operum in tres tomos divisorum . . . volumen tertium* (Venice, 1592), pp. 66–75. For the date of the first edition, see Walker, "Astral Body," p. 127.

[100] Paterno, comm. *Canon* 1.1 (Venice, 1596), fols. 159^v–162^r. For other sixteenth- and early seventeenth-century discussions of the implications for the doctrine of *spiritus* of the absence of the rete mirabile in man, and suggestions for other sites for the manufacture of animal spirits, see Wear, "Galen in the Renaissance," pp. 223–37.

[101] Costeo, *Disq. phys.*, pp. 546–574.

De spiritibus, published by Domenico Bertacchi in 1584.[102] Much of Costeo's endeavor was directed toward explaining away various accusations of inconsistency on the subject of spirits that had been leveled at Galen. However, he also took note of both the anatomical objections to the traditional account of the formation of animal spirits and their transmission to the eye. But Costeo made no attempt to dispute the validity of the anatomical findings; instead, he took the line that even if true these findings in no way imperiled the existence or functions of animal spirits. Thus, of the retiform plexus, he noted that Galen had said only that it was consonant with reason that animal spirits were manufactured there, not that they were so manufactured; if, as the *recentiores* maintained, the retiform plexus was found only in other animals and not in man, the numerous convolutions in the human brain would be an equally suitable site for the manufacture of animal spirits.[103]

As for the solidity of the optic nerves, Costeo claimed that *spiritus* was so fine it could slip through the smallest (imperceptible) cavity. Alternatively, it might be carried to the eyes not by the nerves, but by the arteries; if so, the *spiritus* in the arteries in question would be so refined as to deserve the name "animal" rather than "vital" (as *spiritus* in the arteries were usually called).[104] Here once again Costeo was willing to allow a certain absolute priority to observational, experimental, or sense evidence, to the extent that he sought neither to deny it nor to explain it away; and up to a point he was ready to tailor his theory to fit the evidence, rather than the other way round. Ultimately, however, the anatomical material plays only a subordinate part in a predetermined course of argument, since Costeo's real goal was to save the existence of separate animal spirits.

Santorio, too, presented a modified theory of *spiritus* that took some account of relatively recent anatomical findings. He explicitly denied

---

[102] *Dominici Bertacchii Camporegianensis medici ac philosophi De spiritibus libri quatuor, necnon De facultate vitali libri tres* (Venice, 1584). Bertacchi devoted much of his first book to proving that *spiritus* was not to be identified with soul; in his third book he undertook to refute Argenterio and other recent authors who had written on the subject of spirits. The existence of separate animal spirits was defended by Bertacchi, but his work seems less anatomical in emphasis than that of Costeo.

[103] "Retiformem autem plexum de cuius usu non consentiunt Galeno recentiores, locum esse in quo ii spiritus potissimum fiant non certo demonstrare se ait Galenus, sed rationi tamen consentaneum esse affirmat. . . . Cuius tamen usus, si author non sit ille ipse plexus, non desunt tamen in cerebri universi substantia gyri varii, quibus ille absolvatur." Costeo, *Disq. phys.,* p. 565.

[104] Ibid., p. 566.

the existence of natural spirits[105] and paid little attention to animal spirits. Both the principal accounts of *spiritus* in Santorio's commentary on *Canon* I.I are focused on vital spirits and the transmission of substances in and out of the heart. In one of these passages, Santorio tried to prove that the blood in the vena cava received some *spiritus* directly from the heart because the valves of the heart never closed so tightly as to preclude some transmission of *spiritus* from the right ventricle as well as the left.[106] In the other, he reviewed differing neoteric views on where and how the mixture of blood and vapors constituting *spiritus* took place (supposing the septum to be imperforate).[107] He succinctly described three theories, all of which he dismissed. Of Leonardo Botallo's claim to have found a hitherto unknown channel linking the right ventricle to the left auricle—Botallo had in fact supposedly observed an anomalous instance of an unclosed foramen ovale—Santorio curtly remarked that unknown anatomical organs were figments of the imagination.[108] Another idea, that spirits might be manufactured in the spleen, inspired Santorio to heavy irony: if it were so, excess of melancholy would cause everyone to die in infancy.[109] Unfortunately, he was equally unimpressed with Realdo Colombo's account of the pulmonary transit of the blood and its aeration in the lungs; this was unacceptable to Santorio on the grounds that the return of aerated blood to the heart via the venous artery (pulmonary vein) would conflict with the supposed discharge of smoky vapors from the heart via the same vessel.[110]

Santorio was here clearly responsive to controversies of importance in Paduan anatomical circles, but his goal was to defend Galen. Accordingly, he endorsed the traditional theory that *spiritus* was manufac-

---

[105] Santorio, comm. *Canon* I.I (Venice, 1646), cols. 69–70.   [106] Ibid., col. 407.

[107] Ibid., cols. 1042–44.

[108] "Botalus inquit sanguinem praeparari in dextro sinu et transmitti per ductum incognitum a dextra ad sinistram auriculam cordis, sed cum sit incognitus erit inter figmenta et chimericam imaginationem ponendus." Ibid., cols. 1043–44. On Botallo and his supposed discovery, announced in 1565, see Whitteridge, *Harvey*, p. 64.

[109] "Sed vae nobis si spiritus fierent ex sanguine praeparato in liene; homines enim prae nimia maestitia et melancholia in aetate infantiae decederent e vivis." Santorio, comm. *Canon* I.I (Venice, 1646), col. 1044.

[110] "Columbus anatomicus dicit sanguinem pro generatione spirituum vitalium praeparari in dextro sinu cordis, sed ut fiat vaporosus et aeri permisceatur putat inde refundi ad venam arteriosam et pulmonem; mox a pulmone praeparatum per arteriam venosam transmitti ad sinistrum cordis ventriculum, ubi illico in spiritum vitalem convertitur. Non accipitur haec opinio Columbi de modo generationis spiritus vitalis, quia per arteriam venosam expelluntur fuligines quae resultant post generationem spiritus et non ante, secus ab ipsis fuliginibus sanguinis coinquinaretur et impediretur, ne celerrime ad sinum sinistrum excurreret." Santorio, comm. *Canon* I.I (Venice, 1646), col. 1043.

tured in the left ventricle of the heart from an admixture of inspired air and blood that had crossed through the supposed foramina in the septum. Moreover, he assured his readers that he had personally been able to detect these foramina in dissection, although he supposed that they must be more open in the living body than in the cadaver.[111]

Comparison of the examples that have been cited of the use of anatomy in the commentaries of Costeo and Santorio would appear to suggest that although Santorio almost certainly had a wider knowledge and a more specialized grasp of the subject than did Costeo, the latter was more often ready to admit that neoteric anatomists might on occasion be right. We may redress the balance somewhat by concluding this section with a brief account of one important instance in which Santorio departed radically from Galenic teaching in favor of an explanation and endorsement of the results of very recent scientific work.

In his lectures on *Canon* 1.1, Santorio taught his students that the principal organ of vision was not the crystalline humor (the lens), as Galen and a long line of subsequent medical writers had held, but the retina.[112] Santorio also characterized the crystalline humor as a convex lens,[113] and explained that variations in its curvature were responsible for myopia and longsightedness.[114] He further described an experiment

---

[111] Ibid., col. 1044. The passage is quoted in n. 90, above.

[112] *Quaestio* 123: "An organum formale visionis sit humor crystallinus, vel retina" (ibid., cols. 1060–67). This is certainly not the only instance in which Santorio endorsed new findings in physiology or anatomy. For example, his discussion of the ear and hearing (cols. 1068–70) includes an account of the incus, malleus, and staphes, "tria ossicula a modernis inventa," and the contribution of various sixteenth-century anatomists to the subject. The discovery of the small auricular bones was regarded as important precisely because they were unknown to Galen; see A. Fioretti and G. Concato, "Problemi di storia dell'anatomia dell'orecchio. Nota I: E individuabile lo scopritore dell'incudine e del martello?" *Acta medicae historiae patavina* 3 (1956–57), 47–91, and idem, "Problemi di storia dell'anatomia dell'orecchio. Nota II: Polemiche cinquecentesche intorno alla scoperta della staffa," *Acta medicae historiae patavina* 4 (1957–58), 59–120.

[113] ". . . quod vero retina sit organum formale visionis confirmatur experientia desumpta a lente vitrea, quae est convexa, et valde similis crystallino. Si foramina fenestrae apponatur et inspiciatur extra fenestram candella quae tamen sit in ipso cubiculo, tunc duae videntur candellae. Causa istius apparitionis pendet ex eo quia figura lenticularis est convexa sicuti est figura crystallina, quae figura convexa habet hanc proprietatem quod in ipsa refrangantur radii visorii." Santorio, comm. *Canon* 1.1 (Venice, 1646), cols. 1063–64. ". . . crystallinus est unum vitrum convexum." Ibid., col. 1065.

[114] "Deinde maior vel minor gibbositas crystallini et maior vel minor copia vitrei maxime alterant visionem. Hinc myopes non vident remota, vel ob copiam vitrei vel ob maiorem gibbositate crystallini; hae enim maior gibbositas efficit segmentum spherae minoris, in qua conus brevior sit"—and the opposite for the longsighted. Ibid., col. 1067.

to show that the reception of *species visibilis* required an opaque surface and a darkened environment, conditions obtaining within the eye for the retina, but not for the crystalline humor.[115] Santorio also described various demonstrations and observations relating to lenses, at least one of which he claimed to have performed himself.[116] Moreover, in his *quaestio* on the subject of vision Santorio did not even bother to expound the traditional position, but simply provided his audience with a list of seventeen reasons the principal organ of vision could not be the crystalline or any other part of the eye other than the retina. He brusquely dismissed the conciliatory endeavor of Christopher Scheiner, whose work on optics he otherwise admired, to call attention to the occasions on which Galen had ascribed some role in vision to the retina. According to Santorio, Aristotle, Galen, and Avicenna had all believed the crystalline humor to be the principal organ of sight, and had all been wrong.[117] Nor did Santorio rely on the usual parade of citations of authors, but presented most of the arguments as his own unadorned views.

In fact, Santorio seems to have drawn most of his material from Scheiner's *Oculus*, first published in 1619 (Santorio's commentary appeared in 1625 or 1626);[118] at any rate, Scheiner was the only one of the *recentiores optici* whom Santorio cited by name, and his main arguments are highly simplified, nonmathematical, and abbreviated versions of propositions put forward in Scheiner's technical treatise. Among them, in addition to those mentioned above, is the assertion that if vision were in the lens, objects would be seen reversed from left to right.[119] Of course, it is possible that Santorio was also independently familiar with the work of such earlier writers as Felix Platter, who had asserted in an anatomical opus published in 1583 that the retina was the principal organ of vision; Francesco Maurolico, who in a work pub-

[115] "Quod vero retina et non crystallinus sit formale visionis organum probatur hac experientia. Dum per foramen fenestrae cui apposita sit lens vitrea species visibiles ingrediuntur in cubiculum obscurum, recipiunturque in charta aliquantulum distanti." Ibid., col. 1064.

[116] ". . . sicut observatur domi nostrae, cuius parieti aqua fluminis adiacet: dum per lentem vitream foramini appositam inspicimus obiecta quae sunt trans aquam, illa erecto et non everso situ nobis apparent." Ibid., col. 1065.

[117] Ibid., col. 1067.

[118] *Oculus, hoc est fundamentum opticum* (Innsbruck, 1619). Christopher Scheiner, S.J. (1573–1650) is best known as an astronomer and mathematician; on his career and other writings, see William R. Shea, "Scheiner, Christopher, 1573–1650," *DSB*, 12:151–52.

[119] ". . . quod vero visio non fiat in crystallino patet, quia obiectum dextrum aliquando videretur in loco sinistro et sinistrum in dextro." Santorio, comm. *Canon* 1.1 (Venice, 1646), col. 1062; compare Scheiner, *Oculus*, p. 168.

lished posthumously in 1611 described the crystalline humor as a convex lens, ascribed refractive properties to it, and discussed the effects on vision of variations in lenticular curvature; and Della Porta, whose lengthy work on optics, *De refractione*, appeared in 1593.[120] Like Scheiner, Santorio was much concerned to provide an explanation as to why, if vision took place in the retina, objects were not seen upside down. Santorio put forward as his own idea the notion that the righting of the image was the function of the vitreous humor.[121] There is thus no sign that Santorio had read, or at any rate grasped, Kepler's account of the retinal image, which had appeared in 1604.[122]

Yet the teaching on vision available to beginning medical students at Padua between 1611 and 1625 from Santorio's lectures on *Canon* 1.1 seems nonetheless to have been more advanced than that available during the same period at Basel, where Felix Platter had taught. There, according to H. M. Koelbing, Caspar Bauhin, Platter's younger colleague in anatomy, continued to maintain that the lens was the principal organ of vision in a work published in 1590. The first record of discussion of Platter's ocular physiology at Basel comes in the form of a disputation (not a professorial lecture) by Felix Platter the younger, who was presumably swayed by filial piety, in 1626. Not until 1639 did a student at Basel submit for disputation a study of vision presenting a position that sounds very like that of Santorio: its author claimed the retina as the principal seat of vision and compared the eye to a camera obscura. However, he also asserted that the image on the retina was upright, this result having been achieved by nature's skillful positioning of refractive media within the eye.[123]

Concepts of Disease

For the most part, the lively sixteenth-century discussions about concepts of disease and disease classification and transmission found no

[120] For the general background and development of sixteenth- and early seventeenth-century optics and ocular physiology, I rely on David C. Lindberg, *Theories of Vision from Al Kindi to Kepler* (Chicago, 1976), pp. 173–205, and David C. Lindberg, "Optics in Sixteenth-Century Italy," in *Novità celesti e crisi del sapere*, pp. 131–48.

[121] "Collige mirabilem usum vitrei humoris, qui consistit in erigendis imaginibus, quem usum anatomici et optici (quod sciam) non cognoverunt." Santorio, comm. *Canon* 1.1 (Venice, 1646), col. 1065.

[122] On Kepler's theory of the retinal image see Lindberg, *Theories of Vision*, pp. 193–202.

[123] See H. M. Koelbing, "Ocular Physiology in the Seventeenth Century and Its Acceptance by the Medical Profession," *Analecta Medico-Historica Academiae Internationalis Historiae Medicinae* 3. *The Historical Aspects of Brain Research in the 17th Century*, ed. G. Scherz (Oxford, 1968), pp. 219–24.

echo in the commentaries on *Canon* 1.1. Some brief general comments on the nature of health and sickness occur in Avicenna's overview of the subject matter of medicine in chapter 2 of the first *doctrina*, a section on varieties of complexional imbalance is included in *Doctrina* 3, and a few examples relating to disease and therapy are found from time to time elsewhere in both text and commentaries; but pathology as such was not part of the subject matter of either the work itself or courses based upon it. It was, of course, this state of affairs that prompted Da Monte to lecture in addition on *Canon* 1.2, and others later to advocate the resumption of his practice (see Chapters 4 and 6). Da Monte's lectures on *Canon* 1.2 therefore constitute the single substantial discussion of pathological theory in the body of commentary under review, although Santorio managed to work a couple of questions on the subject into his exposition of *Canon* 1.1. As a consequence, the following summary serves only to call attention to some salient features of the way Da Monte presented the subject to students of *theoria* at Padua in the mid-1540s, and not to any more generally diffused aspect of the teaching of *theoria* from *Canon* 1.

As is well known, the late fifteenth century initiated a period of greatly intensified debate among physicians over the way in which disease should be conceptualized. The description of apparently new diseases, of which syphilis was the most notorious; the question of whether such diseases could be fitted into Galenic classifications; efforts to expand, reinterpret, or supplement the explanation of disease that relied upon variations in temperament and the humors; the consideration of contagion and the means whereby it was transmitted; the effort to find principles of therapy other than those depending on the interaction of the four qualities in remedy and patient—these and similar subjects preoccupied numerous authors, among whom some of the most celebrated are Leoniceno, who wrote the first of a long series of Renaissance treatises on the *morbus gallicus* (1497); Fracastoro, whose *De contagione* was first published in 1546; Fernel, who discussed occult causes of disease in *De abditis rerum causis* (1548); and Paracelsus.[124] Most of the subjects discussed and solutions proposed were far from wholly new; they had antecedents not only in antiquity, but also in the medieval plague tractates—these, too, dealt with a "new" disease—and in the medieval elaborations of the concept of medicaments that worked according to the specific forms of remedy and disease, rather than through the supposedly rational interaction of the primary quali-

[124] See Daniela Mugnai Carrara, "Fra causalità astrologica e causalità naturale. Gli interventi di Nicolò Leoniceno e della sua scuola sul morbo gallico," *Physis* 21 (1979), 37–54; and Nutton, "Seeds of Disease." Regarding Fernel's theories about disease, see further below. I make no attempt to indicate the large literature on Paracelsus here.

ties in remedy and patient. However, in this as in other instances Renaissance physicians appear to have perceived themselves as engaged in a profoundly important reordering of the fundamentals of their discipline, and clearly did contribute, if only by renewed attention they drew to the problems inherent in conceptualizing disease, to beginning the breakdown of traditional categories and ideas.

As a recent scholar has shown, Da Monte's lectures at Padua reflected his active involvement in these debates.[125] To that context certainly belong his set of lectures on *Canon* 1.2, probably delivered in 1545–46, the first half of which constitutes what is in effect a treatise on the classification of disease. These lectures, which deserve much more extended consideration than is possible here, are notable not only for their efforts to rescue an authentically Galenic understanding of disease from what Da Monte considered to be the errors of Giacomo da Forlì and other scholastic physicians (see Chapter 6), but also for Da Monte's critical analysis of terminology and interest in evaluating and in some instances accommodating theories about disease that were not part of the mainstream Galenic tradition.

Da Monte's main framework for classifying diseases remained traditional and Galenic. He followed the division present in Avicenna's text into diseases of *mala temperatura, mala compositio,* and *solutio continuitatis* or *unitatis* (that is, imbalance of the primary qualities, bad arrangement of the organs, and trauma). Furthermore, although he did not rule out occult qualities, he frowned on widespread recourse to them as a principle of explanation in medical practice.[126] Nonetheless, Da Monte managed to find a place within his system for the concept of individual, unique diseases, each marked by symptoms peculiar to itself alone, diseases he termed *pathognomicae*. Thus, within the general category of diseases of *mala temperatura* he placed epilepsy among the *pathognomicae*, explaining that this was because epilepsy was invariably accompanied by constriction of the ventricles of the brain, which occurred in no other disease.[127]

Da Monte was also much aware of the difficulty of distinguishing the concepts of disease, causes of disease, and symptoms of disease. He carefully distinguished between the terms *symptoma, accidens, passio,* and *signum* and warned his students how important and how difficult it was to distinguish between conditions that were the causes of disease and those that were merely its accompanying accidents. Thus, when fever accompanied pleurisy, the fever was only an accident of the pleu-

[125] Nutton, "Seeds of Disease," p. 25.   [126] Ibid.
[127] Da Monte, comm. *Canon* 1.2 (Venice, 1557), p. 42.

risy, and it was the latter that must be treated.[128] Moreover, he objected to the loose use of *morbus* for conditions such as stone in the bladder and anomalies such as the presence of a sixth finger on the hand.[129] Da Monte evidently thought that accuracy in this regard (which was to be practical, not just semantic) was important for therapeutic reasons. He remarked with reference to the example just cited that if his students treated the fever and not the pleurisy they would kill all the pleurisy patients. However, his efforts to point out the ambiguity and imprecision of the ways in which the term "disease" was commonly used are surely also part of the larger context of attempts to rethink traditional modes of description and classification.

On the controversial subject of contagion, Da Monte gave general endorsement to the notion that contagion was the means whereby the *morbus gallicus* and some other diseases were transmitted from person to person, and set out to provide his students with the correct and systematic instruction on the subject that he believed had hitherto been sadly lacking. In his eyes, the numerous other contemporary physicians who addressed the issue talked a lot and understood nothing.[130] Da Monte therefore devoted three lectures to the subject of contagion, introducing them with the admonition "be attentive and don't bother me; since you don't find these things everywhere, and even if they are new they are all based on the foundation and method of the ancients."[131] Although Da Monte acknowledged that he had been unable to find the origin of the actual term "contagion" in any ancient medical writer, he nonetheless set out to show that the concept could be fitted into Galenic medical and Aristotelian philosophical theory. He therefore first considered the established doctrine of consensus or *sympathia*, which dealt with how injury or disease in one part of the body might lead to affections of other parts, and then went on to explain at length that contagion, which occurred between two bodies, involved a corruption of form taking place through an incorporeal alteration of species. This explanation was aimed chiefly against the competing theory that disease was spread by invisible seeds put forward by Da Monte's fellow townsman Girolamo Fracastoro (both men came from Verona), whose ideas Da Monte correctly, and damningly, associated with Epicurus and Democritus.[132] Da Monte linked contagion to complexional

---

[128] Ibid., pp. 33, 50–53.   [129] Ibid., pp. 54–56.   [130] Ibid., p. 428.

[131] "Oportet ergo quod vos sitis attenti, et advertatis neque perturbetis me, quoniam ista non ubique invenietis et si sunt nova, tamen omnia ex fundamentis methodoque antiquorum." Ibid., p. 419. The lectures on contagion occupy pp. 419–57.

[132] Ibid., p. 456. On Fracastoro and Lucretius, see Nutton, "Seeds of Disease," pp. 29–30.

explanations of disease by explaining that (complexional) "disposition" was the reason some people exposed to contagion fell sick and others did not.[133]

The concept of contagion was a powerful explanatory device, welcomed by many physicians, and Fracastoro became famous for his role in propagating it. But once Da Monte (and doubtless others) had found a way to incorporate contagion into the Galenic framework, Fracastoro's radical and essentially non-Galenic central concept of *seminaria* could be explained away as metaphor or ignored. Hence, Fracastoro's ideas, although widely known, were not perceived as nearly as serious a threat or, depending on one's point of view, as viable an alternative to Galenic rational (complexional) pathology as the ideas about occult qualities and disease associated with Fernel. When Santorio, some eighty years later, took up the cudgels against neoteric concepts of disease that threatened the rational basis of Galenic medicine, it was not Fracastoro but Fernel and Argenterio whose ideas, according to Santorio, regrettably pervaded every university in Europe.[134] Fernel's theory of disease of the total substance, which clearly had antecedents in some remarks of Galen himself, as well as in medieval developments of the concept of specific form, was an attempt to account for the special virulence of certain diseases (*morbus gallicus* among them) and poisons. According to Fernel and his followers, such diseases were completely outside the categories of *mala temperatura, mala compositio,* and *solutio unitatis.* Hence they could not be treated by complexional remedies, but demanded specific remedies of their own. Furthermore, such diseases were said to be occult in that they could not be understood by sense or intellect.[135]

Santorio objected to the antirational aspects of this theory and used

---

[133] Da Monte, comm. *Canon* 1.2 (Venice, 1557), p. 437.

[134] *Quaestio* 12: "An praeter tres formas morborum propositas ab Avicenna in hoc textum et a Galeni libro *De differentiis morborum* dentur alia cum Fernelio." Santorio, comm. *Canon* 1.1 (Venice, 1646), cols. 119–28. "Tres Avicennas proponit formas sanitatis et aegritudinis, intemperiem, scilicet, malam compositionem, et unitatem [*sic*; i.e. solutionem unitatis]; et de hac triplici morborum et sanitatum generica forma nullus Graecorum, Arabum, vel antiquorum Latinorum unquam dubitavit; nihilominus Fernelius secundo *De abditis rerum causis* et deinde Argenterius excogitarunt duas alias morborum differentias pertinentes ad partes similares, videlicet morbos materiae partium similarium et morbo formae partium similarium. . . . Occasio agendi de hac re est admodum necessaria; quia haec opinio de morbis formae vagatur per scolas. Imo per totius Europae gymnasia non desunt qui hanc novitatem protegant et defendant." Ibid., cols. 119–22. On the relatively restricted range of Fracastoro's influence in the two or three generations following his own, see Nutton, "Seeds of Disease," p. 29.

[135] On Fernel's theories of disease, see Richardson, "Generation of Disease," pp. 175–

his *quaestio* on the subject as the vehicle for his attack on the idea of occult causes in medicine, taking the position that many things seemed occult that were in fact simply not yet understood, and that recourse to occult causes was a confession of ignorance. However, he also attacked the theory on philosophical grounds as contrary to Aristotle's teaching about *potentiae* and substance, remarking that Fernel's theory was similar to the ideas of Gregory of Rimini, and hence contrary to the views of a formidable series of scholastic theologians: Saint Thomas, Egidius Romanus, Henry of Ghent, and Duns Scotus.[136] And he attempted to counter the assertion that afflictions such as poisoning or rabies could not be or cause complexional disease because there were no *contraria* (i.e., remedies of counterbalancing or opposite complexion) that would counteract and thus cure them, by providing a list of remedies for these conditions drawn from Galen and Pietro d'Abano.[137] Santorio was here at his most antiquarian, scholastic, and it must be admitted, ineffective despite the fact that he was dealing with an issue of current significance to which he attached importance ("It is now time to do something about this"). Never did the claim of Renaissance Galenists to represent rational medicine appear more threadbare than in Santorio's list of complexional remedies for poison copied from Pietro d'Abano. Yet the attack on occult causes with which this list is juxtaposed is another face of the same type of academic Galenism.

On the whole, the courses in *theoria* represented by these commentaries on *Canon* 1.1, and in the case of Da Monte on *Canon* 1.2, emerge as fully in touch with the medical thought of their age. The solid Galenism as regards most aspects of physiological theory displayed by all

---

94. Fernel's disease of the whole substance was also described as disease of form or, as Santorio put it, "hos vero morbos formae dicunt esse in praedicamento substantiae." Santorio, comm. *Canon* 1.1 (Venice, 1646), col. 122.

136 "Tertium argumentum, vel potius fundamentum pro hac opinione, quod desumunt ab altiori scola quam aliqui fortasse putant, videlicet a 2 libro *De anima*, ubi tractatur an potentiae differant a fundamento; isti videntur sequi opinionem Gregorii Ariminensis, qui disputat contra Divum Thomam, Egidium Romanum, Gandavensem, et Scotum." Ibid., col. 124.

137 "Tertio patet, hos morbos quos vocant substantificos non esse in substantia hoc argumento: substantiae nihil est contrarium, sit sic est [*sic*] quod morbi isti occulti habent contrarium, quod inductione probatur. Nonne guaiacum est contrarium lui gallicae, ictui scorpionis ex Galeno 11 *Simplicium* remedium contrarium est integer scorpio? Nonne morsui canis rabidi cinis cancrorum fluvatilium? . . . Similiter pro venenatis boletis oleum de corticibus citri est antidotus praestantissima, et boletis venenatis contraria; lacti coagulato in ventriculo, quod aliquando suffocat infantes ex Conciliatore acetum acre cum drachma assae foetidae contrariatur. Itidem pro nimia dosi scamonei valent quae somnum conciliant. Pro cantaridibus ex Conciliatore decem grana alchengi. . . ." Ibid., cols. 125–26.

the commentators represented the forefront of medicine in the days of Da Monte and Oddo Oddi and was still well within the mainstream in the days of Santorio. Moreover, Galenism in these commentaries cannot be equated with conservatism, mechanical conformity, or imperviousness to other currents in medicine. Attachment to Galen and attention to Avicenna's text did not prevent the commentators from drawing the attention of their students to a wide range of modern developments and controversies. Among major currents of thought and activity affecting sixteenth-century medical ideas, only Paracelsianism (which could in any case have been known only to the later authors) and some aspects of Renaissance occultism seem to have been excluded from the commentators' purview. Moreover, although by and large the nature of their task as teachers and expositors confined the commentators to evaluating arguments advanced by others, those of them who strongly espoused physiological theories of their own did not hesitate to put them forward, if anything more openly than Cardano had introduced his own theories about the elements. Thus, Da Monte instructed his students in his own scheme of classification of the humors and Santorio taught his own theory of insensible perspiration.

Furthermore, the content of these commentaries seems to suggest that in the course of the sixteenth century, to however modest an extent, the combined impact of the at least notional requirement of philological exactitude in the interpretation of Greek texts and of growing recognition of the need for a satisfactory fit between *theoria* and new observational data began to affect standards of precision and concepts of evidence and proof in all categories of medical discourse, not just the works of neoterics. It would be easy to exaggerate the extent of this development in the commentaries, since in every case traditional forms of medical dialectic still occupied a great deal of their authors' attention. Moreover, critical acuity and the appeal to medical experience were by no means always lacking in the medieval commentaries on *Canon* 1.1 and, especially, *Canon* 1.2. Yet the development of new canons of evidence in physiology does seem to be foreshadowed in the skepticism about the evidential basis for complexion theory manifested by Cardano and Costeo, in the enhanced role accorded, in different ways, to anatomy by several of the authors, in Costeo's occasional willingness to give experimental or observational data priority over ancient texts, and of course in Santorio's introduction of instrumentation, physical demonstration, controlled observation, measurement, and recording of results into the actual teaching of medical *theoria*.

The eclectic mix of scholasticism, medical humanism, and attention to contemporary developments in both anatomy and philosophy found in the commentaries on the last four *doctrinae* of *Canon* I.I was by no means peculiar to them, but is characteristic of a good deal of Renaissance academic writing on physiology. However, the commentary genre and the requirements of the course on *theoria* necessarily imposed certain special restraints. The expositions of *Canon* I.I remained bound to the explication of ancient texts, to the insights of the Galenism of the first half of the sixteenth century, and ultimately to carrying on a tradition of physiological scholarship that, despite all the changes in approach and content that had taken place, nonetheless extended back to the thirteenth century. The four most substantial commentaries on the physiological *doctrinae* are those of Da Monte (although Da Monte did not complete the exposition of *Doctrina* 6), the two Oddi, Costeo, and Santorio. Despite the much greater accumulation of references to recent authors and findings in Santorio's work, it would be impossible to claim any steady chronological trend away from scholastic medicine in this sequence of works. On the contrary, Santorio's work is in some respects more scholastic than those of his sixteenth-century predecessors. As will have become apparent, such development as took place from one commentary to the next consisted largely in adding new material without disturbing the underlying base. One final example of this process comes from the realm of metaphor.

Da Monte and Santorio both sought for metaphors with which to convey to their students the idea that the functioning of the body as a whole depended on the satisfactory interaction of many individually functioning parts. Da Monte found it helpful to compare the contribution of various parts of the eye to the process of vision to the cooperative activities of individuals in the Emperor's army, which fought the Lutherans.[138] Santorio compared the body to a musical instrument, in which if one string was too taut or too slack the whole would be out of tune. But Santorio also said that the human body resembled a clock, in which if one wheel malfunctioned the whole clock stopped.[139] This picture of the body as machine occurs immediately after the conclusion of the *quaestio* in which Santorio had insisted on the qualitative and complexional nature of disease. Nothing in the structure, traditions, or recent development of commentary on the *Canon* made juxtaposition

---

[138] Da Monte, comm. *Canon* 1.2 (Venice, 1557), p. 165.

[139] "Merito corpus vivens assimilatur horologio et testudini instrumento musicalis: horologia, quia licet spira chalibia et rotae sint recte dispositae, tamen si unicus alicuius rotulae dens deficiat, omnes horologii operationes deficiunt. Similiter unica operatione animali, aut vitali vel naturali ablata, omnes vel cadunt vel maxime patiuntur. Comparatur similiter corpus vivens testudini, in qua si unica ex multis cordis tensior vel laxior evadat tota perit harmonia." Santorio, comm. *Canon* 1.1 (Venice, 1646), col. 129.

of these two insights inappropriate or required Santorio to choose between them.

Thus, by the late sixteenth century, there seem to have been two options open to teachers of medical *theoria* from *Canon* 1.1. One was that adopted by Paterno, much of whose brief commentary reflects an essential disinclination to engage himself in serious controversy and a desire to pass over most topics with a series of vaguely conciliatory remarks. This was no doubt the type of teaching of *theoria* that at Padua aroused the acerbic criticism of some of the *practici* and their students.

The other, more conscientious, alternative, adopted in different ways by both Costeo and Santorio, involved incorporating into commentary more and more new material while still giving serious attention to the old. This process reached its culmination in Santorio's commentary, in which he made a determined effort to incorporate into one work all the elements called for by an up-to-date commentary on the *Canon*: massive traditional scholastic erudition; wide learning in ancient medical texts and Galenic medicine generally; evaluation of the relative merits of the Gerard of Cremona, Alpago, and Mantino versions of Avicenna's work; presentation and evaluation of an ever-accumulating mass of neoteric physiological and anatomical data and theory; discussion of some therapeutic applications of physiological theory; some description of physiology based on experiment and observation; and his own physiological theories. The result is a worthy monument to his diligence and erudition, as well as to his independent contribution to the development of physiological science, but it is not a textbook from which one can easily envisage learning any system of physiology whatsoever. The almost infinite flexibility of the commentary genre may in the end have been its downfall.

Conclusion

John Aubrey tells us that in 1644 he was contemplating going to study in Italy, following the time-honored practice of generations of young northern Europeans. Whether he had in mind university attendance in a specific discipline, or something more free ranging, we do not know. But before leaving, Aubrey sought out an eminent physician who, some forty-five years earlier, had traveled to Italy for medical studies, and asked his advice about appropriate preparatory reading. And William Harvey proffered the following: "he bid me goe to the fountain head, and read Aristotle, Cicero, Avicenna, and did call the neoteriques shitt-breeches."[1]

No one should be held accountable for sententious advice given to importunate students without any marked gift for serious intellectual endeavor. The essentially dilettantish nature of Aubrey's lively scientific curiosity was doubtless apparent even in his youth; Harvey might have responded differently to another aspirant. As it is, one can only be grateful to Aubrey's mother, who dissuaded him from his Italian enterprise and thus, perhaps, ensured that he left for posterity *Brief Lives*, rather than yet another set of lecture notes on the *Canon* of Avicenna.

Yet the Renaissance exhortation *ad fontes* was seldom as straightforward as it sounds, and Harvey's advice veils some interesting ambiguities. One reading of the recommendations is simply as a vague gesture toward the cultural heritage that was still an indispensable part of the mental baggage of every academically trained medical man (for the mention of Avicenna implies a medical, not just a general educational, context). But they can also be read in a quite specific and practical sense. In a scientific community in which Latin was the language of all serious writing, and discursive prose still the form of much of it, command of Latin style and rhetoric—a likely objective in reading Cicero—was still a real asset. The advice to read Aristotle may reflect Harvey's own interest in Aristotelian physiological concepts and have little or nothing to do with the Aristotle of scholastic philosophy. As for the recommendation of Avicenna, no one who has read thus far will

---

[1] *'Brief Lives,' Chiefly of Contemporaries, Set Down by John Aubrey, Between the Years 1669 & 1696*, ed. Andrew Clark (Oxford, 1898), 1:300.

be any longer surprised to find such advice given to a neophyte as late as the 1640s, even coming from such a source. The most striking feature of Harvey's advice is not the presence of Avicenna, but the absence of Galen, the real fountainhead of medical orthodoxy for the generations up to Harvey's own. And is Harvey's Avicenna the synthesizer of Galen or the compiler of *materia medica*?

The ambiguous nature of this not necessarily reliable anecdote warns one of the difficulty of weighing the significance of the material examined in the previous pages. Some readers may indeed find a certain perversity in the very idea of peering at Renaissance medical culture through the lens provided by the fortuna of one Arabo-Latin textbook and viewing Vesalius and Falloppia refracted through the remarks of commentators on the *Canon*. Yet the story recounted in the preceding pages illustrates activities, concepts, and developments that were by no means peculiar to the use of the *Canon*, but instead were major features of the intellectual and scientific milieu of Renaissance medicine: the impact of medical humanism and of printing, the role of universities and efforts at curricular reform, and the early stages of the spread of a new anatomy and physiology among a broader medical community. And the Renaissance fortuna of the *Canon* has a place not only in the history of medicine more broadly considered, but also in other histories: those of humanist and baroque learning, and of science education in universities during the era of the so-called Scientific Revolution.

If, as has been suggested,[2] our knowledge of sixteenth-century medicine resembles a map on which major topographical features are marked, although their precise outlines and location in relation to one another are not always clear, and the less prominent features of the terrain are only vaguely sketched in, Renaissance manifestations of interest in the *Canon* are only a set of foothills at the periphery. But they are on the same map as the looming and central bulk of such mountain ranges as the Galenic revival and the work of the anatomists. The portions of the *Canon* set as university textbooks were part of a body of literature including both Greek and Arabic elements used to transmit the outlines of physiology and medicine to beginners. As far as lectures on these books are concerned—whether on segments of the *Canon*, or the Hippocratic *Aphorisms*, or the Galenic *Ars*, or on portions of Rasis—it seems likely that common pedagogical goals and conventions produced more resemblances than the distinction between texts of Greek and Arabic origin, or even between lectures on theory and lectures on practice, did differences. (In another category are expositions

---

[2] Nutton, "Medicine in the Age of Montaigne," p. 15.

for medical students of less familiar texts of Greek origin, and in yet another the work on Greek manuscripts and editions of the handful of medical philologists.) One reason for setting before the reader of Part IV so much of the content of some commentaries on *Canon* 1.1 is that this material provides a fairly representative sample of basic Renaissance university medical instruction.

Nor were the mental attitudes likely to be inculcated by study of the *Canon* necessarily out of line with the common assumptions of sixteenth-century medicine. Despite the much-advertised emphasis on practical developments in anatomy and botany and on the close study of the scientific content of Galen's major anatomical works, a great deal of medical learning continued to be acquired in ways that were essentially literary and bookish, whether these are described as scholastic or humanistic. The university medical student began by familiarizing himself with a literature and with historic contexts of disputation, and only subsequently moved on to acquire detailed and specialized information, hands-on experience (whether clinical or anatomical), and, in some cases, new perceptions. The result was a mental climate in which syncretization and attempted reconciliation of new and old was much more commonplace than any real or thoroughgoing repudiation of the past, at least until the middle of the seventeenth century.

We need to differentiate between the small number of genuine scientific innovators and the probably almost equally small number of genuine medical humanists (in the sense of those having the ability to do philological work on Greek medical texts) and the much larger number of educated physicians who retained conventional patterns of thought and an essentially Latin culture. The last group probably included many of those who in the first half of the sixteenth century were loud in fashionable scorn for the Arabs and for the scholastic past. For the late sixteenth century the outlook of this group seems well exemplified by Costeo's endeavor to fit partial acceptance of Vesalian and post-Vesalian anatomy into traditional teaching; his was a typical, not an anomalous, strategy.

Given the constraints of the pedagogical and intellectual context, teaching based on the *Canon* was notably responsive to contemporary trends in medicine (especially anatomy); and equally noteworthy is the freedom with which medical innovators such as Da Monte and Santorio incorporated their own ideas into their lectures. The uses to which *Canon* 1.1 was put thus situate it in the history of the early modern medical textbook, even though the work also helped to perpetuate the ancient concept of medical theory that integrated physiological instruction with philosophy and a smattering of general science.

355

Whether or not Plemp was right to claim that some people in his day thought there had actually been two Avicennas, in a metaphorical sense the Renaissance Avicenna was certainly a split personality. One was the author of systematic summaries of Galenic teaching used as text-books for formal university instruction. It is now possible to have a fairly good idea of the way his work was used in courses on *theoria* and *practica* (the latter thanks to Iain Lonie's study of the use of *Canon* 4. 1 for teaching about fevers).[3] The other Avicenna was the compiler of remedies and *materia medica*, and a much more elusive character. Pharmacology was an area in which Renaissance physicians often acknowledged that the Arabs had added to the Greeks. Faith in *Canon* 2 and 5 seems to have been widespread among working physicians; it certainly extended well beyond the Iberian and Italian academic circles in which the "academic" Avicenna found his chief Renaissance home. Expressions of praise for Avicenna's usefulness for the practitioner almost all relate to his *materia medica*. Moreover, Avicenna's reputation in this regard seems to have survived a number of specific criticisms of misleading or incomprehensible items in his pharmacology. Yet both the pharmacological and the linguistic capacities of the sixteenth century must surely have limited the actual usefulness of *Canon* 2 and 5. Among the many remaining ambiguities about the place of Avicenna in the larger picture of Renaissance medicine is that of the extent to which his pharmacology found any real use or understanding.

In the broader context of Renaissance learning, the *Canon* provides instructive examples of techniques of text editing, of the extent and limitations of language studies, of the impact of printing on a scientific discipline, and of the development and varieties of commentary. Ironically, the history of the Arabo-Latin *Canon* provides powerful confirmation of the central importance of Greek studies in sixteenth-century learning. As far as attempts to purify the Latin text of the *Canon* were concerned, Greek medicine played a more important role than Arabic or Hebrew linguistic studies. The Renaissance editors of the work learned their trade in the school of Greek medical humanism. To the degree that their enterprise involved an attempt to demonstrate Avicenna's dependence on Galen, it was directly parasitical upon Renaissance Galenism, which provided the tools in the shape of the Renaissance editions of Galen and their apparatus.

Printing, indeed, unquestionably had a strong impact on the history of the *Canon* in the West. It greatly facilitated access to Avicenna's text, comparison of different Latin versions, and the identification of Ga-

---

[3] Lonie, "Fever Pathology."

lenic parallels; and one of the great achievements of the early printing industry was the production of the complete *Canon* in its original language. One could argue, legitimately, that the closer knowledge of Avicenna's work made possible by printing contributed, in the long run, to the shift in perspective that changed Avicenna from a current scientific authority into an important figure in the history of medicine. But in the short run, printing surely in this case enhanced the survival value of a medieval textbook tradition.

Commentary was a major vehicle of Renaissance learning and one with many subgenres. Although the philological scholia to the *Canon* produced by seventeenth-century Arabists might repay investigation by historians of European Orientalist learning, most Renaissance commentaries on the *Canon* are school lectures given in medical courses. One goal of this book has been simply to explore a largely unexamined kind of Renaissance writing, in an attempt to understand more clearly what it meant to study or to teach a text and a scientific subject by such a method.

Taken as an example of scientific education in the Renaissance university, the commentaries on the *Canon* can be read in two ways. First, they provide strong confirmation that university education, even in its most traditional aspects, was by no means impervious to change. In the case of sixteenth- and early seventeenth-century Padua, the formal public lectures on set books did not take place in isolated unawareness of the anatomical studies and practical training for which the university was celebrated throughout Europe. And so long as medical theory was conceived of as linked to, and incorporating, aspects of philosophy, good medical teachers made a conscientious effort to keep their pupils informed about—or warned against—current trends in philosophy or sciences other than medicine. Indeed, lectures on *Canon* 1.1 were evidently in some cases given over to teaching philosophy and science as much as to teaching medicine. However deleterious this practice was to the development of physiology as a separate discipline, it provided one more place in the university curriculum where students might expect to receive a little superficial instruction in general science. To an extent, use of *Canon* 1.1 not only perpetuated the old claims for a special relation between medicine and philosophy, but also reinforced the notion that physicians should have some general scientific culture. As purveyors of such culture, the better commentaries make a respectable showing. Moreover, although school commentaries are obviously not the place to look for scientific innovation as such (a generalization to which Santorio's commentary is, on occasion, an exception), some of them, especially those of Costeo and Santorio, communicate a fair

357

amount of information about recent, and nontraditional, scientific work.

Yet the commentaries on the *Canon* also illustrate only too clearly the powerful forces preserving the Aristotelian/Galenic synthesis among those who studied or taught in university faculties of medicine. These forces included not only the weight of ancient authority, but also the fragmentation and discursiveness encouraged by the practice of teaching by commentary, the interwoven medieval and Renaissance pedagogical and disputational traditions, and the apparently endless opportunities for the reconciliation of diverse views offered by sixteenth-century philosophical eclecticism. Santorio's attempt to combine the essentially incompatible procedures of teaching by commentary and teaching by physical demonstration exemplifies not only innovativeness, but also continuing confidence in the adaptability of the existing system of medical learning.

The final collapse of the Aristotelian/Galenic synthesis is thus not reflected in Renaissance commentary on the *Canon*. But the history of the *Canon* in Renaissance Italy reveals something of the complexity of the process whereby the scientific culture and intellectual universe of the medical community began to be transformed.

Latin Editions of the *Canon*
Published after 1500 and Manuscripts
and Editions of Latin Commentaries
on the *Canon* Written after 1500

No complete bibliography of Latin manuscripts and editions of and commentaries on the *Canon* has yet appeared. Two older bibliographies, Felix Willy Eckleben, *Die abendländischen Avicenna-Kommentare* (Leipzig, 1921), and Saïd Naficy, *Bibliographie des principaux travaux européens sur Avicenne* (Teheran, 1953), are a useful starting point, but both are mainly confined to printed works and are incomplete. General bibliographies, namely, *Gesamtkatalog der Wiegendrucke* (Leipzig, 1925–), *TK*, Klebs, and *IA*, yield information for limited categories and time periods. The following checklists of editions of the text and of manuscripts and editions of commentaries written after 1500 are intended merely to illustrate certain aspects of European interest in the *Canon* during the sixteenth and seventeenth centuries. No doubt further research would add a few more items to these lists. It should be noted that the appendices exclude two other categories of early printed books pertaining to Renaissance and early modern interest in the *Canon* (examples of which are included in the general bibliography), namely: (1) sixteenth- and seventeenth-century printings of commentaries written before 1500, and (2) works in which the *Canon* is drawn upon, discussed, or evaluated, but of which it and its author are not the only subjects. A few works in the first category, that is, early sixteenth-century printings of medieval commentaries, are nonetheless included in Appendix 1 because they form part of volumes identified by *IA*, pt. 1, vol. 2, 448–54, s.v. Avicenna, and/or the title page of the work itself, as primarily editions of the text of the *Canon*. Conversely, it should be noted that some volumes printed after 1500 that include portions of the *Canon* text are not listed here because their primary identification in *IA* or on their title pages is as works of medieval commentators.

The principle of following the title pages of the volumes themselves and, where possible, the practice of *IA* also determined the allocation of volumes containing the text of the *Canon* together with commentary written after 1500 between Appendix 1 (editions of the text) and Appendix 2 (commentaries). The reader is, however, once again reminded that in many cases commentaries include portions of the text, and editions are accompanied by scholia, notes, and commentary.

Except where otherwise indicated, the printed works listed in these appendices were consulted at one of the following libraries: BL, NLM, NYAM, WL. Editions or manuscripts that I have not examined personally are indicated by an asterisk.

Names of printers are included to assist in distinguishing the various Renaissance editions of the text, but are omitted for editions of commentaries.

Appendix 1

Latin Editions of the Canon *Published after 1500,*
Arranged by Date of Publication

For Latin, and the one Hebrew, printings of the *Canon* before 1500, see Klebs,
pp. 68–69, and *Gesamtkatalog,* 3, nos. 3314–27. The one early printing of the
complete *Canon* in Arabic is Rome: Typographia Medicea, 1593. Except where
otherwise indicated, the following editions are of Gerard of Cremona's
translation. For additional information regarding editions and versions, see
Chapter 5.

*Tertius Canonis Avicenne cum dilucidissimis expositoribus Gentile Fulginate nec non
Jacobo de Partibus parisiense.* 3 vols. Venice: Bernardinus Benalius, ca. 1505.
Book 3. *IA* 110.580.

*Liber Canonis Avicenne revisus et ab omni errore mendaque purgatus summaque cum
diligentia impressus.* Venice: Bonetus Locatellus for heirs of Octavianus Scotus, 1505. *IA* 110.581.

*[Articella.] In hoc volumine parvo in quantitate, maximo virtute, continentur infra-
scripti codices . . . Textus duarum primarum fen primi Avicenne in theorica. Textus
fen quarte primi, et prime quarti in practica.* Pavia: Bartholomeus de Morandis
for Jacobus de Burgofranco, 1506. . . . *Canon* 1.1–2,4, and 4.1, as part of an
expanded *articella* that includes a humanistic translation of the Hippocratic
Aphorisms. Dedicatory letter by Pietro Antonio Rustico, professor of medical *theoria* at the University of Pavia.

"Nova impressio" of preceding item Venice: Petrus Bergomensus de Qua-
rengis, 1507. *IA* 109.32.

*Liber Canonis Avicenne revisus et ab omni errore mendaque purgatus summaque cum
diligentia impressus.* Venice: Paganinus de Paganinis, 1507; facsimile, Hildesheim, 1964. *IA* 110.582.

Flores Avicenne. Lyon: Claudius Davost for Bartholomeus Trot, 1508. Abbreviation. Preface by Michael de Capella, *artium et medicine magister.* *IA*
110.583.

Primus Avicenne Canon cum argutissima Gentilis expositione. . . . Pavia: Jacobus
de Burgofranco, 1510. Actually includes Books 1 and 2, separately foliated.
I am uncertain as to whether this is to be equated with *IA* 110.585. Appears
to be part of a set with the next entry.

★*Tertius Can. Avicenne cum amplissima Gentilis Fulginatis expositione.* Pavia: Jacobus de Burgofranco for Aloysius de Castello Comensis and Bartholomeus
de Morandis, 1511. *IA* 110.586. NLM has ★two more volumes (Books 4 and
5) of this set, with Gentile's commentary, printed Pavia: Jacobus de Burgofranco, 1511–12 (Durling, *Catalogue,* no. 379).

Flores Avicenne collecti super quinque Canonibus quos edidit in medicina, nec non super decem et novem libris de animalibus cum Canticis eiusdem ad longum positis. Lyon: Gilbertus de Villiers for Bartholomeus Trot, 1514. Reprint of 1508 edition, with additions as indicated. *IA* 110.588.

Articella nuperrime impressa cum quamplurimis tractatibus pristine impressioni super-additis. . . . Lyon: Johannes de la Place, for Bartholomeus Trot, 1515. Includes *Canon* 1.1–2, 4.1,3–5. *IA* 109.35.

Soli Deo. Memoriale medicorum canonice practicantium a Rustico medicine cultore ordinatum. . . . Pavia: Bernardinus de Garaldis, 1517. The first two sets of *canones* (short axioms or rules) are based on *Canon* 1.4 and 4.1 respectively.

Articella nuperrime impressa. . . . Lyon, 1519. Reprint of 1515 collection. *IA* 109.136.

★Textus principis Avicenne ordinem alphabeti in sententia reportatus cum quibusdam additionibus et concordantiis Galieni et quorundam aliorum. . . . Bordeaux: Gaspard Philippe, 1520. *IA* 110.589.

Primus Avicenne Canonis. Avicenne medicorum principis Canonum liber una cum lucidissima Gentilis Fulginatis expositione. . . . Venice: heirs of Octavianus Scotus, 1520. Actually Books 1 and 2, separately foliated. With register of Gentile's *quaestiones*. *IA* 110.591 (where, however, heading of *tabula* is given).

Quartus Canonis Avicenne cum praeclara Gentilis Fulginatis expositione . . . Quintus etiam Canonis cum eiusdem Gentilis Fulginatis lucidissima expositione. . . . Venice: heirs of Octavianus Scotus, 1520. Books 4 and 5 with two other partial commentaries besides that of Gentile. Register of commentator's *quaestiones*. *IA* 110.592 (where, however, heading of *tabula* is given).

Liber Canonis totius medicine ab Avicenna Arabum doctissimo excussus, a Gerardo Cremonensi ab arabica lingua in latinam reductus. Et a Petro Antonio Rustico Placentino in philosophia non mediocriter erudito ad limam ex omni parte ab erroribus et omni barbarie castigatus; necnon a domino Symphoriano Camperio Lugdunensi fecundis annotationibus terminisque arabicis et eorum expositionibus nuper illustratus; una cum eius vita a domino Francisco Calphurnio non minus vere quam eleganter exerpta. Lyon: Jacobus Myt, 1522. *IA* 110.593.

Tertius Canonis Avicennae cum amplissima Gentilis Fulginatis expositione . . . secunda pars Gentilis super tertio Avicennae. . . . Venice: heirs of Octavianus Scotus, 1522. 2 vols., continuously foliated. Book 3, with other partial commentaries besides that of Gentile. Vol. 2, *IA* 110.594.

Praesens maximus codex est totius scientiae medicinae principis Aboali Abinsene cum expositionibus omnium principalium et illustrium interpretum eius. . . . Venice: Philippus Pincius for L.A. Junta, 1523. 5 vols. Includes commentaries by Gentile da Foligno, Jacques Despars, Dino del Garbo, Taddeo Alderotti, Ugo Benzi, etc. *IA* 110.595.

Habes humane lector Gabrielis de Tarrega Burgdalensis civitatis medici regentis et ordinarii opera brevissima theoricam et prathicam [sic] medicinales scientie. . . . The third treatise in the collection is *Textus Avicenne per ordinem alphabeti in sententia per eundum reportatus. Cum quibusdam additionibus et concordantiis Galieni et quorundam aliorum antiquorum.* Bordeaux: Johannes Guyart, 1524? (the

Textus Avicenne is undated, but other treatises have colophons dated 1520 and 1524). It is possible that this is to be identified with *IA* 110.589 (see above).

Articella nuperrime impressa. . . . Lyon, 1525; reprint of 1515 and 1519 collection. *IA* 109.138.

Principis Avicennae libri Canonis necnon De medicinis cordialibus et Cantica ab Andrea Bellunensi ex antiquis Arabum originalibus ingenti labore summaque diligentia correcti atque in integrum restituti, una cum interpretatione nominum arabicorum, quae partim mendosa partim incognita lectores antea morabantur. Opus plane aureum ac omni ex parte absolutum. Venice: L.A. Junta, 1527. With Alpago's textual emendations to the *Canon* (in the margin) and glossary. *IA* 110.598.

Flores Avicennae. . . . Lyon: Gilbertus de Villiers for Bartholomeus Trot, 1528. Reprint of 1514 edition. *IA* 110.599.

Avicennae quarta fen primi libri De universali ratione medendi, nunc primum M. Jacobi Mantini medici hebrei opera latinitate donata. Venice: L.A. Junta, 1530. *Canon* 1.4. *IA* 110.600.

Avicennae Arabis medicorum ob succinctam brevitatis copiam facile principis quarta fen primi De universale ratione medendi, nunc primum M. Jacobi Mantini medici hebraei latinitate donata, et in studiosorum utilitatem ab phisicae studiosis quibusdam, germanis typis tradita. Ettlingen: Valentinus Kobian, 1531. *Canon* 1.4. Bound with *Galeni Pergameni dissectionis venarum arteriarumque commentarium* . . . *Antonio Fortolo Ioseriensi interprete* (Basel, 1529) and other works. Rome: Biblioteca Nazionale. *IA* 110.601.

Avicennae arabis medicorum ob succinctam brevitatis copiam facile princeps quarta fen primi De universali ratione medendi. Interprete Jacob Mantino medico hebraeo. Paris: Claudius Chevallonius, 1532. *Canon* 1.4. *IA* 110.602.

Avicennae arabis inter omnes medicos cum ex stemmate, tum ob succinctam brevitatis copiam, facile principis quarta fen primi de universali ratione medendi per M. Jacob Mantinum medicum hebreum latinate donata, denuo germanis typis nuper multo emendatior in lucem edita. The Hague: Valentinus Kobian, 1532. *Canon* 1.4. *IA* 110.603.

Articella nuperrime impressa. . . . Lyon: Johannes Moylin, 1534. Reprint of the same collection as the Lyons editions of 1515, 1519, and 1525. *IA* 109.140.

Caput illud aureum Avicennae 29 tertii fen primae tractatus primi de canonibus universalibus curationis dolorum capitis, nuper ab eximio artium et medicinae doctore Jacobo Mantino hebraeo latinitate donatum ante hac non excussa. Printed with *Methodus universae artis medicae* . . . *Cornelio a Baersdorp Goseri autore* (Bruges, 1538), at sig. Vii^r-[Vv^v]. Dedicatory letter from Mantino to Hadrianus Brant of Germany.

Avicennae primi libri fen prima nunc primum per Magistrum Jacobum Mantimam [sic] *medicum hebreum ex hebraico in latinum translata* (n.p.,n.d.; WL catalogue suggests Venice, ca. 1540). *Canon* 1.1. *IA* 110.604.

Avicennae liber Canonis, De medicinis cordialibus, et Cantica, cum castigationibus Andreae Alpagi Bellunensis philosophi ac medici clarissimi, una cum eiusdem nominum arabicorum interpretatione. Quibus recens quamplurimae accesserunt ab *eodem ex multis Arabum codicibus excerptae huiusmodi asterisco* notatae. . . .* Venice: Junta, 1544. Paolo Alpago's second edition of his uncle's work. The second part of the volume (containing glossaries and biography of Avicenna) is separately paginated. Decorated title page, and illustrations. *IA* 110.606.

**Primi libri fen prima nunc primum per Jacobum Mantinum ex hebraico in latinam translata et diligentius nuper emendata.* Padua: Bernardius Bindonus and Jacobus Fabrianus, 1547. *Canon* 1.1. *IA* 110.608.

Prima primi Canonis Avicennae sectio, Michaele Hieronymo Ledesma Valentino medico et interprete et enarratore. Valencia: Johannes Mey of Flanders, 1547. The date is from the title page; on fol. 118ʳ is the date 1548.

Prima fen quarti Canonis Avicennae de febribus. . . . Paris: Poncetus le Preux, 1549. *Canon* 4.1. *IA* 110.610.

**Quarta fen primi de universali ratione medendi. Interprete Jacob Mantino medico hebreo.* Paris: M. Juvenis, 1555. *Canon* 1.4. *IA* 110.611.

Avicennae liber Canonis, De medicinis cordialibus, et Cantica, iam olim quidem a Gerardo Carmonensi ex arabico sermone in latinum conversa, postea vero ab Andrea Alpago Bellunensi, philosopho et medico egregio, infinitis pene correctionibus ad veterum exemplarium arabicorum fidem in margine factis, locupletissimoque nominum arabicorum ab ipso interpretatorum indice decorata, nunc autem demum a Benedicto Rinio Veneto, philosopho et medico eminentissimo, eruditissimis accuratissimisque lucubrationibus illustrata. Qui et castigationes ab Alpago factas suis quasque locis aptissime inseruit. Et quamplurimas alias depravatas lectiones in margine ingeniosissime emendavit. Et locos in quibus auctor ipse vel eandem sententiam, eandemve medicamenti unius compositionem iterat, vel oppositas inter se sententias ponit, vel aliquid denique ab Hippocrate, Aristotele, Dioscoride, Galeno, Paulo, Aetio, Alexandro, Serapione, Rasi, Halyabate, Alfarabio mutuatur diligentissime indicavit. Plurimis etiam arabicis vocibus nunquam antea expositis, latinum nomen invenit. Indicemque latinum medicamentorum simplicium in secundum librum composuit. . . . Venice: Junta, 1555. The volume also includes Alpago's translations of Avicenna, *De removendis nocumentis* and *De syrupo acetoso,* and Massa's life of Avicenna. Alpago's glossary and the "old" glossary are separately foliated at the end of the volume. Bound with *Index in Avicennae libros nuper Venetiis editos . . . Julio Palamede Adriensi medico auctore.* Venice: Junta, 1557. *IA* 110.612.

Avicennae medicorum Arabum principis liber Canonis, De medicinis cordialibus, et Cantica . . . ab Andrea Alpago Bellunensi . . . correctionibus . . . decorata . . . , a Benedicto Rinio . . . lucubrationibus illustrata. . . . Basel: Joannes Hervagios, 1556. A reissue of the edition of Venice, 1555. The copy at NYAM has a few manuscript marginalia in Arabic on fol. *5ᵛ and elsewhere. On the copy at NLM the imprint date has been altered by hand to 1576 (see Durling, *Catalogue,* no. 386). *IA* 110.613. Reissued in facsimile, Teheran, 1976.

Avicennae liber Canonis, De medicinis cordialibus, Cantica, De removendis nocumentis in regimine sanitatis, De syrupo acetoso. . . . Venice: Junta, 1562. The Alpago-Rinio version (see items published in 1555 and 1556, above), with additional emendations by Rinio. Palamede's index appears at the end of the volume. *IA* 110.616.

Avicennae principis et philosophi sapientissimi libri in re medica omnes, qui hactenus ad nos pervenere, id est libri Canonis quinque, De viribus cordis, De removendis nocumentis in regimine sanitatis, De sirupo acetoso, et Cantica, omnia novissime post aliorum omnium operam a Joanne Paulo Mongio Hydruntino, et Joanne Costaeo Laudensi recognita. . . . Venice: Vincentius Valgrisius, 1564. WL copy is in 2 vols. BL copy has Arabic manuscript annotations. *IA* 110.618.

Avicennae medicorum Arabum facile principis libri tertii fen secunda, quae latine ex synonymo hebraico . . . *Ophan reddi potest, intuitus sive rotundus sermo secundus, qui est de aegritudinibus nervorum, tractatu uno contentus, ad fidem codicis hebraici latinus factus. Interprete Johanne Quinquarboreo Aurilacensi, literarum Hebraicarum et Caldaicarum professore regio.* . . . Paris: M. Iuvenis, 1570. *Canon* 3.2. *IA* 110.620.

Avicennae medicorum arabum facile principis libri tertii fen primae tractatus quartus, in quo accurate et cogitate scribit ille de aegritudinibus capitis et noxa multa illarum in functionibus sensus et moderaminis sive partis rectricis, in linguam latinam conversus et a salebris ac mendis, quibus scatebat, ad fidem codicis hebraici correcti et emendati maxime, in integrum restitutus ac perpurgatus. Interprete Johanne Quinquarboreo. . . . Paris, 1572. Bound with preceding item in BL copy. *Canon* 3.1.4.

Principis Avicennae liber primus de universalibus medicae scientiae praeceptis. Andrea Gratiolo Salodiano interprete. Adiectis utilissimis eiusdem interpretis scholiis Hippocratis et Galeni praecipue loca commonstrantibus. . . . Venice: Franciscus Zilettus, 1580. *Canon* 1. *IA* 110.622.

Avicennae liber Canonis, De medicinis cordialibus, Cantica, De removendis nocumentis in regimine sanitatis, De syrupo acetoso. . . . Venice: Junta, 1582. A reprint of the Alpago/Rinio edition of 1562. *IA* 110.623. The NLM copy is bound with *Index in Avicennae libros . . . Julio Palamede . . . auctore.* 2nd edition, Venice: Junta, 1582.

⋆*Libri tertii fen primae tractatus quintus, de aegritudinibus cerebri, ad fidem hebraici exemplaris, latinus factus et passim restitutus ac emendatus. Interprete Johanne Quinquarboreo.* . . . Paris: Dionysius a Prato, 1586. *Canon* 3.1.5. *IA* 110.625.

Avicennae Arabum medicorum principis. Ex Gerardi Cremonensis versione, et Andreae Alpagi Bellunensis castigatione. A Joanne Costaeo, et Joanne Paulo Mongio annotationibus iampridem illustratus. Nunc vero ab eodem Costaeo recognitus, et novis alicubi observationibus adauctus . . . Additis nuper etiam librorum Canonis oeconomiis, necnon tabulis Isagogicis in universam medicinam ex arte Humain [sic], *id est Joannitii Arabis. Per Fabium Paulinum Utinensem.* . . . 2 vols. Venice: Junta, 1595. Revised edition of the Costeo and Mongio version of 1564. Includes illustrations previously used in the Junta edition of 1544 (see above). *IA* 110.627.

Avicennae . . . ex Gerardi Cremonensis versione, et Andreae Alpagi Bellunensis castigatione. A Joanne Costaeo et Joanne Paulo Mongio annotationibus iampridem illustratus. Nunc vero ab eodem Costaeo recognitus. . . . 2 vols. Venice: Junta, 1608. A reprint of the preceding item with minor typographical alterations.

Liber secundus de canone Canonis a filio Sina studio sumptibus ac typis Arabicis Petri Kirsteni. Breslau, 1609 or 1610. Arabic text of *Canon* 2, with Kirsten's Latin translation and Arab-Latin vocabulary, and philological scholia.

Avicennae summi inter medicos nominis fen I, libri 1 Canonis. Vicenza: apud Orlandum Iadram, 1611. *Canon* 1.1, abbreviated. Bound with *Ars medica.*

Avicennae summi inter Arabes medici fen I, libri Canonis in usum Gymnasii Patavini. Editio correctior. Padua, 1636. *Canon* 1.1, abbreviated.

Schola medica in qua Hippocratis, Galeni, Avicennaeque medicinae facile principum pro tyronibus habentur fundamenta. . . . Venice, 1647. *Canon* 1.1 (with *Ars medica* and *Aphorisms*), abbreviated. Preface from Vicenza, 1611, edition.

Avicennae Arabum medicorum summi fen I libri I Canonis, Gerardo Cremonense interprete, in usum Gymnasii Patavini. Nova editio castigatior. Padua: Paulus Frambottus, 1648. *Canon* 1.1, with *Ars medica, Aphorisms,* and *Prognostics* (tr. Leoniceno).

Clarissimi et praecellentissimi doctoris Abualj Ibn-Tsina, qui hactenus perperam dictus est Avicenna, Canon medicinae, interprete et scholiaste Vopisco Fortunato Plempio. Tomus 1, librum primum et secundum Canonis exhibens, atque ex libro quarto tractatum de febribus. Louvain: Hieronymus Nempaeia, 1658. *Canon* 1, 2, and 4.1.

Abugalii filii Sinae sive, ut vulgo dicitur, Avicennae philosophorum ac medicorum Arabum principis, De morbis mentis tractatus, editus in specimen normae medicorum universae ex arabico in latinum de integro conversae et a barbarorum inscitia spurcitiaque vindicatae. Interprete Petro Vatterio. . . . Paris, 1659. Excerpts from *Canon* 3.1.

Avicennae quarti libri Canonis, fen prima de febribus. Nova editio caeteris accuratior. Padua: Matthaeus Cadorinus, 1659. *Canon* 4.1. Edited by Girolamo Santasofia, holder of first extraordinary chair in medical theory, Padua.

Georgii Hieronymi Velschii Exercitatio de vene medinensi ad mentem Ebnsinae, sive De dracunculis veterum. Specimen exhibens novae versionis ex Arabico. . . . Augsburg: Theophilus Coebelius, 1674. *Canon* 4.3.21–22 (Arabic edition and Latin translation)

Appendix 2

Latin Commentaries on the Canon
Written after ca. 1500

Commentaries and lectures in manuscript, arranged alphabetically
by location of libraries

Surviving sets of lectures obviously represent only a small portion of those once in existence. For example, I have been able to find no trace of the commentaries on portions of the *Canon* attributed to Emilio Campilongo, Albertino Bottoni, Niccolò Trivisano, Bernardino Trivisano, Francesco Frigimelica, and Antonio Fracanzano, all teachers at Padua in the sixteenth century, in J. F. Tomasini, *Bibliothecae patavinae manuscriptae publicae et privatae* (Udine, 1639), 96, 101, 107–16, or of that by Girolamo Vergerio (d. 1678) noted in N. C. Papadopoli, *Historia Gymnasii Patavini* (Venice, 1726), 1:371–72 (which, indeed, may have appeared in print, since the other commentaries on the *Canon* by Paduan professors listed by Papadopoli are all printed editions). The manuscripts in the following list were located by consulting the printed catalogues of selected major individual libraries (including many that yielded no results); Paul Oskar Kristeller, *Iter Italicum: A Finding List of Uncatalogued or Incompletely Catalogued Humanistic Manuscripts of the Renaissance in Italian and Other Libraries*, vols. 1 and 2, *Italy*; vol. 3, *Australia to Germany* (vol. 3 being unindexed at the time of consultation) (London and Leiden, 1963–), which fortunately includes significant amounts of medical, and indeed scholastic, material; Paul Oskar Kristeller, *Latin Manuscript Books before 1600: A List of the Printed Catalogues and Unpublished Inventories of Extant Collections* (new ed., New York, 1960), and microfilms of various handwritten catalogues listed therein at the Library of Congress; F. Edward Cranz, *A Microfilm Corpus of the Indices to Printed Catalogues of Latin Manuscripts before 1600 A.D.* (New London, Conn., 1982), and the additional microfilms of handwritten catalogues deposited by Professor Cranz in the library of Connecticut College. For Italy, I have also been through the volumes (one hundred, at the time of consultation) of the *Inventari dei manoscritti delle biblioteche d'Italia* begun by G. Mazzatinti (vol. 1, Turin, 1887). As anyone who has worked in the field knows, none of this endeavor is any guarantee of completeness. In particular, my search in smaller collections has been more thorough for Italy than for other parts of Europe. It seems probable, however, that the following list is representative of the surviving material.

(Manuscripts not personally inspected are marked ★; manuscripts inspected only in microfilm are marked †.)

*Berlin (East), Preussische Staatsbibliothek. Codices Electorales Recentiores 102, lat. qu. 137. Notebook with lectures of Bernardino Paterno, written by a German student at Padua. Contents include, no. 3, "Paternus in primam fen Avicennae" (fols. 48–180), dated 1578–79. See Valentin Rose, *Die Handschriften-Verzeichnisse der königlichen Bibliothek zu Berlin. Vol. 13. Verzeichnis der lateinischen Handschriften*, vol. 2, pt. 3 (Berlin, 1905), 1380.

Bologna, Archivio di Stato. Riformatori dello Studio. *Dispute e ripetizioni di scolari per ottenere letture d'università*, 1487–1527. Separate sheets, with modern numbering, in one *busta*. Proposed topics for student disputations (in various fields, not just medicine), to obtain a lectureship set up for the benefit of poor students. There is usually one medical disputation a year, more in other fields. Those specifically mentioning Avicenna in their titles are: 17, Pompeius Emihenus de Faventia, 1487–88; 89, Antonius Serzanensis (Sergianensis), 1495–96; 104–5, Albertus Budrius, 1496. Various other disputations are apparently based on unacknowledged tags from the *Canon*.

———, Biblioteca Comunale dell'Archiginnasio. A 922. 173 unnumbered folios. *Curtius super prima primi Avicennae*. 63 numbered lectures on the first three *doctrinae* of *Canon* 1.1 (at end: "quam legit anno 1528"), followed by a series of additions by Franciscus Cassianus, with Corti's responses thereto.

———, Biblioteca Universitaria. Lat. 14 (10), I.1^r-I.5^r. Alessandro Achillini, notes or syllabus for a course on *Canon* 1.4, 1509.

———, Biblioteca Universitaria. Lat. 582(1077). *Miscellanea medica*, vol. 1. item 4, "Lectiones matutinae super quartam fen primi libri principis nostri Avicennae habitae anno domini 1654 . . . a me Nicolao Betto Florentiola lectore publico," fols. 1–27 (8 numbered lectures).

*Escorial, Real Biblioteca. L III 30, medical lectures by professors at Salamanca written by a bachelor, 1674–76; includes, item 6, fols. 109–62, Eduardo Fernandez, comm. *Canon* 1.4. I cite this manuscript from P. Guillermo Antolín, *Catálogo de los códices latinos de la Real Biblioteca del Escorial* (5 vols., Madrid, 1910–23), 2:46–48.

*———, Real Biblioteca. q II 17, 1548–50. *Augustini Lopez theoricae in fen I–IV libri primi, & fen I, II libri quarti Canonis Avicennae*. I cite this manuscript from Antolín, *Catálogo*, 2:256.

London, BL. Sloane 3133, *Practicae medicae vectigal Julii Mancini*. A mostly practical medical miscellany of recipes, consilia, etc. Fols. 412^r–435^r: *Compendium primae fen Avicennae fragmentum*, dated (435^r), Siena, 15 September 1617.

*———, WL. 300. Aurelius Gallina, comm. "in Avicennam." Milan, 1603–1604. I overlooked the opportunity to see this manuscript and cite it from S.A.J. Moorat, *Catalogue of Western Manuscripts in Medicine and Science in the Wellcome Historical Medical Library. I. Manuscripts Written before 1650 A.D.* (London, 1962).

———, WL. 129. Fols. 2^r-16^r, *Aloisii Bellacati in quartam fen de febribus* [*Canon* 4.1], 1563; fols. 121^r–224^r, *Nicolai Curti super Avicennae fen quartam de febribus* [*Canon* 4.1].

————, WL. 454. Fols. 19ʳ–40 [Agostino Lopez (fl. 1548–50)], annotations on *Canon* 1.2. Fol. 19ʳ, "Incipiunt annotationes super fen secunda Canonis primi Avicene dicavit dominus licentiatus Augustinus Lupus a quo ego primo incepi audire medicinam."

————, WL. 602. Unnumbered folios. Notebook containing lectures of Bernardino Paterno (with a few by Mercuriale and Capodivacca), including as the first item *Publice lectiones excellentissimi Bernardini Paterni profitentes theoricam primo loco ordinariam in Patavino Gymnasio in prima fen primi libri Avicennae. Anno 1578.* 43 numbered lectures, inc. "Ut vestrae utilitati in primis consulam."

————, WL. 3453. a. 1716. Commonplace book of J. L. Marmi, vol. 9. The first 43 unnumbered folios consist of handwritten excerpts copied from one of the printed editions of Santorio, comm. *Canon* 1.1.

————, WL. 4353. Notebook of Joannes Gambius. On flyleaf: "Ego Joannes Gambius Patavinus doctor philosophie collegi hanc fen sub lectionem Jeronimo Santasophia, eodem dictante anno a Christi nativitate 1651." The commentary on *Canon* 1.1 takes up the whole book.

————, WL. 4354. Notebook of Joannes Gambius containing *Lectiones in Galeni Artem medicinalem*, Padua, 1652. On the last three leaves are notes for a proem to lectures on *Canon* 1.1 in a different hand, dated 1670.

Mantua, Biblioteca Comunale. 83 (A III 19). *Lectiones excellentissimi D. Bernardini Paterni super quartam fen primi Canonis Avicennae MDLI.* The lectures contain numerous sections consisting primarily of tabular representations and outlines. However, the manuscript is a *reportatio*, not Paterno's own draft or notes, as on fol. 173ᵛ occurs "Vidi in actu practico Paternum semper praecipere ne dormiatur post assumptum pharmacum aut leve aut validum"—a glimpse of the practice of a professor who spent most of his career teaching *theoria*.

————, Biblioteca Comunale. 600 (E III 28). Student notebook of Pietro Francesco Occlerio (signature p. 11 and elsewhere). P. 1: "Lectiones medicae D. Horatii Augenii dictatae in scholis Taurini, scriptore et auditore Occlerio Tridenense." P. 11: "Libellus Avicennae de febribus in quo sunt omnes lectiones D. Horatii Augenii publice perlectae ac nobis summo studio inscriptis in scola traditae anno . . . 1590." Augenio's commentary on *Canon* 4.1 ends p. 554.

Milan, Biblioteca Ambrosiana. A 180 Inf., 301 fols. *Excellentissimi artium et medicinae doctoris D. Nicolai Boldoni lectiones in quartam fen primi Canonis Avicennae quas aggressus est anno 1555. . . . .*

————, Biblioteca Ambrosiana. A 215 Inf. 862 pp. *In quartam librum Canonis Avicennae fen 1.* At top left-hand corner of p. 1: Nicolai Boldoni. P. 1: "anno superiori vobis tractationem eam Avicennae explicuerimus quae precepta universalia curandi in se continet"—a reference to the preceding entry, which dates this commentary 1556.

Milan, Biblioteca Ambrosiana. S 84 Sup., fols. 336^r–357^r, 5 numbered lectures on *Canon* 1.1; fol. 336^r: "Excellentissimi D. Nicolai Curtii Brixiensis substituti in loco theorice medicinae ordinariae in loco excellentissimi Bassiani Landi in primam fen primi Avicennae. Lectio prima die 8 Januarii, 1563."

Modena, Biblioteca Estense. Alpha U 7 19 (Lat. 542), Notebook inscribed on flyleaf "Alexandri Ferri Regiensis Ferrarie 1620 Patavii 1626," later the property of Prospero Magati. Fols. 1^r–97^r, *Liber primus continens doctrinam mixtam quae tamen maiori . . . spectat ad primam fen primi libri Canonis Avicennae.* 32 numbered lectures.

Padua, Biblioteca Comunale. CM 414, vol. 1. Three separately paginated sets of lectures on the three basic books in *theoria* by Girolamo Capodivacca (title page of first set), of which the second set is *In prima fen primi libri Avicennae lectiones.* 171 pages, 43 numbered lectures, going up to *Canon* 1.1.4, completed 1563.

———, Biblioteca del Seminario Vescovile. 160. Sixteenth century. Notebook "Ad usum Aloysii de Barlisa(?)." Fols. 3–118, *Epitome tertii libri Avicennae*; fols. 123^r–142^v, *Epitome quarti libri Avicennae.*

———, Biblioteca del Seminario Vescovile. 291. Sixteenth-century miscellany on fevers, including works by Dr. Fernandez and Dr. Luis Rodriguez. Fols. 3^r–159^v (Fernandez), *Commentaria super fen primum libri quarti Canonis Avicennae.*

Paris, Bibliothèque Nationale. Lat. 7080. Fol. 81^r, "Sequitur aliqua excerpta ex practica magistri Johannis Spirinki super primam fen tertii Canonis." The excerpts from the commentary appear to end fol. 116^v. At fol. 177^r is the date 29 August 1531.

———, Bibliothèque Nationale. Lat. 7084. Notebook containing handwritten excerpts from printed medical books. Fols. 74^r–128^v, "Ex Joh. Bapt. Montani lectionibus in primi libri Canonis Avicennae primum fen, Venetiis Valgris. 1558 [*sic*, presumably 1557; page nos. of the excerpted passages are noted]." Signature of A. Dudith, fol. 71^r. On the last folio (169^r) is an inscription that is hard to decipher, but may read "Donzell. [i.e., Hieronymus Donzellinus] Crac. Kal. Mar 1584." Girolamo Donzellini, a physician who practiced at various times in Brescia, Verona, and Venice, was for many years involved in smuggling Protestant books into Italy and spent long periods in exile in northern Europe (where he presumably knew Dudith). Donzellini was executed for heresy in Venice in 1587 (Grendler, *Roman Inquisition*, pp. 108–10).

Parma, Biblioteca Palatina. 1501. 230 fols. plus 8 unnumbered leaves at the beginning. Fol. 1^r, *Principium Canonis Avicennae excellentissimi artium et medicinae doctoris Dom. Francisci Cass[i]ani theoricam ordinariam legentis in almo Ticinensis studio scripta sub anno 1534.* Cassiani's commentary on *Canon* 1.1 occupies the entire volume except for a list on the unnumbered folios at the beginning of parallels and differences between Avicenna and Galen, drawn from Matteo Corti's commentary on *Canon* 1.1.

Perugia, Biblioteca Comunale Augusta. Conv. Sopp. 978 (M I), 305 fols., seventeenth century. Anon. *In prima fen primi libri Avicennae expositio.* Inc. "Divinus ille Plato. . . ." Ends at *Canon* 1.1.4.

Rome, Biblioteca Lancisiana. 50. *Miscellanea et elencus omnium operum M.A. Severini MSS.* The list of Severini's works appears to be autograph; at fol. 76ʳ: "In Avicennae tractatum de ulceribus metaphrasis. Item in Avicennae de vulneribus generatim." (The works themselves may be among the Severini manuscripts in the Biblioteca Lancisiana, but the Severini collection was not available for consultation during my visit there.)

———, Biblioteca Lancisiana. 127. Notes or drafts for lectures at the Sapienza (University of Rome) by Carolus Vallesius, with many insertions and loose pages. Fols. 299ʳ–413ᵛ, commentary on *Canon* 1.1; variant drafts for the opening of a commentary on this book are also found on earlier folios, e.g. 293ʳ: "praelecturus institutiones medicae ex oraculis Avicennae in hac Romane Sapientiae." On fol. 228ʳ are the dates 1659 and 1660.

———, Biblioteca Lancisiana. 129. Notes or drafts for lectures at the Sapienza by Carolus Vallesius. Unbound sheets in gatherings. Fol. 3ʳff. "In fen primam quarti Canonis Avicennae."

★Salamanca, Biblioteca de la Universidad. Isidro Aldaba Galceran, *In Avicennam de febribus.* Seventeenth century, 438 pp. Cited from *Catálogo de los libros manuscritos, que se conservan en la Biblioteca de la Universidad de Salamanca. . . .* (Salamanca, 1855), pp. 11–12.

★———, Biblioteca de la Universidad. Fulgentio de Benavente. *Commentaria supra primam canonis Avicenae,* reported by Duarte Fernandez. Cited from *Catálogo de los . . . manuscritos . . . de la Universidad de Salamanca,* p. 26.

★———, Biblioteca de la Universidad. Gaspar Fernandez. *Commentaria de febribus in librum quartum Canonis Avicenae.* 1625, 279 pp. Cited from *Catálogo de los . . . manuscritos . . . de la Universidad de Salamanca,* p. 29.

★———, Biblioteca de la Universidad. Godinez. *In Avicennam.* 1585. Cited from *Catálogo de los . . . manuscritos . . . de la Universidad de Salamanca,* p. 32.

Siena, Biblioteca Comunale. C IX 11. *Reportationes* of lectures on the *Canon* and Averroes, *Colliget* by Matteo Corti. Fols. 6ʳ–106ᵛ: *M. Curtii expositio super prima fen primi Canonis Avicennae 1529;* fol. 7ʳ: date of copying 1537 and "E.D.M. Curtii expositio super prima fen primi Canonis Avicennae quam notavit E. D. Justinianus Finettus [Sinettus?] Luponensis Patavii"; 69 numbered lectures follow, to fol. 90. Fol. 90ᵛ "Quae sequuntur addita sunt alia eiusdem Curtii lectura anni 1527 quae deerant huic lecturae, habita a D. H. Stephanello"; 17 numbered lectures follow, to fol. 106ᵛ. Fols. 108ʳ–15ʳ, *Curtius super prima quarti Avicennae;* fol. 114r, 1536. Fols. 115ʳ–208ᵛ, "E.D.M. Curtius expositio publice in ticinensi gimnasio legentis practicam ordinariam . . . super fen prima quarti Canonis 1536." Fols. 211–37ʳ, *Expositio super septimo Colliget Averrois E. Matthei Curtii 1527.*

———, Biblioteca Comunale. C IX 18. Fols. 1ʳ–129ᵛ, *Lectiones . . . Hieronymi Capivacci in primam fen libri quarti Avicennae . . . habitae publice in Patavino*

Gymnasio. 77 numbered lectures delivered between 3 November 1579 and 20 June 1580.

†Turin, Biblioteca Nazionale. K3 II 4. Mazzatinti 28:154 describes this manuscript as containing a commentary on the *Canon* by Girolamo Mercuriale. The first 200 folios do indeed contain a commentary on *Canon* 1.1.1–4, but it is anonymous, and the incipit, "Ut vestrae utilitati in primis consulam . . . ," matches that of Paterno's commentary on the same text in WL 602. This manuscript survived the fire that destroyed many of the Turin manuscripts in the early twentieth century, but was badly water-damaged. Parts of the microfilm—which I am informed by Dr. Giuseppe Dondi, the director of the Biblioteca Nazionale, is more legible than the original—are indecipherable. Dr. Dondi also confirms the absence of any ascription to an author in the original. There seems to be no other record that Mercuriale, who usually taught *practica* for which *Canon* 1.1 was not a text, produced a commentary on the *Canon*; most likely, this is another copy of Paterno's commentary.

Vatican City, Biblioteca Apostolica del Vaticano. Barb. lat. 269. *Iatrophysica seu ratiocinationes ad Avicennae Canonem digestae a Matthia Naldio.* Seventeenth century. Naldio d. 1682.

———, Biblioteca Apostolica del Vaticano. Reg. lat. 1271. *Horatii Augenii commentariorum in primam quarti Avicennae liber primus.* The manuscript is divided into seven books on fevers, all of which are presumably part of the commentary. 1591. The sequence of subjects seems to differ from that in his *De febribus . . . libri septem . . .* (Frankfurt, 1605), which does not take the form of a commentary, but the two works may nevertheless be related. *De febribus* was written between 1568 and 1572.

Venice, Biblioteca Marciana. Lat. VII 23 (3491). *Josephi del Papa medicinae tractatus aliquot ad usum scholae accommodati, videlicet de temperamentis, de humoribus, de differentiis partium, de rebus praeter naturam, de methodo medendi. In quibus cum veterum tum recentiorum medicinae principium sententiae enarruntur, expenduntur, atque adinvicem comparantur.* At fol. 4ᵛ: "Liber primus fen prima doctrina prima caput primum de definitione medicinae." The commentary, on the first five *doctrinae* of *Canon* 1.1, ends on fol. 37ʳ. The author lived from 1649 to 1735 and taught at Pisa early in his career.

———, Biblioteca Marciana. Lat. VII 68 (9693). Lectures by Girolamo Capodivacca, inc., fol. 2ʳ: "Lectio 12. Medicamenta evacuantia caput erant reprimentia." Possibly on *Canon* 2.

Verona, Biblioteca Civica. 1507 (Biadego 580). *Excellentissimi domini Johannis Baptistae Montani Veronensis in primum primi Avicennae doctissima interpretatio.* 73 numbered lectures to fol. 124ᵛ. A second set of numbered lectures on the same text, beginning with no. 62, starts on fol. 126ʳ and ends with lecture no. 75 on fol. 147ʳ. Two lectures numbered 57 and 58 follow on fols. 147ʳ–50ʳ. Fols. 153ʳ–167ʳ, *Excellentissimi domini Jo. Baptistae Montani Veronensis in quartam primi Avicennae.*

Printed commentaries, arranged chronologically by date of publication (but with second and subsequent editions of the same work immediately following the first)

Corso, Bartolomeo. *Apologia . . . cum apta expositione vel clara declaratione illorum Avicenne verborum quorum fuit contentio et altercatio.* Rome, 1519. On *Canon* 1.3.1.

Rustico, Pietro Antonio. *Qui atrocem horres pestem pestilentemque times febrem ecce dicta principis Avicenne de pestilentia seu peste . . . ordinata, exposita, discussa a Rustico medicine cultore. . . .* Printed with Baviera, Baverio, *Consilia Baverii.* Pavia, 1521. On portions of *Canon* 4.

————. *Qui venenosa formidas apostemata et pestiferos paves bubones ecce dicta Avicene arabis de igne persico pruna vel carbone . . . ordinata, exposita, discussa a Rustico medicine cultore. . . .* Printed with preceding item. Based on portions of *Canon* 4.

Legio, Leonardo. *Propositiones seu flosculi ex Galeni libros per . . . D. Magistrum Leonardum Legium . . . collecte . . . Eiusdem magistri Leonardi ex expositione capituli aurei Avicenne introductorium medicorum. . . .* Venice, 1523. The commentary on *Canon* 3.1.2.29 is separately foliated. The author identified himself as a professor at Pavia.

Degli Emanuelli, Bartolomeo. *Adnotationes super dicta Gentilis de Fulgineo dicta ab illo super definitione de febre data ab Avicenna in primo capitulo libri eius quarti in tractatu primo de febribus. . . .* Rome, 1524. A brief supercommentary on Gentile's commentary on *Canon* 4.1.

Luiz, Antonio. *Expositio . . . in diffinitionem quam de humoribus Avicenna consignat.* Fols. 89ᵛ–93ʳ in his *De re medica opera. . . .* Lisbon, 1540.

Forte, Angelo. *De calamitoso errore Avicennae, unde communium medicorum orrenda malefitia inter homines cotidie pullulant.* Venice, 1542. An attack on *Canon* 1.1.4 (humors) and also on academic physicians; not a school commentary.

Santo, Mariano. *Ad communem medicorum chirurgicorum usum commentaria nuper in lucem aedita in Avicennae textum. . . .* Venice, 1543. On *Canon* 4.3.1.

Milich, Jacob. *Oratio . . . de Avicenna vita.* Printed with his *Oratio de consideranda sympathia et antipathia in rerum natura. . . .* Wittenberg, 1550.

Da Monte, Giambatista. *De differentiis medicamentorum. . . .* Edited by Kaspar Peucer. Wittenberg, 1551. Corresponds to part of his commentary on *Canon* 1.4. According to the NLM card catalogue, an earlier edition of this work appeared Venice, 1550, edited by Lucas Stengel, under the title *★Metaphrasis summaria eorum quae ad medicamentorum doctrinam attinent.* It was also reissued as part of his *★Explicatio locorum medicinae. . . .* Paris, 1554 (Durling, *Catalogue*, no. 3242).

Pellenegra, Filippo. *Contradictiones Avicennae. . . .* Venice, 1552.

Ingrassia, Giovanni Filippo. *De tumoribus praeter naturam tomus primus. . . . Occasione sumpta ab Avicenna verbis, Arabum medicorum principis, tertia fen, quarti libri, tractatu primo, cuius interim universum primum caput in hoc tomo elucidatur. . . .* Naples, 1553. On *Canon* 4.3.1.

*Ingrassia, Giovanni Filippo. *Avicennae caput de fractura cranii ab ipso correptus* in Jo. Paschalis, *De morbo gallico* (handwritten catalogue of printed books, Biblioteca Lancisiana, Rome). Presumably on *Canon* 4.5.3.1.

Da Monte, Giambatista. *In primam fen libri primi Canonis Avicennae explanatio.* . . . Edited by Valentinus Lublin. Venice, 1554. On *Canon* 1.1.

————. *In primi libri Canonis Avicennae primam fen profundissimi commentaria. Adiecto nuper secundo quod nunquam ante fuerat typis excussum de membris capite.* . . . Edited by J. M. Durastante. Venice, 1557. A reprint of the previous item, with an additional chapter, also presumably by Da Monte.

————. *In quartam fen primi Canonis Avicenne lectiones.* . . . Edited by Valentinus Lublin. Venice, 1556. On *Canon* 1.4. Fols. 33ʳ–67ʳ of this edition correspond to Parts 1–3 of Da Monte's *De differentiis medicamentorum* (Wittenberg, 1551).

————. *Lectiones . . . in secundam fen primi Canonis Avicennae.* . . . Venice, 1557. On *Canon* 1.2.

Betti, Antonio Maria. *In quartam fen primi Canonis Avicennae commentarium.* . . . Bologna, 1560. IA 118.243. On *Canon* 1.4.

*————. Another edition of the previous item. Bologna, 1562. IA 118.244.

————. *In IIII fen primi Canonis Avicennae commentarius doctissimus, nunc primum in lucem editus. Impressus anno LX, sed hucusque (immerito) incognitus.* . . . Bologna, 1591. Another edition of the same.

Oddi, Oddo. *In primam totam fen primi libri Canonis Avicennae dilucidissima et expectatissima expositio.* . . . Venice, 1575. On *Canon* 1.1. Portions by Marco Oddi.

————. *In primam totam fen primi libri Canonis Avicennae dilucidissima et expectatissima expositio. Nunc tertio in lucem edita.* . . . Padua, 1612. I do not know where, or when, the second edition was published.

Luca, Constantino. *In Avicennae caput de phlebotomia expositio.* Pavia, 1584. Apparently on part of *Canon* 1.4. The author was a professor at Pavia.

Da Monte, Giambatista. *Medicina universa.* . . . Edited by Martin Weindrich. Frankfurt, 1587. Excerpts from Da Monte's works arranged as a continuous narrative; substantial sections from his commentaries on the *Canon* are incorporated (for example, pp. 103–26 on the elements; p. 187 also corresponds to a passage in the commentary on *Canon* 1.1).

Costeo, Giovanni. *Disquisitionum physiologicarum . . . in primam primi Canonis Avicennae sectionem libri sex.* . . . Bologna, 1589. On *Canon* 1.1.

Paterno, Bernardino. *Bernardini Salodiensis, philosophi et medici clarissimi, qui in praecipuis Italiae gimnasiis ac demum Patavino totos quinquaginta annos rem medicam ad veterem Hippocratis et Galeni disciplinam summa cum laude interpretatus est, explanationes in primam fen primi Canonis Avicennae.* . . . Edited by Bernardino Gaio. Venice, 1596. On *Canon* 1.1.

Trincavella, Vettor. *Explanationes in primam fen quarti Canonis Avicennae habitae Patavii MDLIII ac in commentarii formam redactae.* In his *Opera*, 2nd edition, Venice, 1599. Vol. 3 of 3 vols. in 2. Separately foliated. On *Canon* 4.1.

Massaria, Alessandro. *Practica medica.* . . . Trèves, 1607. Book 7, *De febribus,* pp. 314–446, is a commentary on *Canon* 4.1. Other editions of Massaria's *Practica medica* were published Frankfurt, 1601; Venice, 1622; and *Lyon, 1622 (British Library, *General Catalogue of Printed Books*).

Capodivacca, Girolamo. *Practicae medicinae liber sextus de febribus.* In his *Opera omnia*, section 4, pp. 814–912. Frankfurt, 1603. A commentary on *Canon* 4.1. Other editions of his *Opera omnia* were published *Venice, 1597; *Venice, 1598; *Venice, 1599 (*IA* 131.679–81); and Venice, 1606.

Garcia Carrero, Pedro. *Disputationes medicae super fen primam libri primi Avicennae etiam philosophis valde utiles. . . .* Alcalá de Henares, 1611. 1398 folio pages.

Colle, Giovanni. *Elucidarium anatomicum et chirurgicum ex Graecis, Arabibus et Latinus selectum, una cum commentariis in quartum librum Avicennae, fen tertiam. . . .* Venice, 1621. On *Canon* 4.3.

Ponce Santa Cruz, Antonio. *Disputationes in primam primi Avicennae.* In his *Opuscula medica et philosophica . . .* , fols. 1ʳ–305ʳ. Madrid, 1624. The title of the work on the *Canon* given here is taken from the title page of the collection; the work itself is headed *Lectiones primariae in primam primi Avicennae*.

Santorio, Santorio. *Commentaria in primam fen primi libri Canonis Avicennae. . . .* Venice, 1626. Biblioteca Comunale degli Intronati, Siena. I am unclear as to whether this should be regarded as a separate edition from the copy in the British Library, which appears identical as regards title, publisher, place, contents, dedication, and typography, but bears the date 1625. On *Canon* 1.1.

———. *Commentaria in primam fen primi libri Canonis Avicennae. . . .* Venice, 1646. Another edition of the previous item.

———. *Opera. . . .* 4 vols., Venice, 1660. Vol. 3 contains the commentary on *Canon* 1.1. Biblioteca Nazionale, Rome.

Garcia Carrero, Pedro. *Disputationes medicae et commentaria in fen primam libri quarti Avicennae. . . .* Bordeaux, 1628. 1122 folio pages.

Stefano, Giovanni. *Paraphrasis Joannis Stephani physici et almi Venetorum Medicorum et Philosophorum Collegii Prioris in primam fen libri quarti Avicennae de febribus studiose perpolita.* Venice, 1646. Bibliothèque Nationale, Paris. The paraphrase falls somewhere between a commentary and a revised version of the Latin text of *Canon* 4.1.

———. *Opera universa, cum medicinae ac philosophiae tum cultoris literaturae studiosis apprime utilia. . . .* Venice, 1653. Another edition of the preceding item at pp. 242–96. On pp. 88–223 is Stefano's *Paraphrasis in novem fen libri III Avicennae continens universos capitis affectus*. The handwritten catalogue of printed books of the Biblioteca Lancisiana, Rome, includes another edition of each paraphrase, both published *Venice, 1649.

Scarabicio, Sebastiano. *De ortu ignis febriferi historia physica medica ad Avicennae ordinem. . . .* Padua, 1655. Organization follows *Canon* 4.1.

Cardano, Girolamo. *Commentaria in quatuor primas Principis primae sectionis doc[t]rinas, seu Floridorum libri duo.* In his *Opera*. Lyon, 1663. Facsimile, London and New York, 1967. 9:453–567. On *Canon* 1.1.1–4.

Salio Diverso, Pietro. *In Avicennae librum tertium de morbis particularibus . . . annotationes luculentissimae, opus posthumum, nunc primum in lucem edita.* Padua, 1673. The author seems to have flourished in the first half of the sixteenth century. On *Canon* 3.

Patin, Charles. *De Avicenna oratio habita in Archi-Lycaeo Patavino die x Novembris 1676.* Padua, 1678.

Morgagni, G. Battista. *Commento ad Avicenna* [sic]. In his *Opera postuma*, edited by Adalberto Pazzini, vols. 4, 5, and 6 (Rome, 1969, 1975, 1981). On *Canon* 1.1. Latin commentary, with modern Italian translation. The commentary remained in manuscript until this edition.

Selected Bibliography

What follows is neither a comprehensive bibliography of the subject nor a complete listing of all works consulted or examined for this book. It mainly consists of items cited in the footnotes. The reader should, however, note that (1) versions of the *Canon* and commentaries produced after 1500 are not included here, but listed separately in the appendices; (2) reference works and collections named in the list of abbreviations at the front of the volume and the introductory remarks to the appendices are not repeated in the bibliography, nor are individual articles or treatises within them; (3) the listing of works printed before 1700 includes a few additional samples, not discussed in text or notes, of books that indicate some, but not exclusive, reliance on Avicenna in their titles; (4) the final section of the bibliography, "Other Works," is a limited selection from items cited in the notes. Only works to which I was able to obtain access by April 1986 are included.

Manuscripts

AAUP, *filze* 242, rotuli, 1520–1733, some including names of prescribed books; 507, fols. 89–108, documents relating to university reform, early eighteenth century; 651, rotuli and lists of lecturers and salaries, some including names of prescribed books, 1579–1604; 667, includes documents relating to the establishment of a chair for lectures on *Canon* 1.2, 1600–1602 (basis of Bertolaso,"Cattedra de pulsibus"); 669, 231ʳ–237ʳ, lists of lecturers and documents relating to the chair for lectures on *Canon* 3, 1518–1733, fols. 335ʳ–55ʳ, same for professorship of *teoria extraordinaria* on holidays, 1602–1719; 722, letters and decrees of Riformatori dello Studio and reports of *bidelli* on lectures delivered, 1672–1740s; 727, index to decrees of Venetian Senate and Moderators of the University relating to the University, 1406–1686, with notices of documents having to do with lectures on the *Canon* at 111, 177, 199, 279, 299, 300, 372.

ASB, Assunteria di Studio, Serie di annue lezione, *busta* 1, 319ʳ–600ʳ, lecture topics, mostly from the 1640s.

ASB, Assunteria di Studio, Diversorum: Letture. 1 *busta* of material relating to condition and reform of lectureships; first folder, marked 1735–37, contains letters of M. Bazzani and G. B. Beccari concerning the restablishment of lectures on *Canon* 1.1.

ASF, Stamperia Orientale Medicea, *filze* 1–6, records of the Medici press; included are correspondence of G. B. Raimondi and legal documents pertain-

377

ing to the production and distribution of the 1593 edition of the *Canon* in Arabic.

ASP, Università, A II 2, rotuli (some giving names of prescribed books) and other university documents, 1543–47; A II 3, same, 1547–64; III 1, reports on the state of the university and proposals for reform, 1734–40; G 77 (sixteenth century and early seventeenth century) and G 78 (to 1700), first 2 vols. of a 3-vol. collection of university documents, compiled in the eighteenth century by G. Fabroni, including many rotuli and lists of lecturers and salaries, some with names of prescribed books.

ASV, Riformatori dello Studio di Padova, *busta* 419, includes correspondence relating to the establishment of a chair for lectures on *Canon* 1.2, 1601–1602.

———, Riformatori dello Studio di Padova, *busta* 452, includes printed rotuli and course descriptions, including that of Lorenzo Bacchetto.

Bologna, Biblioteca Universitaria, MSS Aldrovandi 136, vol. XIII, fols. 6ʳ–57ʳ, vocabulary of transliterated Arabic plant and drug names compiled by Aldrovandi from the *Canon* and Alpago's glossary.

Florence, Biblioteca Medicea Laurenziana, Ashburnham 1260. Thirteenth and fourteenth centuries. 39 fols. French medical compendium based on the *Canon*. Inc. "Ici commence l'Avicen en romance."

———, BNC, Magl. III,81; II III 13 (Magl.III, 130); II III 14 (Magl. III,129); II III 15 (Magl. III, 119); II III 20 (Magl. III, 117), notebooks of G. B. Raimondi containing vocabularies, book lists, passages of partial translation from Arabic into Latin, and other material relating to the printing of the *Canon* in Arabic in 1593 by the Stamperia Orientale Medicea.

Padua, Biblioteca Comunale, BP 1223, fifteenth century, humanist miscellany; at fol. 160, supposed letter of Avicenna to Saint Augustine, inc. "Avicenna physicus et phylosophus Aurelio Augustino salutem. Apparuisti compatriota noster."

*Paris, Bibliothèque Nationale, arab. 2897, Arabic text with interlinear Latin translation and Latin marginalia. *Canon* 1, with translation by Ramusio, 1484. Description supplied by Charles B. Schmitt (see also Kristeller, *Iter* 3: 576).

———, Bibliothèque Nationale, lat. 6852, sixteenth century, lectures of Matteo Corti on Book 2 of the Hippocratic *Aphorisms* and, separately foliated, *Canon* 4.1 (the latter identified as given at Pavia). Evaluation of Arab medicine in preface to Hippocratic commentary, fols. 1ʳ⁻ᵛ.

Pisa, Biblioteca Universitaria, 234, notebook of Giulio Angeli of Barga, containing philosophical and medical excerpts and the catalogue of his personal library (ed. L. Zampieri, 1981 [see "Other Works" section of Bibliography]); 333–44, Giulio Angeli's lecture notes, 1578–94 (mostly lectures on the Hippocratic *Aphorisms* and Galenic *Ars*).

*Uppsala, University Library, uncatalogued, Waller 653 D:3. 1478. 67 fols. North Italian vernacular medical compendium based on the *Canon*. Inc. "Questo sie uno fioreto trato de Avicena." Photocopy of some folios supplied by Per-Gunnar Ottosson.

Vatican City, Biblioteca Apostolica Vaticana, Vat. lat. 5108, fifteenth-century humanist miscellany, with so-called letter of Avicenna to Augustine at fol. 107^v. Inc. "Aicenna [*sic*] medicinae professor beatissimo Augustino episcopo salutem dicit. Apparuisti compatriota noster."

Venice, Biblioteca Correr, Dona dalle Rose 212, miscellany of letters and documents relating to the *studio* of Padua, 1584–1606. Includes, 41^r–42^v, report of Antonio Rosato, *bidello*, on lectures given 1583–84; 63^r, 64^r, two dogal letters, 1591, concerning the chair for lectures on *Canon* III; 105^r, 122^r, printed rotuli for 1599 and 1603–1604, giving names of lecturers and books.

———, Biblioteca Correr, Cicogna 301 8, item 32, *Catalogo di scrittori medici veneziani, 1473–1760*. Includes various commentators on and editors of the *Canon*.

———, Biblioteca Marciana, lat. VI 59 (2548), fifteenth century, *Liber de simplicibus Benedicti Rinii medici et philosophi veneti*.

Works Printed before 1700

Most of the works in this category were consulted at the following libraries: NLM, NYAM, WL, BL, and Special Collections, Columbia University, New York. The National Library of Medicine, History of Medicine Division, supplied me with microfilms of a number of early printed books, for which I am grateful.

Amatus Lusitanus. *Curationum medicinalium . . . tomus primus continens centuria quatuor. . . .* Venice, 1566.

Arcolano, Giovanni. *De febribus . . . In Avicennae IV Canonis fen primam dilucida atque optima expositio nunc denuo accuratissime expurgata ac duplici Avicennae textu exornata, altero antiquo, quem sequutus est Arculanus; altero quem post Andreae Alpagi Bellunensis castigationes et locorum citationibus illustravit. . . .* Padua, 1685.

———. *Expositio perutilis in primam fen quarti Canonis Avicenne una cum adnotamentis prestantissimi viri domini Symphoriani Champerii. . . .* Lyon 1518.

Argenterio, Giovanni. *De febribus liber.* In his *Opera. . . .* Hanover, 1610. Cols. 2171–322. Follows the arrangement of *Canon* 4.1.

———. *Operum in tres tomos divisorum volumen primum tres in Artem medicam Galeni commentarios complectens. . . .* Venice, 1592.

Astario, Biagio. *De curis febrium libellus utilis. . . .* Bound with Marco Gatinaria, *De curis egritudinum particularium. . . .* Venice, 1521.

Avicenna. *Opera philosophica Venise, 1508.* Facsimile, Louvain, 1961.

Benzi, Ugo. *Expositio . . . super primo Canonis Avicennae. . . .* Venice, 1498. Klebs 998.2.

Bertacchi, Domenico. *De spiritibus libri quatuor necnon De facultate vitali libri tres.* Venice, 1584.

Bertocci, Alfonso. *Methodus generalis et compendiaria ex Hippocratis, Galeni, et Avicennae placitis deprompta ac in ordinem redacta. . . .* Lyon, 1558.

Boissard, Jean Jacques, and De Bry, Theodore. *Bibliotheca seu thesaurus virtutis et gloriae in qua continentur illustrium eruditione et doctrina virorum effigies et vitae.* Frankfurt, 1628. No. 48, portrait and biography of Gilbert Fusch of Limburg.

Bovio, Giacinto. *Flores medicinales, seu sententiae, authoritates et rationes ex Hippocrate, Galeno, Avicenna, et aliis summis authoribus . . . collectae. . . .* Venice, 1668.

Brissot, Pierre. *Apologetica disceptatio qua docetur per quae loca sanguis mitti debeat. . . .* Paris, 1525. Facsimile, Brussels, 1973.

Capodivacca, Girolamo. *In primum Aphorismorum Hippocratis librum doctissima et dilucidissima explanatio, in scholis per ordinarias lectiones tradita. . . .* Printed with his *Tractatus de foetus formatione. . . .* Venice, 1599.

Cardano, Girolamo. *Contradicentium medicorum liber continens contradictiones centum octo.* Venice, 1545.

———. *De libris propriis eorum usu liber recognitus.* In his *Opera,* 1:96–150. Lyon, 1663. Facsimile, New York and London, 1967.

———. *De malo recentiorum medicorum medendi usus libellus. . . .* Venice, 1536.

———. *De subtilitate libri XXI. . . .* Basel, 1560.

———. *In Cl. Ptolomaei . . . Quadripartitae constructionis libros commentaria. . . .* Lyon, 1555.

———. *Liber de libris propriis, eorumque ordine et usu, ac de mirabilibus operibus in arte medica factis.* In his *Opera,* 1:60–95. Lyon, 1663. Facsimile, New York and London, 1967.

Castelli, Pietro. *Optimus medicus.* In Conring, Herman, *In universam artem medicam . . . introductio. . . .* Helmstadt, 1687. Castelli's work is dated 1637.

Cesalpino, Andrea. *Quaestionum peripateticarum libri V . . . Daemonum investigatio peripatetica.* Printed together in one volume. Venice, 1593.

Champier, Symphorien. *De medicine claris scriptoribus. . . .* Lyon, ca. 1506.

———. *Officina apothecariorum. . . .* Lyon, 1532.

———. *Practica nova in medicina . . . ex traditionibus Grecorum, Latinorum, Arabum, penorum ac recentium autorum. . . .* Lyon, 1517.

———. *Symphonia Galeni ad Hippocratem, Cornelii Celsi ad Avicennam, una cum sectis antiquorum medicorum ac recentium. . . . Item Clysteriorum campi contra Arabum opinionem, pro Galeni sententia. . . .* [Lyon, 1528].

Clavius, Christopher. *In sphaeram Joannis de Sacro Bosco commentarius.* Rome, 1570.

Cop, Guillaume, tr. *Galeni de affectorum locorum notitia libri sex. . . .* Paris [1513].

Crato, Johann, of Krafftheim. *Consiliorum et epistolarum medicinalium liber. . . .* Compiled by Peter Monau. Frankfurt, 1591. Books 3 and 4, Frankfurt, 1671. Books 5 and 6, Frankfurt, 1671.

Cremonini, Cesare. *De calido innato et semine pro Aristotele adversus Galenum.* Leiden, 1634.

Dalechamps, Jaques. *Chirurgie françoise.* Lyon, 1570.

Da Monte, Giambatista. *In nonum librum Rhasis ad Mansorem regem Arabum expositio.* Edited by Valentinus Lublin. Venice, 1554.

——. Preface in *Galeni Opera ex sexta Juntarum editione.* Venice, 1586. Vol. 1, sig. [A8^r]–b2^r.

Del Garbo, Dino. *Expositio super 3^a et 4^a fen Avicenne et super parte quinte.* . . . Ferrara, 1489. Usually known as Dino's *Chirurgia.* Klebs 336.1.

——. *Super quarta fen primi Avicenne preclarissima commentaria que Dilucidatorium totius practice generalis medicinalis scientie nuncupatur.* . . . Volume includes his *Expositio . . . super canones generales de virtutibus medicinarum simplicium secundi Canonis Avicenne.* Venice, 1514.

Del Garbo, Tommaso. *Summa medicinalis.* . . . Venice, 1506.

Dondi, Jacopo. *Tractatus de causa salsedinis aquarum et modo conficiendi salis ex eis.* In *De balneis omnia quae extant apud Graecos, Latinos, et Arabos.* . . . Venice, 1553. Fol. 109^{r-v}.

Dos Reys Tavares, Emmanuel. *Controversias philosophicas et medicas ex doctrina de febribus.* . . . Lisbon, 1667.

Falloppia, Gabriele. *De metallis atque fossilibus.* In his *Omnia, quae adhuc extant, opera.* Venice, 1584.

——. *Observationes anatomicae.* . . . Venice, 1561.

Fernel, Jean. *Universa medicina.* . . . Paris, 1554; Lyon, 1581; Frankfurt, 1593.

Ferrari, Ognibene. *De regulis medicinae ex Hippocrate, Galeno et Avicenna . . . libri tres.* . . . Venice, 1573.

Fracastoro, Girolamo. *Homocentricorum, sive de stellis liber unus.* In his *Opera omnia.* . . . 2nd edition. Venice, 1574. Fols. 1^r–48^r.

Fries, Lorenz. *Defensio medicorum principis Avicennae.* Strasbourg, 1530.

Fuchs, Leonhart. *Paradoxorum medicinae libri tres, in quibus sane multa a nemine hactenus prodita Arabum aetatisque nostrae medicorum errata non tantum indicantur, sed . . . confutantur.* . . . Paris, 1555.

Fusch, Gilbert. *Modus et ordo quibus possint medicinae studiosi Avicennam, medicum Arabem, cum Hippocrate, Galeno, caeterisque medicis Graecis conciliare, et errata, si quae deprehendantur, ad illorum regulam expendendo, facile in integram restituere.* . . . Lyon, 1541.

Gentile da Foligno. *Quaestiones et tractatus extravagantes.* . . . Venice, 1520.

Gesner, Konrad. *Bibliotheca universalis, sive catalogus scriptorum locupletissimus in tribus linguis, Latina, Graeca, et Hebraica.* . . . Zurich, 1545. Article on Avicenna.

Giacomo da Forlì. *Expositio et quaestiones in primum Canonem Avicennae.* Venice, 1547.

Gryll, Lorenz. *Oratio de peregrinatione studii medicinalis.* . . . Printed with his *De sapore dulci et amaro libri duo.* . . . Prague, 1566.

Gui de Chauliac. *Cyrurgia Guidonis de Cauliaco et Cyrurgia Bruni, Theodorici, Rolandi, Rogerii, Bertipalie, Lanfranci.* Venice, 1498. Klebs 494.1.

Guinter, Johann, of Andernach. *De medicina veteri et nova tum cognoscenda, tum faciunda commentarii duo.* Basel, 1571.

Haly Abbas. *Liber totius medicine.* Lyon, 1523.

Houllier, Jacques. Preface to his *De materia chirurgica*. In his *Omnia opera practica*. . . . Geneva, 1623.

Kirsten, Peter. *Grammatices Arabicae. Liber I. Sive orthographia et prosodia arabica.* Breslau [1608].

―――. *Vitae Evangelistarum quatuor: nunc primum ex antiquissimo codice manuscript arabico Caesario erutae*. . . . Breslau [1608].

[Landi, Bassiano, and others.] *Novae Academiae Florentinae opuscula adversus Avicennam et medicos neotericos, qui Galeni disciplina neglecta, barbaros colunt.* . . . Venice, 1533.

Lange, Johann. *Epistolarum medicinalium volumen tripartitum*. Hanover, 1605. Book 1, letter 44, and Book 3, letter 6.

Le Coq (Gallus), Pascal. *Bibliotheca medica*. Basel, 1590. Facsimile reprint in Obinu, Giovanni Maria, *La "Biblioteca medica" di Pasquale Le Coq (Gallus), sec. XVI (edizione anastatica)*. Scientia Veterum 151, 152, 1970.

Leoniceno, Nicolò. *De Plinii et plurium aliorum medicorum in medicina erroribus libri quatuor*. In his *Opuscula*, fols. 1ʳ–61ᵛ. Basel, 1532.

Manardo, Giovanni. *Epistolarum medicinalium libros XX*. . . . Basel, 1540.

Massa, Nicolò. *Epistolarum medicinalium tomus alter*. . . . Venice, 1558.

Mercado, Luis. *De constitutione et fabrica corporis humani, ab elementis usque ad ipsius integritatem*. In his *Operum tomus primus*. . . . Frankfurt, 1620.

Minadoi, Giovanni Tommaso. *Historia della guerra fra Turchi e Persiani*. . . . Rome, 1587.

Montuo, Sebastiano. *Dialexeon medicinalium libri duo*. . . . Lyon, 1537. A defense of Avicenna, against Leonhard Fuchs.

Nifo, Agostino. *Expositiones in Aristotelis libros Metaphysices*. Venice, 1559. Facsimile, Frankfurt, 1967.

Ocellus Lucanus. *De universi natura libellus Ludovico Nogarola . . . interprete*. . . . Venice, 1559.

Oddi, Oddo. *In primam Aphorismorum Hippocratis sectionem elaboratissima et lucidatissima expositio*. . . . Edited by Marco Oddi. Padua, 1564.

Paolino, Fabio. *Praelectiones Marciae, sive Commentaria in Thucydidis Historiam.* . . . Venice, 1603. Passage about proposed translation of *Canon*, Book 1, p. 181.

Patin, Charles. *Circulationem sanguinis a veteribus cognitam fuisse, Oratio habita in Archi-Lyceo Patavino, Die iii Novembris MDCLXXXV*. Padua, 1685.

―――. *Lyceum patavinum, sive icones et vitae professorum Patavii, MDCLXXXII publice docentium*. Padua, 1682.

Pianeri (Planerius), Giovanni. *Febrium omnium simplicium divisio et compositio ex Galeno et Avicenna excerpta et in arbores, ut facilius intelligatur, redacta*. Venice, 1574. The *arbores* are elaborate tables.

Petrus Hispanus, comm. Isaac Judeus. *Liber dietarum universalium*. In *Omnia opera Ysaac*. . . . Lyon, 1515.

Pictorius, Georg. *Medicinae tam simplices quam compositae . . . ex Hippocrate, Galeno, Avicenna, Aegineta, et aliis*. . . . Basel, 1560.

Pietro d'Abano. *Conciliator*. . . . Venice, 1548, 1565 (facsimile, Padua, 1985).

Raphael, A. F. *In funere Bernardini Paterni . . . oratio.* Padua, 1592.

Riccobono, Antonio. *De gymnasio patavino . . . commentariorum libri sex.* Padua, 1598.

Rinio, Benedetto. *De morbo gallico. . . .* In vol. 2 of *De morbo gallico omnia quae extant. . . .* 2 vols. Venice, 1566.

Rolfinck, Werner. *Liber de purgantibus vegetabilibus.* Jena, 1667. Includes a few passages from the *Canon* in Arabic.

Rorario, Niccolò. *Contradictiones, dubia, et paradoxa in libros Hippocratis, Celsi, Galeni, Aetii, Aeginetae, Avicennae, cum eorumdem conciliationibus. . . .* Venice, 1566.

Santorio, Santorio. *Ars . . . De statica medicina aphorismorum. . . .* Leipzig [1626].

Scaliger, Julius Caesar. *Exotericarum exercitationum liber XV de subtilitate ad Hieronymum Cardanum. . . .* Frankfurt, 1592.

Scaligerana, Thuana, Perroniana, Pithoeana, et Colomesiana. . . . Amsterdam, 1740. Entry on Avicenna.

Scheiner, Christopher. *Oculus, hoc est fundamentum opticum. . . .* Innsbruck, 1619.

Schenk, Georg. *Biblia iatrica sive bibliotheca medica. . . .* Frankfurt, 1609.

Sennert, Daniel. *Institutionum medicinae libri V. . . .* Wittenberg [1632].

Statuta almae universitatis D. artistarum et medicorum patavini gymnasii. . . . Venice, 1589.

Statuta almae universitatis D.D. philosophorum et medicorum cognomento artistarum patavini gymnasii. . . . Padua, 1607.

Statuta dominorum artistarum achademiae patavinae. Padua, n.d. Hain 15015 (microfilm at Columbia University supplied courtesy of William H. Scheide).

Sylvius, Jacobus (Jacques de la Boë). *Opera medica. . . .* Geneva, 1630.

Tomasini, Jacopo Filippo. *Bibliothecae patavinae manuscriptae publicae et privatae. . . .* Udine, 1639.

―――. *Illustrium virorum elogia iconibus exornata.* Padua, 1630.

Torrigiano de' Torrigiani, Pietro (Turisanus). *Plusquam commentum in Microtegni Galieni. . . .* Venice, 1512.

Vallés, Francisco. *Controversariarium medicarum et philosophicarum . . . editio tertia. . . .* Frankfurt, 1590.

Van Beverwijck, Jan. *Medicinae encomium.* Rotterdam, 1644.

Vesalius, Andreas. *De humani corporis fabrica libri septem.* Basel, 1543.

Vincent of Beauvais. *Speculum naturale,* books 10–14, 28–30. In his *Speculum quadruplex, naturale, doctrinale, morale, historiale. . . .* Douai, 1624.

Other Works

Abel, Günter. *Stoizismus und Frühe Neuzeit.* Berlin and New York, 1978.

Adelmann, Howard B. *Marcello Malpighi and the Evolution of Embryology.* Vols. 1 and 2. Ithaca, N.Y., 1966.

Agrimi, Jole, and Crisciani, Chiara. *Medicina del corpo e medicina dell'anima: Note sul sapere del medico fino all'inizio del secolo XIII.* Milan, 1978.

Antonioli, Roland. *Rabelais et la médecine.* Etudes Rabelaisiennes, vol. 12. Geneva, 1976. Travaux d'humanisme et de Renaissance, no. 143.

Avicenna. *Avicenna Latinus. Liber De anima seu Sextus de naturalibus I-II-III.* Edited by Simone Van Riet. Louvain and Leiden, 1972.

Baader, Gerhard. "Die Bibliothek des Giovanni Marco da Rimini: Eine Quelle zur medizinischen Bildung im Humanismus." *Studia codicologica.* Edited by Kurt Treu. Texte und Untersuchungen zur Geschichte der Altchristlichen Literatur, 124, pp. 43–97. Berlin, 1977.

———. "Jacques Dubois." In Wear et al., eds. *The Medical Renaissance of the Sixteenth Century.* Cambridge, 1985.

———. "Medizinisches Reformdenken und Arabismus im Deutschland des 16. Jahrhunderts." *Sudhoffs Archiv für Geschichte der Medizin und der Naturwissenschaften* 63 (1979).

Bacon, Roger. *De erroribus medicorum.* In his *Opera hactenus inedita.* Fasc. 9. Edited by A. G. Little and E. Withington. Oxford, 1928.

Baldini, Ugo. "L'astronomia del Cardinale Bellarmino." In *Novità celesti e crisi del sapere. Atti del Convegno Internazionale di Studi Galileiani.* Edited by P. Galluzzi. Supplemento agli *Annali dell'Istituto e Museo di Storia della Scienza,* Anno 1983, fasc. 2.

Beaujouan, Guy. "Fautes et obscurités dans les traductions médicales du Moyen Age." *Revue de synthèse,* 3rd ser., 89 (1968):145–52.

Bertolaso, Bartolo. "La cattedra 'De pulsibus et urinis' (1601–1748) nello Studio Padovano." *Castalia: Rivista di storia di medicina* 16 (1960), 109–17.

———. "Ricerche d'archivio su alcuni aspetti dell'insegnamento medico presso la Università di Padova nel Cinque- e Seicento." *Acta medicae historiae patavina* 6 (1959–60), 23–34.

Bertolotti, A. "Le tipografie orientali e gli orientalisti a Roma nei secoli XVI e XVII." *Rivista europea* 9 (1878), 217–68.

Bianchi, Vicenzo. *Le opere a stampa di Matthaeus Curtius.* Pavia, n.d.

Boerhaave, Herman. *Institutiones medicae.* Leiden, 1707; Naples, 1751.

Bonamici, F. "Sull'antico statuto della Università di Pisa: Alcune preliminari notizie storiche." *Annali delle università toscane* 30 (1911).

Bono, James J. "The Languages of Life: Jean Fernel (1497–1558) and Spiritus in Pre-Harveian Bio-Medical Thought." Ph.D. diss., Harvard University, 1981.

Borsetti Ferranti Bolani, Ferrante. *Historia almi Ferrariae Gymnasii.* Ferrara, 1735.

Brugi, Biagio. "Un parere di Scipione Maffei intorno allo Studio di Padova sui principi del Settecento." *Atti del R. Istituto Veneto di Scienze, Lettere ed Arti* 69 (1909–10), part 2, pp. 575–91.

Buck, August, and Herding, Otto, eds. *Der Kommentar in der Renaissance.* Boppard, 1975.

Burke, Michael E. *The Royal College of San Carlos: Surgery and Spanish Medical Reform in the Late Eighteenth Century.* Durham, N.C., 1977.

Bylebyl, Jerome J. "Disputation and Description in the Renaissance Pulse Controversy." In Wear et al., eds., *The Medical Renaissance of the Sixteenth Century*. Cambridge, 1985.

———. "Medicine, Philosophy, and Humanism in Renaissance Italy." In *Science and the Arts in the Renaissance*, edited by John W. Shirley and F. David Hoeniger, pp. 27–49. Washington, 1985.

———. "The School of Padua: Humanistic Medicine in the Sixteenth Century." In *Health, Medicine and Mortality in the Sixteenth Century*, edited by Charles Webster. Cambridge, 1979.

Camerini, Paolo. *Annali dei Giunti*. I. *Venezia*. Part 1. Florence, 1962.

Capello, Arcadio. *De vita clarissimi viri Sanctorii Sanctorii*. Venice, 1750. Includes *Oratio a Sanctorio Sanctorio habita in Archilyceo Patavino dum ipse primarium theoricae medicinae explicandae munus auspicaretur, anno salutis 1612.*

Carafa, J. *De professoribus gymnasii romani*. Rome, 1751.

Carugo, Adriano. "L'insegnamento della matematica all'Università di Padova prima e dopo Galileo." In *Storia della cultura veneta*, vol. 4, part 2, pp. 151–99. Vicenza, 1984.

A Catalogue of Printed Books in the Wellcome Historical Medical Library. Vol. 1, *Books Printed before 1641*. Vols. 2 and 3. *Books Printed from 1641 to 1850, A–L*. London, 1962, 1966, 1976.

Cencetti, Giorgio. *Gli archivi dello Studio Bolognese*. Bologna, 1938.

Cervetto, G. *Di Giambatista da Monte e della medicina italiana nel secolo XVI*. Verona, 1839.

Copenhaver, Brian P. "Scholastic Philosophy and Renaissance Magic in the *De vita* of Marsilio Ficino." *Renaissance Quarterly* 37 (1984), 523–54.

———. *Symphorien Champier and the Reception of the Occultist Tradition in Renaissance France*. The Hague, Paris, New York, 1978.

Coury, Charles. "The Teaching of Medicine in France from the Beginning of the Seventeenth Century." In *The History of Medical Education*, edited by C. D. O'Malley. UCLA Forum in Medical Sciences, no. 12, pp. 121–72. Los Angeles, 1970.

Cranz, F. Edward, and Schmitt, Charles B. *A Bibliography of Aristotle Editions, 1501–1600*. 2nd ed. Bibliotheca Bibliographica Aureliana 38*. Baden-Baden, 1984.

Cunningham, Andrew. "Fabricius and the 'Aristotle Project.' " In Wear et al., eds., *The Medical Renaissance of the Sixteenth Century*. Cambridge, 1985.

Dallari, Umberto, ed. *I rotuli dei lettori legisti e artisti dello studio bolognese dal 1384 al 1799*. 4 vols. Bologna, 1888–1924.

d'Alverny, M. T. "Andrea Alpago, interprète et commentateur d'Avicenne." *Atti del XII Congresso internazionale di filosofia*. Florence, 1960, 9:1–6.

———. "Avicenne et les médecins de Venise." In *Medioevo e Rinascimento: Studi in onore di Bruno Nardi*. Florence [1955], 1:178–98.

———. "Les traductions d'Avicenne (Moyen Age et Renaissance)." In *Avicenna nella storia della cultura medioevale*. Problemi attuali di scienza e di cultura dell'Accademia Nazionale dei Lincei. Quaderno no. 40, pp. 71–87. Rome, 1955.

d'Alverny, M. T. "Les traductions d'Avicenne. Quelques résultats d'une enquête." *Vᵉ Congrès Internationale d'Arabisants et d'Islamisants, Bruxelles 31 août–6 septembre, 1970, Actes.* Pp. 151–58.

Dannenfeldt, Karl H. "The Renaissance Humanists and the Knowledge of Arabic." *Studies in the Renaissance* 2 (1955), 96–117.

Deer, Linda A. "Academic Theories of Generation in the Renaissance: The Contemporaries and Successors of Jean Fernel (1497–1558)." Ph.D. diss., Warburg Institute, University of London, 1980.

del Gaizo, Modestino. "Ricerche storiche intorno a Santorio Santorio ed alla medicina statica." *Resoconto della R. Accademia Medico-Chirurgica di Napoli.* Naples, 1889.

Dooley, Brendan. "Science Teaching as a Career at Padua in the Early Eighteenth Century: The Case of Giovanni Poleni." *History of Universities* 4 (1984), 115–51.

Dulieu, Louis. "L'arabisme médical à Montpellier du XIIᵉ au XIVᵉ siècle." *Les cahiers de Tunisie* 3 (1955), 86–95.

———. *La médecine à Montpellier. II. La Renaissance.* Avignon, 1979.

Durling, Richard J. *A Catalogue of Sixteenth-Century Printed Books in the National Library of Medicine.* Bethesda, Md., 1967.

———. "A Chronological Census of Renaissance Editions and Translations of Galen." *Journal of the Warburg and Courtauld Institutes* 24 (1961), 230–305.

———. "Linacre and Medical Humanism." In *Linacre Studies: Essays on the Life and Work of Thomas Linacre, ca. 1460–1524,* edited by Francis Maddison, Margaret Pelling, and Charles Webster, pp. 76–106. Oxford 1977.

Edwards, William F. "Niccolò Leoniceno and the Origins of Humanist Discussion of Method." In *Philosophy and Humanism: Renaissance Essays in Honor of Paul Oskar Kristeller,* edited by Edward P. Mahoney, pp. 283–305. New York, 1976.

Eisenstein, Elizabeth, L. *The Printing Press as an Agent of Change.* 2 vols. Cambridge, 1979.

Estes, Leland L. "The Medical Origins of the European Witch Craze: A Hypothesis." *Journal of Social History* 17 (1983), 271–84.

Ettari, L. S., and Procopio, M. *Santorio Santorio: La vita e le opere.* Monografie dei "Quaderni della Nutrizione," no. 4. Istituto Nazionale della Nutrizione, Città Universitaria. Rome, n.d.

Fabroni, Angelo. *Historiae academiae pisanae.* Pisa, 1792.

Facciolati, J. *Fasti Gymnasii Patavini.* Vol. 2. Padua, 1757.

Favaro, Antonio, "Indice dei rotuli dello Studio di Padova." *Monografie storiche sullo Studio di Padova.* [Venice, 1922].

———, ed. *Atti della Nazione Germanica Artista nello Studio di Padova.* 2 vols. Venice, 1911–12. Monumenti storici pubblicati dalla R. Deputazione Veneta di Storia Patria, vols. 19 and 20. Serie prima: Documenti, vols. 14 and 15.

Federici Vescovini, Graziella. *"Arti" e filosofia nel secolo XIV. Studi sulla tradizione aristotelica e i "moderni."* Florence, 1983.

Feingold, Mordechai. *The Mathematicians' Apprenticeship: Science, Universities and Society in England, 1560–1640.* Cambridge, 1984.

Fichtner, Gerhard. "Padova e Tübingen: La formazione medica nei secoli XVI e XVII." *Acta medicae historiae patavina* 19 (1972–73), 43–62.

Fracastoro, Girolamo. *Hieronymi Fracastorii De contagione et contagiosis morbis et eorum curatione, libri III.* Translated by Wilmer C. Wright. New York and London, 1930.

Franceschini, Adriano. *Nuovi documenti relativi ai docenti dello studio di Ferrara nel secolo XVI.* Deputazione Provinciale Ferrarese di Storia Patria. Serie Monumenti, 6. Ferrara, 1970.

French, Roger. "Berengario da Carpi and the Use of Commentary in Anatomical Teaching." In Wear et al., eds., *The Medical Renaissance of the Sixteenth Century.* Cambridge, 1985.

————. "Gentile da Foligno and the *via medicorum.*" In *The Light of Nature: Essays in the History and Philosophy of Science Presented to A. C. Crombie,* edited by J. D. North and J. J. Roche. Archives internationales d'histoire des idées, 110. Dordrecht, 1985.

Fück, Johann. *Die arabischen Studien in Europa bis in den Anfang des 20. Jahrhunderts.* Leipzig, 1955.

Galen. *Burgundio of Pisa's Translation of Galen's Peri Kraseon "De complexionibus."* Edited by R. J. Durling. Galenus latinus 1. Berlin and New York, 1976.

————. *On the Doctrines of Hippocrates and Plato.* Edited and translated by Philip De Lacey. Corpus medicorum graecorum 5, 4, 1, 2. 2 vols. Berlin 1978.

————. *On the Natural Faculties.* Translated by A. J. Brock. Loeb Classical Library. Reprint. Cambridge, Mass., and London, 1979.

————. *On the Usefulness of the Parts of the Body.* Translated by Margaret T. May. Ithaca, N.Y., 1968.

Garcia Ballester, Luis. "Arnau de Vilanova (c. 1240–1311) y la reforma de los estudios médicos en Montpellier (1309): El Hipócrates latino y la introducción del nuevo Galeno." *Dynamis* 2 (1982), 97–158.

————. "The Circulation and Use of Medical Manuscripts in Arabic in Sixteenth-Century Spain." *Journal for the History of Arabic Science* 3 (1979), 183–99.

————. *Los Moriscos y la medicina. Un capítulo de la medicina y la ciencia marginadas en la España del siglo XVI.* Barcelona, 1984.

Garin, Eugenio. *Lo zodiaco della vita: La polemica sull'astrologia dal Trecento al Cinquecento.* Rome and Bari, 1976.

Garosi, Alcide. *Siena nella storia della medicina, 1240–1555.* Florence, 1958.

Giese, Ernst, and von Hagen, Benno. *Geschichte der medizinischen Fakultät der Friedrich-Schiller-Universität Jena.* Jena, 1958.

Goerke, Heinz. "Die medizinische Fakultät von 1472 bis zur Gegenwart." In *Die Ludwig-Maximilians Universität in ihren Fakultäten.* Vol. 1. Berlin, 1972.

Gohlman, William E., ed. and tr. *The Life of Ibn Sina: A Critical Edition and Annotated Translation.* Albany, N.Y., 1974.

Goltz, Dietlinde. *Studien zur Geschichte der Mineralnamen in Pharmazie, Chemie und Medizin von den Anfängen bis Paracelsus. Sudhoffs Archiv: Zeitschrift für Wissenschaftsgeschichte.* Beiheft 14. Wiesbaden, 1972.

Gonzalez Castrillo, Rafaela. *Rhazes y Avicenna en la Biblioteca de la Faculatad de Medicina de la Universidad Complutense.* Madrid, 1984. A bibliography of thirty early printed editions of or related to works of Rhazes, and sixty-five of or related to medical writings of Avicenna. The collection was not assembled in a single university during the sixteenth century. Most of the items relating to the fortuna of the *Canon* after 1500 are the same as editions listed from exemplars in different collections in the notes, appendices, and bibliography of the present book. The only relevant items not so included are the following short works, said to show the use of Avicenna by Spanish authors (I have not examined these treatises): 7. *Articella,* edited by Pedro Pomar. Lyon: Johannes Moylin, 1534 (contents apparently different from another *Articella* issued by Moylin in the same year and listed in Appendix 1). 85. Carbon, Damián. *Libro del arte de las comadres o madrinas y del regimiento de las preñadas y paridas y de los niños.* Mallorca, 1541. 88. Lobera de Avila, Luis. *Vergel de sanidad.* Alcalá de Henares, 1542. 90. Gomez, Alfonso. *Libellus de humorum praeparatione.* Hispali, 1546. An attack on Arab medicine.

Grafton, Anthony. *Joseph Scaliger: A Study in the History of Classical Scholarship.* I. *Textual Criticism and Exegesis.* Oxford, 1983.

———. "Teacher, Text, and Pupil in the Renaissance Class-Room: A Case Study from a Parisian College." *History of Universities* 1 (1981), 37–70.

Granjel, Luis S. *Historia general de la medicina española.* II. *La medicina española renacentista.* Salamanca, 1980.

Grant, Edward. *In Defense of the Earth's Centrality and Immobility: Scholastic Reaction to Copernicanism in the Seventeenth Century.* Transactions of the American Philosophical Society, 74, part 4. Philadelphia, 1984.

———. *Much Ado about Nothing: Theories of Space and Vacuum from the Middle Ages to the Scientific Revolution.* Cambridge, 1981.

Grendler, Paul F. *The Roman Inquisition and the Venetian Press, 1540-1605.* Princeton, 1977.

Grmek, M. D. *L'introduction de l'expérience quantitative dans les sciences biologiques.* Conférence donnée au Palais de la Découverte le 7 avril, 1962. Paris, 1962.

———. *Santorio Santorio i Njegovi aparati i instrumenti.* Zagreb [1952]. With English summary.

Gruner, Christian Gottfried. *De variolis et morbillis fragmenta medicorum Arabistarum. . . .* Jena, 1790. Includes portion of Biagio Astario's commentary on *Canon* 4.1.

Hameed, Hakim Abdul. "Gerard's Latin Translation of Ibn Sīna's *Al-Qanun.*" *Studies in Islam* 8 (1971), 1–7.

Harris, C.R.S. *The Heart and the Vascular System in Ancient Greek Medicine: From Alcmaeon to Galen.* Oxford, 1973.

Hutchinson, Keith. "What Happened to Occult Qualities in the Scientific Revolution?" *Isis* 73 (1982), 233–53.

Illgen, H. Otto. *Die abendländischen Rhazes-Kommentatoren des XIV bis XVII Jahrhunderts.* Leipzig, 1921.

Jacquart, Danielle. "De *crasis* à *complexio*: Note sur le vocabulaire du tempérament en Latin médiéval." Centre Jean Palerme, Mémoires 5, *Textes médicaux latins antiques.* Edited by G. Sabbah, pp. 71–75. Saint-Etienne, 1984.

————. *Le milieu médical en France du XIIe au XVe siècle.* Geneva, 1981.

————. "La réception du *Canon* d'Avicenne: Comparaison entre Montpellier et Paris au XIIIe et XIVe siècles." *Actes du 110e Congrès national des sociétés savantes, Montpellier, 1985. Section d'histoire des sciences et des techniques.* II. *Histoire de l'école médicale de Montpellier,* pp. 69–77. Paris, 1985.

————. "Le regard d'un médecin sur son temps: Jacques Despars (1380?–1458)." *Bibliothèque de l'Ecole des Chartes* 138 (1980), 35–86.

Jarcho, Saul. *The Concept of Heart Failure: From Avicenna to Albertini.* Cambridge, Mass., 1980.

Jones, J. R. "The Arabic and Persian Studies of Giovan Battista Raimondi, ca. 1536–1614." M.Phil. diss., Warburg Institute, University of London, 1981.

Kaufman, D. "Jacob Mantino. Une page d'histoire de la Renaissance." *Revue des études juives* 28 (1893), 30–60, 207–38.

Kibre, Pearl. "Arts and Medicine in the Universities of the Later Middle Ages." In *Les universités à la fin du Moyen Age,* edited by Jacques Paquet and Jozef Ijsewijn, pp. 213–27. Louvain, 1978.

————. *Hippocrates Latinus: Repertorium of Hippocratic Writings in the Latin Middle Ages.* New York, 1985.

King, Lester S. *The Road to Medical Enlightenment, 1650–1695.* London and New York, 1970.

Klein-Franke, Felix. *Die klassische Antike in der Tradition des Islam.* Darmstadt, 1980.

Koelbing, H. M. "Ocular Physiology in the Seventeenth Century and Its Acceptance by the Medical Profession." *Analecta Medico-Historica Academiae Internationalis Historiae Medicinae* 3. *The Historical Aspects of Brain Research in the 17th Century.* Edited by G. Scherz. Oxford, 1968.

Kristeller, Paul Oskar. "Bartholomaeus, Musandinus and Maurus of Salerno and Other Early Commentators on the 'Articella' with a Tentative List of Texts and Manuscripts." *Italia medioevale e umanistica* 19 (1976), 57–87.

————. "Philosophy and Medicine in Medieval and Renaissance Italy." In *Organism, Medicine, and Metaphysics,* edited by S. F. Spicker, pp. 29–36. Dordrecht, 1978.

Lasswitz, Kurd. *Geschichte der Atomistik.* Vol. 1. Hamburg and Leipzig, 1890. Reprint. Hildesheim, 1963.

Lind, L. R. *Studies in Pre-Vesalian Anatomy: Biography, Translations, Documents.* Philadelphia, 1975.

Lindberg, David C. "Optics in Sixteenth-Century Italy." In *Novità celesti e crisi del sapere. Atti del Convegno Internazionale di Studi Galileiani,* edited by P. Galluzzi, pp. 131–48. Supplemento agli *Annali dell'Istituto e Museo di Storia della Scienza*, Anno 1983, fasc. 2.

―――. *Theories of Vision from Al-Kindi to Kepler*. Chicago, 1976.

Lockwood, Dean P. *Ugo Benzi: Medieval Philosopher and Physician, 1376–1439*. Chicago, 1951.

Lohr, Charles H. "Renaissance Latin Aristotle Commentaries," *Studies in the Renaissance* 21 (1974), 228–89. *Renaissance Quarterly* 28 (1975), 689–741; 29 (1976), 714–45; 30 (1977), 681–741; 31 (1978), 532–603; 32 (1979), 529–80; 33 (1980), 623–734; 35 (1982), 164–256.

Lonie, Iain M. "Fever Pathology in the Sixteenth Century: Tradition and Innovation." In *Theories of Fever from Antiquity to the Enlightenment*, edited by W. F. Bynum and V. Nutton. *Medical History* Supplement no. 1. London, 1981.

―――. "The 'Paris Hippocratics': Teaching and Research in Paris in the Second Half of the Sixteenth Century." In Wear et al., eds., *The Medical Renaissance of the Sixteenth Century*. Cambridge, 1985.

López Piñero, José Maria. *Ciencia y técnica en la sociedad española de los siglos XVI y XVII*. Barcelona, 1979.

Lowry, Martin. *The World of Aldus Manutius: Business and Scholarship in Renaissance Venice*. Oxford, 1979.

Lucchetta, Francesca. "Girolamo Ramusio." *Quaderni per la storia dell'Università di Padova* 15 (1982), 1–60.

―――. *Il Medico e filosofo bellunese Andrea Alpago († 1522) traduttore di Avicenna. Profilo biografico*. Padua, 1964.

Maclean, Ian. "The Interpretation of Natural Signs: Cardano's *De subtilitate* versus Scaliger's *Exercitationes*." In *Occult and Scientific Mentalities in the Renaissance*, edited by Brian Vickers. Cambridge, 1984.

―――. *The Renaissance Notion of Woman: A Study in the Fortunes of Scholasticism and Medical Science in European Intellectual Life*. Cambridge, 1980.

McVaugh, Michael. "The 'humidum radicale' in Thirteenth-Century Medicine." *Traditio* 30 (1974), 259–83.

Mahoney, Edward P. "Philosophy and Science in Nicoletto Vernia and Agostino Nifo." In Poppi, ed., *Scienza e filosofia all'Università di Padova nel Quattrocento*. Padua and Trieste, 1983.

―――. "Albert the Great and the *Studio Patavino* in the Late Fifteenth and Early Sixteenth Centuries." In *Albertus Magnus and the Sciences: Commemorative Essays, 1980*, edited by James A. Weisheipl, O.P., pp. 537–63. Toronto, 1980.

Middleton, W. Knowles. *A History of the Thermometer and Its Use in Meteorology*. Baltimore, 1966.

Moraux, Paul. "Galien comme philosophe: la philosophie de la nature." In *Galen: Problems and Prospects*, edited by Vivian Nutton. London, 1981.

Mugnai Carrara, Daniela. "Fra causalità astrologica e causalità naturale. Gli interventi di Nicolò Leoniceno e della sua scuola sul morbo gallico." *Physis* 21 (1979), 37–54.

———. "Una polemica umanistico-scolastica circa l'interpretazione delle tre dottrine ordinate di Galeno." *Annali dell'Istituto e Museo di Storia della Scienza di Firenze* 8 (1983), 31–57.

———. "Profilo di Nicolò Leoniceno." *Interpres* 2 (1978), 169–212.

Nardi, Bruno. *Saggi sull'Aristotelismo padovano dal secolo XIV al XVI.* Florence, n.d.

Nauert, Charles G. "Humanists, Scientists and Pliny: Changing Approaches to a Classical Author." *American Historical Review* 84 (1979), 72–85.

Nutton, Vivian. "Humanist Surgery." In Wear et al., eds., *The Medical Renaissance of the Sixteenth Century.* Cambridge, 1985.

———. "John Caius and the Eton Galen: Medical Philology in the Renaissance." *Medizinhistorisches Journal* 20 (1985), 227–52.

———. "John Caius and the Linacre Tradition." *Medical History* 23 (1979), 373–89.

———. "Medicine in the Age of Montaigne." In *Montaigne and His Age*, edited by K. Cameron, pp. 15–25. Exeter, 1981.

———. "Montanus, Vesalius and the Haemorrhoidal Veins." *Clio medica* 18 (1983), 33–36.

———. " 'Qui magni Galeni doctrinam in re medica primus revocavit'; Matteo Corti und der Galenismus im medizinischen Unterricht der Renaissance." Paper delivered to the Heidelberger Tagung der Senatskommission der DFG für Humanismusforschung, September 1985.

———. "The Seeds of Disease: An Explanation of Contagion and Infection from the Greeks to the Renaissance." *Medical History* 27 (1983), 1–34.

Ohl, Ronald E. "The University of Padua, 1405–1509: An International Community of Students and Professors." Ph.D. diss., University of Pennsylvania, 1980.

Ongaro, Giuseppe. "La medicina nello Studio di Padova e nel Veneto." In *Storia della cultura veneta*, vol. 3, part 3, pp. 75–134. Vicenza, 1981.

Opelt, Ilona. "Zur Übersetzungstechnik des Gerhard von Cremona." *Glotta* 38 (1960), 135–70.

Ottosson, Per-Gunnar. *Scholastic Medicine and Philosophy: A Study of Commentaries on Galen's Tegni (ca. 1300–1450).* Naples, 1984.

Pagel, Walter. "Medical Humanism—A Historical Necessity in the Era of the Renaissance." In *Linacre Studies: Essays on the Life and Work of Thomas Linacre, ca. 1460–1524*, edited by Francis Maddison, Margaret Pelling, and Charles Webster, pp. 375–86. Oxford, 1977.

———. *Paracelsus: An Introduction to Philosophical Medicine of the Era of the Renaissance.* Basel and New York, 1958.

———. *William Harvey's Biological Ideas.* Basel and New York, 1967.

Palmer, Richard. "The Control of Plague in Venice and Northern Italy, 1348–1600." Ph.D. diss., University of Kent at Canterbury, 1978.

———. "Medical Botany in Northern Italy in the Renaissance." *Journal of the Royal Society of Medicine* 78 (1985), 149–57.

Palmer, Richard. "Nicolò Massa, His Family and His Fortune." *Medical History* 25 (1981): 385–410.

———. *The Studio of Venice and Its Graduates in the Sixteenth Century.* Padua and Trieste, 1983.

Papadopoli, N. C. *Historia Gymnasii Patavini.* . . . Vol. 1. Venice, 1726.

Pardi, Giuseppe. *Lo studio di Ferrara nei secoli XV° e XVI° con documenti inediti.* Ferrara, 1903.

Park, Katharine. *Doctors and Medicine in Early Renaissance Florence.* Princeton, N.J., 1985.

Pesenti, Tiziana. "Generi e pubblico della letteratura medica padovana nel Tre- e Quattrocento." *Università e società nei secoli XII–XVI. Atti del nono Convegno Internazionale di studio tenuto a Pistoia nei giorni 20–25 settembre 1979*, pp. 523–45. Bologna, 1983.

———. *Professori e promotori di medicina nello Studio di Padova dal 1405 al 1509: repertorio bio-bibliografico.* Padua and Trieste, 1984.

Piaia, Gregorio. *Vestigia philosophorum: il medioevo e la storiografia filosofica.* Rimini, 1983.

Picotti, Giovan Battista. "Per la storia dell'Università di Pisa." In his *Scritti vari di storia pisana e toscana.* Pisa, 1968.

Pittion, J.-P. "Skepticism and Medicine in the Renaissance." In *Skepticism from the Renaissance to the Enlightenment*, edited by R. H. Popkin and C. B. Schmitt. Wolfenbüttel, 1986.

Poppi, Antonino, ed. *Scienza e filosofia all'Università di Padova nel Quattrocento.* Padua and Trieste, 1983.

Richardson, Linda Deer. "The Generation of Disease." In Wear et al., eds., *Medical Renaissance of the Sixteenth Century.* Cambridge, 1985.

Richler, Benjamin. "Manuscripts of Avicenna's *Kanon* in Hebrew Translation: A Revised and Up-to-date List." *Koroth* 8 (1982), 145*–68*.

Rodriguez Cruz, Agueda Maria. *Historia de las Universidades Hispanoamericanas período hispánico.* 2 vols. Bogotá, 1973.

Roger, Jacques. *Jean Fernel et les problèmes de la médecine de la Renaissance.* Les Conférences du Palais de la Découverte, ser. D., no. 70. Paris, 1960.

———. "La situation d'Aristote chez les anatomistes padouans." In *Platon et Aristote à la Renaissance. XVIᵉ Colloque International de Tours*, pp. 217–24. Paris, 1976.

Rossetti, Lucia, ed. *Acta Nationis Germanicae Artistarum (1616–1636).* Padua, 1967.

Saltini, G. E. "Della Stamperia Orientale Medicea e di Giovan Battista Raimondi." *Giornale storico degli archivi toscani* 4 (1860), 257–308.

Sarton, George. "Query No. 134—Was any attempt made by the editors of the late Latin editions of Avicenna's *Canon* to modernize it?" *Isis* 43 (1952), 54.

Scapini, Aldo. *L'archiatra mediceo e pontificio Matteo Corti (secolo XVI) e il suo commento all'Anatomia di Mondino di Liuzzi.* Scientia Veterum, no. 142. Pisa, 1970.

Schipperges, Heinrich. *Die Assimilation der arabischen Medizin durch das lateinische Mittelalter. Sudhoffs Archiv für Geschichte der Medizin und der Naturwissenschaften,* Beiheft 3. Wiesbaden, 1964.

Schmitt, Charles. "Aristotelian Textual Studies at Padua: The Case of Francesco Cavalli." In Poppi, ed., *Scienza e filosofia all'Università di Padova nel Quattrocento.* Padua and Trieste, 1983.

―――. *The Aristotelian Tradition and Renaissance Universities.* London, 1984. Collection of previously published papers; see especially "Aristotelianism in the Veneto and the Origins of Modern Science: Some Considerations on the Problem of Continuity," "Renaissance Averroism Studied through the Venetian Editions of Aristotle-Averroes (with Particular Reference to the Giunta Edition of 1550–1552)," "Cesare Cremonini: un aristotelico al tempo di Galilei," and "Philosophy and Science in Sixteenth-Century Italian Universities."

―――. "Aristotle among the Physicians." In Wear et al., eds., *The Medical Renaissance of the Sixteenth Century.* Cambridge, 1985.

―――. *Aristotle and the Renaissance.* Cambridge, Mass., and London, 1983.

―――. *Studies in Renaissance Philosophy and Science.* London, 1981. Collection of previously published papers; see especially "Philosophy and Science in Sixteenth-Century Universities: Some Preliminary Comments" and "The Faculty of Arts at Pisa in the Time of Galileo."

Schmitz, Rudolf, and Keil, Gundolf, eds. *Humanismus und Medizin.* Weinheim, 1984.

Scienze, credenze occulte, livelli di cultura: Convegno Internazionale di Studi (Firenze, 26–30 giugno 1980). Istituto Nazionale di Studi sul Rinascimento. Florence, 1982.

Secco Stuardo, Girolamo. "Lo studio di Ferrara a tutto il secolo XV." *Atti della Deputazione Ferrarese di Storia Patria* 6 (1894), 25–294.

Sherrington, Charles. *The Endeavor of Jean Fernel.* Cambridge, 1946.

Simeoni, Luigi. *Storia dell'Università di Bologna. II. L'età moderna.* Bologna, 1940.

Siraisi, Nancy G. *Arts and Sciences at Padua.* Toronto, 1973.

―――. *Taddeo Alderotti and His Pupils: Two Generations of Italian Medical Learning.* Princeton, N.J., 1981.

Smith, Wesley D. *The Hippocratic Tradition.* Ithaca, N.Y., 1979.

Solerti, Angelo. "Documenti riguardanti lo studio di Ferrara nei secoli XV e XVI conservati nell'Archivio Estense." *Atti della Deputazione Ferrarese di Storia Patria* 4 (1892), 5–51.

Someda da Marco, Pietro. *Medici Forojuliensi dal sec. XIII al sec. XVIII.* Udine, 1963.

Soppelsa, Marialaura. *Genesi del metodo galileiano e tramonto dell'Aristotelismo nella scuola di Padova.* Padua, 1974.

Steinschneider, Moritz. *Die europäischen Übersetzungen aus dem Arabischen bis Mitte des 17. Jahrhunderts.* Sitzungsberichten der Kais. Akademie der Wissenschaften in Wien. Philosphisch-Historische Klasse, 149. Vienna, 1904.

Steinschneider, Moritz. *Die hebräischen Übersetzungen des Mittelalters und die Juden als Dolmetscher*. Berlin, 1893. Facsimile, Graz, 1956.

Temkin, Owsei. "The Classical Roots of Glisson's Doctrine of Irritation." In his *The Double Face of Janus and Other Essays in the History of Medicine*, pp. 290–316. Baltimore, 1977.

―――. *Galenism: Rise and Decline of a Medical Philosophy*. Ithaca, N.Y., and London, 1973.

Todd, Robert B., *Alexander of Aphrodisias on Stoic Physics*. Leiden, 1976.

Ulvioni, P. "Astrologia, astronomia e medicina nella Repubblica Veneta tra Cinque- e Seicento." *Studi Trentini di scienze storiche* 61 (1982), 1–69.

Vaccari, Pietro. *Storia della Università di Pavia*. 2nd ed. Pavia, 1957.

Vasoli, Cesare. "La cultura dei secoli XIV–XVI." *Atti del primo convegno internazionale di recognizione delle fonti per la storia della scienza italiana: i secoli XIV–XVI*, edited by Carlo Maccagni. Domus Galileiana, Pisa. Pubblicazioni di storia della scienza. Florence, 1967. Sezione 5, vol. 1.

Visconti, Alessandro. *La storia dell'Università di Ferrara*. Bologna, 1950.

von Schnurrer, C. F. *Bibliotheca Arabica*. Halle, 1811.

von Wegele, Franz X. *Geschichte der Universität Wirzburg* [sic]. Würzburg, 1882. Facsimile, 1969.

Walker, D. P. "The Astral Body in Renaissance Medicine." *Journal of the Warburg and Courtauld Institutes* 21 (1958), 119–33.

Wear, A., French, R. K., and Lonie, I. M., eds. *The Medical Renaissance of the Sixteenth Century*. Cambridge, 1985.

Wear, Andrew. "Galen in the Renaissance." In *Galen: Problems and Prospects*, edited by Vivian Nutton, pp. 229–62. London, 1981.

―――. "William Harvey and the 'Way of the Anatomists.'" *History of Science* 21 (1983), 223–49.

Weisser, Ursula. "Ibn Sīnā und die Medizin des arabisch-islamischen Mittelalters—Alte und neue Urteile und Vorurteile." *Medizinhistorisches Journal* 18 (1983), 283–305.

Westman, Robert S. "The Comet and the Cosmos: Kepler, Mästlin and the Copernican Hypothesis." In *Colloquia Copernicana*. I. *Etudes sur l'audience de la théorie héliocentrique*, pp. 7–30. Studia Copernicana 5. Wroclaw, 1972.

Whitteridge, Gweneth. *William Harvey and the Circulation of the Blood*. London and New York, 1971.

Wickersheimer, Ernest. "Die 'Apologetica epistola pro defensione Arabum medicorum' von Bernhard Unger aus Tübingen (1533)." *Sudhoffs Archiv für Geschichte der Medizin und Naturwissenschaften* 38 (1954), 322–28.

―――. "Laurent Fries et la querelle de l'arabisme en médecine (1530)." *Les cahiers de Tunisie* 9 (1955), 96–103.

Wightman, William P. D. "Quid sit methodus? 'Method' in Sixteenth-Century Medical Teaching and Discovery." *Journal of the History of Medicine and Allied Sciences* 19 (1964), 360–76.

Zambelli, Paola. "Scienza, filosofia, religione nella Toscana di Cosimo I." In *Florence and Venice: Comparisons and Relations*. II. *Cinquecento*, pp. 3–52. Florence, 1980.

Zampieri, Laura. *Un illustre medico umanista dello Studio pisano: Giulio Angeli*. Pisa, 1981.

Zanier, Giancarlo. *Medicina e filosofia tra '500 e '600*. Milan, 1983.

———. *Ricerche sulla diffusione e fortuna del "De incantationibus" di Pomponazzi*. Florence, 1975.

———. "Ricerche sull'occultismo a Padova nel sec. XV." In Poppi, ed., *Scienza e filosofia all'Università di Padova nel Quattrocento*. Padua and Trieste, 1983.

Index

Early editions of the *Canon* are indexed under the names of editors, translators, or printers (a list of editions is to be found in Appendix 1). Commentaries on the *Canon* are indexed under the names of their authors (a list of Renaissance commentaries is to be found in Appendix 2). Bodily parts are gathered as subentries under the general heading *anatomy*; physiological concepts (Renaissance and modern) and processes are indexed as subentries under *physiology*. Renaissance and modern concepts and terminology relating to disease, conditions, and symptoms are grouped under the general heading *pathology*. Forms of treatment are collected under the heading *therapy*. Frequently occurring names (e.g., Avicenna, Galen, Da Monte, Santorio) are indexed selectively; some names referred to only incidentally are not indexed. Bibliographic citations in the notes are not indexed.

Nancy G. Siraisi is Professor of History at Hunter College and the Graduate School of the City University of New York. She is the author of *Arts and Sciences at Padua* (Pontifical Institute of Mediaeval Studies) and *Taddeo Alderotti and His Pupils* (Princeton), for which she received the American Association for the History of Medicine's Welch Medal.

Library of Congress Cataloging-in-Publication Data

Siraisi, Nancy G.
Avicenna in Renaissance Italy.

Bibliography: p.
Includes index.
1. Medicine—Study and teaching—Italy—History.
2. Avicenna, 980–1037. Qānūn fī al-ṭibb. 3. Medicine—Italy—
15th–18th centuries. 4. Renaissance—Italy. I. Title.
R791.A6S57 1987 610'.7'1145 86–30687
ISBN 0–691–05137–2 (alk. paper)

DATE DUE

HIGHSMITH   #LO-45220